MANAGING
SPINAL CORD INJURY

A Guide to Living Well After
Spinal Cord Injury

Edited by
SUZANNE L. GROAH, M.D., M.S.P.H.

NRH Press
Washington, D.C.

Paperback, wirebound and CD-Rom editions published by
NRH Press
National Rehabilitation Hospital
Publication Office
102 Irving Street, N.W.
Washington, D.C. 20010

Trade paperback ISBN 0-9661676-3-5
Wirebound ISBN 0-9661676-4-3
CD-Rom ISBN 0-9661676-5-1

****

Hardcover edition published by
ABI Professional Publications
P.O. Box 149
St. Petersburg, FL 33731

ISBN 1-886236-37-2

Acknowledgments

Publication of *Managing Spinal Cord Injury: A Guide to Living Well After Spinal Cord Injury* would not have been possible without the contributions and support of many people at the National Rehabilitation Hospital (NRH) and elsewhere. In particular, I extend my sincere appreciation to all of the chapter authors for sharing their knowledge and expertise, and to the former NRH patients and other consumers who shared their personal experiences and perspectives about living with spinal cord injury. I also thank NRH President and Chief Executive Officer Edward A. Eckenhoff and NRH Senior Vice President and Medical Director Edward S. Healton, MD, MPH, for their support of NRH Press and the development of this book. In addition, I am indebted to Robert S. Hartmann for his unwavering commitment to the book; to Susan R. Farrer for her support in planning and help in managing the project from start to finish; and to Arthur Brown, our publisher, for his expertise and assistance in bringing the book to fruition, and to my father, William Groah, for his time, assistance, and comments in reviewing this manuscript. Lastly, without the love and support of my husband, Steve Fox, and children, Abby and Zach, this book would not have been possible.

Suzanne L. Groah, M.D., M.S.P.H.
Editor

Managing Spinal Cord Injury was made possible in part through a grant from the United States Department of Education, National Institute on Disability and Rehabilitation Research, grant #H133B031114

Contributors

Pamela Ballard, M.D.
Clinical Director, Spinal Cord
Injury Program
National Rehabilitation Hospital
Washington, D.C.

Kianda Bell, B.A.
Former Research Data Analyst
Center for Health & Disability
Research
National Rehabilitation Hospital
Washington, D.C.

P. Carol Bullard-Bates, Ph.D.
Clinical Psychologist and
Neuropsychologist
National Rehabilitation Hospital
Washington, D.C.

William A. Butler, O.T.R./L
Former Senior Occupational
Therapist
National Rehabilitation Hospital
Washington, D.C.

Lisa DiNapoli, P.T.
Physical Therapist
National Rehabilitation Hospital
Washington, D.C.

Lori Eisen, P.T.
Physical Therapist
National Rehabilitation Hospital
Washington, D.C.

**Matthew W. Elrod, P.T., M.Ed.,
N.C.S.**
Program Coordinator,
Neuroscience Research Center
National Rehabilitation Hospital
Washington, D.C.

Samuel A. Gordon, Ph.D.
Clinical Psychologist
National Rehabilitation Hospital
Washington, D.C.

**Suzanne L. Groah, M.D.,
M.S.P.H.**
Director, Consultation Liaison
Service
Director, Spinal Cord Injury
Research
National Rehabilitation Hospital
Washington, D.C.

Lauro S. Halstead, M.D., M.P.H.
Former Director, Spinal Cord
Injury Program
Founder and Former Director, Male
SCI Fertility Program
National Rehabilitation Hospital
Washington, D.C.

Ashley M. Harmon, M.S., C.R.C.
Case Manager/Rehabilitation
Counselor
National Rehabilitation Hospital
Washington, D.C.

Jennifer Hendricks, LIC.S.W.
Care Coordination Manager
National Rehabilitation Hospital
Washington, D.C.

Cara Hosler-Smythe, P.T.
Physical Therapist
National Rehabilitation Hospital
Washington, D.C.

Gwyn C. Jones, Ph.D.
Senior Research Associate
Center for Health & Disability
Research
National Rehabilitation Hospital
Washington, D.C.

Joan Parchem Joyce, C.T.R.S., M.S.
Therapeutic Recreation Specialist
National Rehabilitation Hospital
Washington, D.C.

Lindsey Kanski, O.T.
Occupational Therapist
National Rehabilitation Hospital
Washington, D.C.

Thilo Kroll, Ph.D.
Senior Research Associate
Center for Health & Disability
Research
National Rehabilitation Hospital
Washington, D.C.

Marion Levine, M.Ed., C.R.C.
Vocational Rehabilitation
Coordinator
National Rehabilitation Hospital
Washington, D.C.

Alison Lichy, P.T., M.P.T.
Research Physical Therapist
National Rehabilitation Hospital
Washington, D.C.

John A. Noiseux, M.S., A.T.P.
Rehabilitation Engineering
Specialist
National Rehabilitation Hospital
Washington, D.C.

Marianne Oursler, P.T.
Physical Therapist
National Rehabilitation Hospital
Washington, D.C.

Judi Rogers, O.T.R./L.
Pregnancy and Birthing Specialist,
and Parenting Equipment
Specialist
Through The Looking Glass
Berkeley, CA

Neepa Shah, OT.R./L.
Occupational Therapist
National Rehabilitation Hospital
Washington, D.C.

John E. Toerge, D.O.
Chief, Rehabilitation Medicine
Service
Georgetown University Hospital
Washington, DC

Chair, Physical Medicine and
Rehabilitation Department
Washington Hospital Center
Washington, DC

Vice President for Medical Affairs
National Rehabilitation Hospital

Christi Tuleja, M.S., O.T.R.
Parenting With A Disability
Specialist
Through The Looking Glass
Berkeley, CA

Consumer Essay Contributors

Steven Ferguson
Jennifer Sheehy Keller
Robert Marsteller
Reverend Rob McQuay
Tim Strachan
Steven A. Towle
LaShonne T. Williams-Fraley

Contents

Foreword

Edward A. Eckenhoff

Each year in the United States, 11,000 people—more than half of them below the age of 30—sustain spinal cord injuries (SCI) from motor vehicle crashes, falls, acts of violence, sports or diving accidents, and other causes. In an instant of time, most aspects of these individuals' lives—from how they get around and dress themselves to how they work, play, and relate to others—change dramatically, often for the rest of their lives.

I know, because I've been there myself. More than 40 years ago, when I was a 20-year-old college student, I was thrown from a car and paralyzed from the waist down. In a split second and without warning, I lost the ability to walk and to do much of what I had always taken for granted in my everyday life. I was fortunate throughout my recovery to have the strong support and encouragement of my family and friends, as well as from a dedicated, skilled team of medical rehabilitation professionals. With their help, I was able to maintain a positive outlook and to learn new skills that enabled me to return to an active, rewarding life.

Since my injury and rehabilitation four decades ago, though, the opportunities for persons with spinal cord injury have increased significantly. Better medical treatment and rehabilitation, greater access to public facilities and services, and new technology—ranging from high-tech power wheelchairs to sophisticated environmental control units—have enabled persons with SCI to lead more productive, self-determined lives. Not only can we live independently, we can also enjoy successful careers, return to school, have families, take part in recreation activities and competitive sports, travel, and do so much more than we could in the past.

Recent years have also brought many exciting advances in our understanding of SCI that are paving the way for improved treatment and rehabilitation in the future. For example, neuroscience researchers have developed a growing body of knowledge about what happens when the spinal cord is injured, how the damage might be minimized, and what eventually might be the keys to regenerating cells and repairing the spinal cord's function.

In addition, rehabilitation experts are working to develop new clinical strategies and technologies that hold promise for restoring function, reducing spasticity, relieving pain, improving bladder function, and enhancing the fertility of men with SCI. For example, researchers are testing the use of innovative treadmill systems to retrain leg muscles, and the use of sophisticated functional electrical stimulation systems to control limb muscles, stimulate reaching and gripping, and help exercise paralyzed muscles. Investigators also are exploring the benefits of electrical stimulation to reduce spasticity, developing pump systems and other new drug approaches to treat pain, and designing implants to improve bladder control.

Moreover, rehabilitation professionals are refining applications of high-speed telecommunications and video technology to provide "telerehabilitation" services. These services allow us to offer consultations, clinical interventions, and training to people in "remote" locations—whether at a patient's home down the street, at a rehabilitation hospital in another state, or at a facility halfway around the world.

As both an SCI survivor and a medical rehabilitation hospital administrator, I am excited about these research advances, which hold so much promise for reducing disability and further improving the lives of persons with SCI in the 21st century. I am also excited about how far post-injury treatment has come and how much we can offer to maximize the quality of life of persons with SCI today.

Within this context, the National Rehabilitation Hospital staff is pleased to publish Managing Spinal Cord Injury: A Guide to Living Well with Spinal Cord Injury. The third book produced NRH Press, Managing Spinal Cord Injury was written mainly for SCI survivors and their families, although health care professionals will also find it useful as they treat and advise persons with SCI. In the pages that follow, the authors recommend practical strategies for confronting the physical, emotional, psychological, and social effects of spinal cord injury. We recognize that there truly is no "cookbook" approach to living well with SCI, but we hope to share in this volume some valuable ingredients for living well and to reinforce what readers have learned in the process of medical rehabilitation.

The authors of Managing Spinal Cord Injury include rehabilitation and disability experts from the National Rehabilitation Hospital and other organizations. They also include a number of insightful persons with SCI who reflect on their experiences and offer personal perspectives about living with disability. We thank all of the authors for sharing their knowledge and expertise. In addition, we are indebted to the editor, Dr. Suzanne Groah, a member of the NRH Medical Staff and an expert in spinal cord injury rehabilitation, for her energy and commitment to making this book a reality.

As you read this book, we hope that the authors' collective wisdom and advice will empower you to set and attain your goals, take steps to remain healthy and active, and make the most of your personal and community resources. Whether you are recently injured or are months or years post-injury, we believe that Managing Spinal Cord Injury will offer new ideas and useful information that will help you to live as independently, actively, and productively as possible in the years to come.

Edward A. Eckenhoff
President and Chief Executive Officer
National Rehabilitation Hospital

Introduction

Suzanne L. Groah, M.D., M.S.P.H.

Since the National Rehabilitation Hospital (NRH) opened in 1986, we have seen many positive changes affecting the lives of people with spinal cord injury (SCI) and other disabling conditions. Improvements in trauma care and medical rehabilitation are saving more lives and improving outcomes among persons with SCI. Medical rehabilitation services have improved because of new research, use of advanced technology in both clinical care and everyday life, and the field's increased understanding of the outcomes of what we do and what works best.

During the past several decades, we have also witnessed tremendous advances in society's awareness about, and attitudes toward, persons with all types of disabilities. Because of the Americans with Disabilities Act of 1990 and other laws—as well as the persistence of many advocates nationwide—it is not unusual to see persons with disabilities working and learning side by side with able-bodied persons in the workplace and classrooms; to see curb cuts on street corners and automatic door openers, ramps, and accessible restrooms in shopping malls, office buildings, and public facilities; and to see persons with disabilities using public transportation, competing in sports, and actively engaged in other activities.

All of these changes are offering persons with disabilities greater independence and access to life's opportunities, as well as greater power to make informed choices about their own futures. Despite the improvements we have seen in medical care and in society as a whole, there is no doubt that people with SCI face tremendous challenges from the moment of injury onward. Physical, emotional, psychological, social, vocational, financial, and other changes must be confronted, both during the initial stages of recovery and often for the rest of one's life. However, with advances in today's excellent rehabilitative care, community-based services, and technology, many people have demonstrated that independence and high quality of life are possible, regardless of the extent and level of injury.

We hope that this book, *Managing Spinal Cord Injury: A Guide to Living Well with Spinal Cord Injury*, will help those who are newly injured and those who are months or even years post-injury to adapt and adjust to the many changes brought about by SCI. The third volume published by NRH Press, *Managing Spinal Cord Injury*, was planned and written to offer persons with SCI and their families practical information and advice, useful tools, and helpful resources for coping with the aftermath of spinal cord injury. More than 25 medical rehabilitation experts at NRH and elsewhere have contributed their wealth of knowledge to this book. Each of the authors was carefully selected because of his or her expertise about a particular aspect of rehabilitation and successful living with spinal cord injury. The first portion of *Managing Spinal Cord Injury* offers practical information about the aftermath of SCI. Chapter 1 reviews facts about SCI, describes the different types of SCI, and discusses the typical physical changes experienced after SCI. Chapters 2 through 4 build on what is taught during rehabilitation, by offering advice about doing activities of daily living, adjusting to the psychological and emotional changes that come with SCI, and setting goals and solve problems.

The second portion of this guide looks at issues associated with independence and quality of life. Chapters 5 and 6 discuss what to consider when planning to return home from the rehabilitation hospital and how to find and work with peer mentors. Chapter 7 explains health insurance and financial support options, while Chapters 8 and 9 describe considerations when returning to school or work, and the value of technology for everything from self-care to computer access. Chapter 10 then explores the importance of physical activity and recreation and offers tools to help persons with SCI return to enjoyable, fulfilling leisure activities.

Subsequent chapters cover focus on three issues that are foremost on the minds of many people with SCI—sexuality, fertility, and parenting. Chapter 11 addresses sexual identity, returning to your sexual relationships, sexual dysfunction, and fertility issues. Chapters 12 and 13 offer advice for parenting after an SCI and tips regarding pregnancy and childbirth.

The next two chapters address the aging process after SCI. Chapter 14 highlights some typical changes that occur with aging, describes how the aging process might be different because of SCI, and advises readers about healthy aging. Chapter 15 focuses more specifically on shoulder problems and how to prevent them. Finally, Chapter 16 offers thoughtful observations by an experienced medical rehabilitation specialist about living with SCI.

The appendices found at the back of this book also provide useful information for persons with SCI and those who are involved in their lives. Appendix A offers reflections about living with SCI from "veteran" SCI survivors who have graciously offered their insights and advice about everything from relationships and parenting to spirituality and substance abuse. These richly written essays offer the writers' firsthand perspectives and complement the content of the book chapters. Appendix B provides a glossary of important words and terms used throughout this guide. These terms are highlighted in bold type where they are first used in each chapter. Finally, Appendix C presents a detailed list of SCI and disability organizations, periodicals, and online resources, as well as articles and other material recommended by the chapter authors. Readers no doubt will find many of these resources to be useful as they seek out further information or take steps to connect with others with SCI.

More than two years in development and writing, *Managing Spinal Cord Injury* offers a wealth of information and resources for living well with SCI. In keeping with NRH's credo of "Adding Life to Years," we hope that this guide will enable readers to live productively and fully, to maintain good health, to be as independent as possible, and to achieve their personal goals and aspirations.

Suzanne L. Groah, M.D., M.S.P.H., Editor

1
Understanding Spinal Cord Injury

PAMELA BALLARD
SUZANNE L. GROAH

"Nothing completely prepares you for the reality that awaits you. . . . You can't help but ask questions such as: What is it going to be like? How will I be able to live like this? How are others going to react to me? Will life ever be normal again?" —Tim

Spinal cord injury (SCI) is a complex condition that can affect nearly every aspect of your life—from how you get around and do routine tasks to how you interact with your family and friends. The changes you experience and the ways in which those changes affect your life depend greatly on not only the type and extent of your injury, but also your personality (for example, whether you like to do everything yourself or are willing to let others help you). It also depends on your determination. As you continue on your journey with your SCI, it is helpful to know as much as you can about your injury and how it affects your physical abilities, health, emotional well-being, and relationships with other people. The more you know about your injury, the better prepared you will be to adapt to its effects and prevent complications, both now and in the future.

This chapter will help you understand your SCI and some of the physical changes you may confront. In this chapter, you will learn:

• What the spinal cord is
• What spinal cord injury is
• About different types of spinal cord injury
• Some common physical changes that occur after spinal cord injury

WHAT MAKES UP THE NERVOUS SYSTEM?

The nervous system is the electrical system of the body, carrying messages that control most, if not all, information about bodily functions. The nervous system is divided into three major divisions, based on the location of the nerves (Figure 1.1), as follows:

- Central nervous system—the brain and spinal cord
- Peripheral nervous system—the peripheral or spinal nerves
- Autonomic nervous system—sympathetic nervous system and parasympathetic nervous system

The brain and spinal cord make up the central nervous system. Taken together, the nerves that branch off the brain and spinal cord to go to all of the parts of the body are called the peripheral nervous system. The autonomic nervous system is made up of the sympathetic nervous system and the parasympathetic nervous system, which work together to control most organ functions such as sweating, heart rate, blood pressure, digestion of food, bowel movements, emptying your bladder, and more.

WHAT IS THE SPINAL CORD?

The spinal cord is a soft, rope-like structure that is made up of millions of nerves. It runs from the base of the brain to the lower part of the back. Its purpose is to carry information between the brain and, by way of the peripheral nerves, to other parts of the body, such as the arms, legs, and all of the organs in the body. Some of the nerves in the spinal cord send messages telling a particular body part to move in a certain way. Other nerve fibers send messages about heat, cold, or pain. Some tell your bladder or bowel to "hold on a little longer," or "it's OK to go now." Still others control your body's involuntary (autonomic) activities, such as your blood pressure, body temperature, and sweating. In addition, information from various parts of your body travels back to the brain by way of the spinal cord.

Here's an example of how the brain, spinal cord, and peripheral nerves work together: When you sit down, your brain sends messages down the spinal cord and then to the peripheral nerves going to the muscles, telling your legs to bend and your arms to stabilize your body. Then, if you accidentally sit on a tack, peripheral nerves from your rear end send a message via the spinal cord, telling your brain that there is something painful down there. The cycle repeats itself, with the brain sending another message down the spinal cord and through the peripheral nerves, telling the legs to stand back up. Your nervous system is able to control many of these sequences for different body parts and functions continually throughout the day.

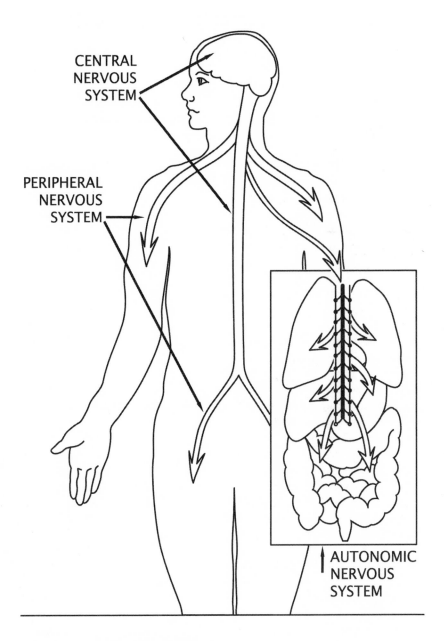

CENTRAL NERVOUS SYSTEM

PERIPHERAL NERVOUS SYSTEM

AUTONOMIC NERVOUS SYSTEM

Figure 1.1. The Nervous System

The nervous system carries messages that control information about bodily functions. It includes the central, peripheral, and autonomic nervous systems.

HOW DOES MY BODY PROTECT THE SPINAL CORD?

The spinal cord is surrounded and protected by 29 vertebrae—the small back bones that make up the spinal column. The vertebrae are stacked one on top of another and each has a hole, creating a canal through which the spinal cord passes. The vertebrae are cushioned from one another by spongy material called disks. Ligaments (very tough and strong ropes) hold the vertebrae in the proper alignment.

SPINAL CORD ANATOMY 101

To understand the effects of a SCI, you first need to understand the spinal cord's anatomy, or its structure. The spinal cord emerges from the base of the skull and ends at the lower part of the back. The peripheral nerves (also called spinal nerves) are paired and travel to various parts of the body. There are 31 pairs of spinal nerves, which are numbered according to sections of the spinal column (Figure 1.2).

The sections of the spine are:

- The cervical or neck section (C1 to C8), which includes 8 nerves and 7 vertebrae in the neck area.
- The thoracic or chest section (T1 to T12), which includes 12 nerves and 12 vertebrae in the chest and abdomen (belly) area.
- The lumbar or low back section (L1 to L5), which includes 5 nerves and 5 vertebrae in the lower back.
- The spinal cord ends at the L2 level. Beyond this point, a collection of many nerves form the cauda equina, or "horse's tail," which is just what the bundle of nerves looks like.
- The sacral section (S1 to S5) includes the lowest nerves exiting the spinal cord in the pelvic area (area of the buttocks). The sacrum is actually several vertebral bones that are fused, or attached, to form one large bone with 5 nerves emerging from holes in each side of the bone.

WHAT CAUSES SPINAL CORD INJURY?

An SCI is damage to the spinal cord from trauma or an accident. Approximately 11,000 new cases of SCI (caused by trauma) occur each year in the United States. Approximately 243,000 people in the United States are living with SCI today. Traumatic SCI might occur because of the following:

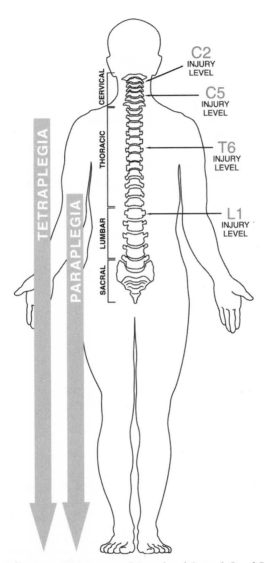

Figure 1.2. The Spinal Nerves and Levels of Spinal Cord Injury
The higher on the spinal cord an injury occurs, the greater the effect on movement, sensation, and other body functions. Tetraplegia refers to an injury to the cervical (neck) section of the spinal cord. It can involve either partial or complete loss of movement and/or feeling in the head, neck, shoulders, upper chest, arms, and legs. Paraplegia refers to an injury in the thoracic, lumbar, or sacral sections of the spinal cord. It can involve either partial or complete loss of movement or feeling in the chest, stomach, hips, legs, and feet.

- Car, truck, or motorcycle crash
- Fall
- Act of violence such as gunshot or stab wound
- Sports injury

Often we speak of SCI resulting from trauma or injury, although with the aging of the population in general, we are seeing more and more other "non-traumatic" causes of SCI. We tend to know more about traumatic injuries because more research has been done in that area. When a disease causes a SCI, we often refer to this as **myelopathy** ("myelo" means spinal cord and "pathy" means disease). Some diseases that cause SCI include:

- Multiple sclerosis
- Blood vessel disorders leading to bleeding around the spinal cord or a lack of blood supply to the spinal cord
- Tumors (benign or cancerous)
- Infections
- Developmental disorders
- Arthritis

While we don't know the exact frequency of these types of SCI, we know from experience that they are responsible for more and more injuries. Whatever the cause, trauma or disease, the spinal cord is so sensitive to damage that an injury to it or a disease process that involves it often results in some type of paralysis (or weakness) and sensory loss (loss of feeling). The sections below give an overview of the effects of SCI.

So, what exactly happens when my spinal cord is damaged?

The spinal cord is one of the most fragile organs of the body. That's why there are so many bones and ligaments that protect it. When an injury to the back or neck causes a vertebra to break or a ligament to tear, the backbone can pinch the spinal cord. Similarly, a tumor or infection may put pressure on the spinal cord or even cause a vertebra to break. This pinching or pressure may cause bruising, swelling, or bleeding of the spinal cord.

Only rarely is the spinal cord actually severed or cut. This type of injury to the spinal cord may temporarily or permanently impair some or all of the communication between the brain and various parts of the body. Then, the ability of the nervous system to send and receive messages back and forth between the brain and your arms, legs, bowel, bladder, and other body organs is lost to some degree. In turn, the ability to move, feel, and control involuntary (autonomic) body functions can be impaired. An important point to

can lead to life-threatening complications. However, bowel problems can be managed to prevent complications.

To understand the bowel changes you might experience, it helps to understand the **digestive system**. Your gastrointestinal tract includes your mouth, esophagus (swallowing tube), stomach, small intestine, and large intestine. Together, the small and large intestines make up your bowel. The digestive system breaks down food and liquid into nutrients for your body to use. Water and nutrients are absorbed back into the body and waste products are eliminated from your body in your stool. For the most part, your body's ability to absorb water and nutrients is unchanged because of the SCI. On the other hand, your body's ability to move the stool through the colon and eliminate waste products from your body through a bowel movement is affected.

Normally, when you feel stool is in your rectum, you have the sensation that you are going to have a bowel movement. You squeeze the muscle called the "anal sphincter" that functions to keep stool in your body. Then, when you are ready to move your bowels, you relax the sphincter and the stool leaves your body resulting in a bowel movement. However, as we've learned already, sensation and muscle function (including the muscles around the anus) can change after SCI, and you may develop what doctors call a **neurogenic** bowel.

Your **rehabilitation team** may have suggested that you follow a bowel care program so that you can gain control of your bowel function again. The overall goal of your bowel care program is the safe, predictable, and efficient elimination of stool with few to no bowel accidents, which, in turn, will go far in preventing any other bowel-related complications. Important components of a bowel care program are to:

- Maintain a consistent schedule. This means making sure that you follow your bowel care program regularly and without failure, usually daily or every other day.
- Find the "right" time during the day. You may tend to have bowel movements more in the morning or at night. Listen to your body because it might be best to schedule your bowel care during those times.
- Find the best position (lying down or sitting up). Gravity often helps move things along, so if you can, you may want to consider being upright for your bowel care.
- Eat a healthy diet. Make sure you are getting enough fiber in your diet and pay attention to foods or spices that disrupt your bowel care.
- Drink enough water. Fluids help move things along, but you need to balance this with your bladder management.

- Find out if you need medications, and if so, which one(s) work for you.
- Learn the right way to do manual evacuation of stool, digital stimulation, and put in suppositories and/or enemas.

Bowel care may not seem like the most important aspect of recovery after your SCI, but as time goes on, most people report that bowel and bladder function are more important to them than being able to walk. Also, bowel problems are a leading cause of social isolation and increase the need for assistance from others. People with SCI report that the three major bowel complaints are **constipation**, pain, and **incontinence**. So, as you go forward following your SCI, you will want to make sure that you take good care of your bowels to avoid these problemss.

Finally, it's always a good idea to revisit and reevaluate your bowel program periodically. Ask yourself the following questions:

- *How long does my bowel care take?* Roughly more than one hour total or more than 30 minutes for a suppository to work is too long.
- *Are you having bowel accidents?* More than a rare accident is too many.
- *How often are you emptying your bowels?* Don't get lazy with those bowels. Most people need to do this at least two to three times per week.
- *Do you have pain and/or bleeding from hemorrhoids?* This might be due to constipation.
- *Are you constipated?* Signs of constipation can include bloating, pain, mucous leaking from your rectum, and long delays in your bowel care regimen.
- *Are you taking other medicines that might affect your bowel care?* These medicines might include pain killers and antibiotics.
- *Are you satisfied with your bowel care program?* If not, call your SCI specialist to discuss things you can do differently.

Even though at some point you may be satisfied with your bowel care program, you may find it may slowly change over time. Ask yourself these questions above every so often to head off small problems before they become larger ones.

Because of the impact that bowel problems have on people after SCI, researchers are currently conducting experiments in which electrodes are implanted around the nerves controlling the bowel and bladder so that you can just push a button on a remote control to cause you to have a bowel movement or empty your bladder.

A very good resource for the down and dirty details of bowel care is the Paralyzed Veterans of America's book entitled *Neurogenic Bowel: What You Should Know. A Guide for People with Spinal Cord Injury.*

What About Colostomy?

Sometimes, either immediately after SCI or even years down the road, you may hear about a colostomy for bowel care. "Ostomy" means an artificial, or surgically created, opening from the urinary or digestive tract to the outside of the body. A "colostomy" is either a temporary or permanent opening made by a surgeon in which a portion of the large intestine, or colon, is brought to the skin of the abdomen, forming an opening through which stool passes. The stool is then collected on the outside of your abdomen in a collection bag, which is hidden by clothing.

Having a colostomy sometimes makes what has been difficult bowel care easier because there is no need to insert a suppository, perform digital stimulation, or wait sometimes hours for a bowel movement. Some recent studies have shown that people with long-term SCI who choose a colostomy are satisfied and report that their **quality of life** has improved as a result. If you feel that you've tried everything (changing the time, frequency, position, your diet and fluids, medications, etc.), you may want to speak with your health care provider to see if a colostomy is a good option for you. Also, it's always helpful to speak with other people who are living with a colostomy to find out what it's like.

BLADDER CHANGES

Not being able to urinate and having difficulty urinating are also common problems after SCI. These problems can lead to complications such as a **urinary tract infection**, bladder stones, sepsis (blood poisoning), kidney failure, and even death. Until several decades ago, many people with SCI developed very early bladder and kidney disease, often leading to permanent problems or even death. With improved medical management of the bladder and kidney and improved bladder care techniques, survival after SCI has improved dramatically. Careful bladder management can help prevent such complications. Your rehabilitation team can help you evaluate and reevaluate your bladder care program through your lifetime.

Understanding the **urinary system** (Figure 1.3) can help you better manage your bladder function. The urinary system is divided into the upper tracts and the lower tracts. The kidneys and the ureters (small tubes that connect the kidneys and the bladder) make up the upper tracts. The bladder and the urethra (the tube through which urine leaves the body) make up the lower tracts. Women's urinary systems differ from men's in that women have shorter urethras. Women often get more bladder infections because the bacteria have a shorter distance to travel to the bladder from outside the body.

Wastes and excess water are filtered through your kidneys and turned into urine. The urine flows from the kidneys through the ureters to the bladder. Your bladder is able to stretch and hold urine until it is time to urinate. When you urinate, your bladder contracts, the sphincter (muscle that controls outflow of urine) opens, and the urine flows out through the urethra.

Normally, urination is under voluntary and involuntary nervous system control (through the autonomic nervous system). When the amount of urine in the bladder reaches a certain critical volume, messages are sent to the sacral nerves in the spinal cord, telling your brain that your bladder is full. You then decide whether to hold the urine longer or to urinate. If you decide it is time to urinate, messages are sent down the spinal cord to the urinary system, your bladder contracts, and the sphincter opens to release the urine.

A neurogenic bladder develops if your spinal cord is damaged and messages cannot travel between the brain and the bladder. The most common type of bladder problem after SCI is the inability to void, or empty the bladder, either partially or totally. If you cannot empty your bladder, serious health dangers could result, such as bladder and/or kidney infection or urine backing up from the bladder into the kidneys, which can cause permanent kidney damage.

There are a variety of options for bladder management after SCI, which is an important factor in the long-term health of your bladder and kidneys. Table 1.2 summarizes the options for bladder management.

It's a good idea to check in periodically (every one to two years) with your SCI specialist and/or your urologist about your bladder health. Depending on your type of bladder management, you may need any of a variety of tests to make sure your bladder is healthy. These tests may include any combination of the following:

- Urinalysis and/or urine culture to check for infection or bacteria in the urine
- Bladder X-ray or CT to check for bladder stones
- Creatinine blood test to check kidney function
- Creatinine urine test to check kidney function
- Kidney ultrasound to check for kidney stones
- Renogram (a more high-tech kidney X-ray involving radioactive dye) to test kidney function
- Cystogram (a test in which dye is put in your bladder through your urethra) to check the size and shape of your bladder as well as for a condition called vesicoureteral reflux, resulting from too much pressure in the bladder
- Cystoscopy, in which the urologist takes a look into your bladder for stones, changes in the bladder, or even cancer

Table 1.2. Options for Bladder Management

Type of Bladder Management	What Is It?	Who Does It?	Pros and Cons
Voiding on your own	Emptying your bladder unassisted	Usually if you have a very incomplete SCI (ASIA D or E)	•Promotes good bladder and kidney health •Ease, though it may take more time to empty bladder
Voiding + intermittent catheterization	Voiding partially on your own and emptying the remainder with a catheter	Usually if you have a very incomplete spinal cord injury (ASIA C or D)	•Promotes good bladder and kidney health. •Requires carrying catheter supplies
Voiding + Valsalva maneuver or Credé maneuver	Valsalva maneuver is bearing down to push out urine and/or stool. Crede maneuver is applying pressure to the lower abdomen with your hands to push urine out of the bladder	Usually if you have had a sphincterotomy or have a very weak bladder (as with a very low SCI)	•Can be associated with serious bladder and kidney health problems if improperly done (this is generally no longer recommended)
Intermittent catheterization	Inserting a small catheter into your urethra every 4-6 hours to empty the urine	Anyone with an SCI who cannot fully empty their bladder on their own	•Relatively safe •Fewer associated complications than indwelling catheterization •Need to time catheterizations, monitor fluid in-take, carry supplies •May require assistance from others if hand function is impaired •More difficult for women to catheterize while seated
Indwelling catheterization (usually a urethral or "foley" catheter or a suprapubic catheter)	A bladder catheter remains in the bladder either through the urethra or through a site in the lower abdomen below the umbilicus (suprapubic site)	Anyone with SCI who cannot fully empty their bladder on their own AND does not have the ability to manage intermittent catheterization OR has failed intermittent catheterization	•Associated with more long-term bladder and kidney complications, such as stones, kidney scars and bladder cancer. •Urine is collected in a bag that is worn or carried. •No need to monitor fluid intake

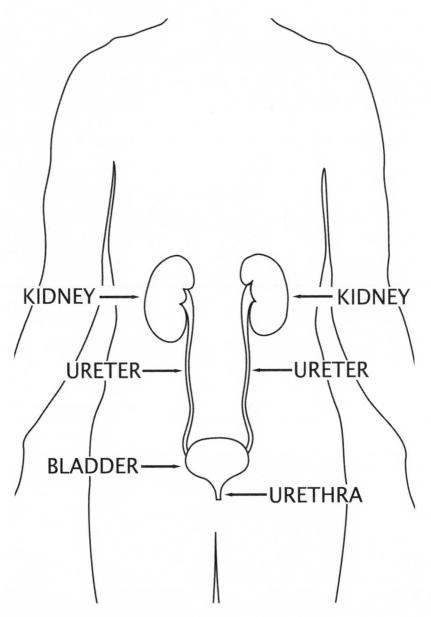

Figure 1.3. The Urinary System
The urinary system, also called the urinary tract, filters the body's blood. This system gets rid of waste products and excess water in the form of urine.

When you see your urologist, make sure to ask which tests you need and how often you may need them.

THE AFFECT OF SPINAL CORD INJURY ON THE HEART

Your **circulatory system** (Figure 1.4) includes your heart, arteries, veins, and capillaries. It is designed to send nutrients from absorbed from food in the gastrointestinal tract and oxygen from the lungs to other parts of your body. Because the nervous system helps control the function of your heart and other parts of the circulatory system, its function is often affected after SCI. The heart pumps blood to the walls of your lungs where it gathers up oxygen. The blood then returns to the heart and is pumped into the arteries and then to the capillaries, which are tiny blood vessels found throughout your body tissues. Blood flowing through the capillaries delivers oxygen and nutrients to the tissues and gathers waste products from the tissues. The blood flows from the capillaries into the veins, which return the blood to the heart. On the way, the blood gets filtered by the kidneys, which remove wastes by excreting it in the urine. There, the cycle begins again.

Spinal cord injury can affect your circulation in two important ways. First, it can change your blood pressure (the force with which your blood goes to the blood vessels). After an SCI, some nerves stop sending the messages to keep your arteries tight. As a result, your blood pressure may stabilize at a level that is lower than before the injury. As a result of this change in circulation, orthostatic hypotension (decreased blood pressure which may cause you to become lightheaded when you sit or stand up) might occur. This change can also cause your heart rate to slow, which may cause dizziness or lightheadedness.

Second, SCI can change how well blood flows from your body to your heart. The muscles affected by the injury no longer flex and relax as they did before your injury, and the blood does not move throughout your body as well as before. These circulation changes may cause edema (swelling) in your legs and hands, depending on the level of your injury, and blood clots in your legs or lungs. When a blood clot stays in the veins in your leg it's called a thrombus. Swelling, redness, and/or pain most often in a leg can be a sign of a blood clot.

In some cases, a piece of a blood clot called an **embolus** might break off and move through the veins up toward the heart and lungs. If a blood clot lodges in one of your lungs (called a **pulmonary** embolus), it can be deadly. Signs of an embolus in your lungs (a pulmonary embolus include shortness of breath, dizziness, coughing up more phlegm than usual, and coughing up blood.

Usually, you are at risk for a blood clot or embolus for a few months

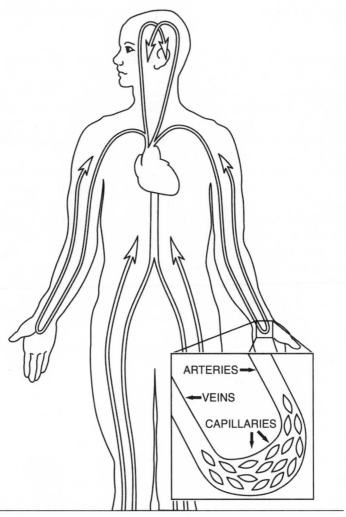

Figure 1.4. The Circulatory System
The circulatory system includes the heart, arteries, veins, and capillaries. It sends nutrients absorbed from food in the gastrointestinal tract and oxygen from the lungs to other parts of the body.

immediately after your SCI. You are also at risk for blood clots beyond that time if you've had surgery or if you have been bedridden for a period of time (for example, as caused by a **pressure sore**, broken bone, etc). If you think you might have a blood clot or an embolus, you should see your doctor immediately because it can be life-threatening.

BREATHING CHANGES AFTER SPINAL CORD INJURY

Spinal cord injury also may affect your ability to breathe because certain muscles may not be as strong or work as well as before the injury. In general, exhaling (breathing out) usually takes little to no energy or effort. Inhaling (breathing in) requires different muscles and uses more energy. Inhaling is obviously very important because this is the way you get oxygen to all parts of your body. Muscles that help you inhale include the diaphragm, your neck muscles, and the intercostals muscles (muscles between your ribs). In general, the lower your SCI, the better your lung function will be.

The diaphragm is the main breathing muscle, which gets its nerve supply primarily from C4 (remember our anatomy?). Therefore, a person with a complete injury above the C4 level will most likely need a ventilator (breathing machine) to help with breathing. Someone who has a C4 injury may need to use a ventilator to breathe, either temporarily or permanently. In our experience, most healthy, young, nonsmokers with a C4 injury will eventually be able to breath without the assistance of a ventilator. On the other hand, many people with C4, C5, C6 or even lower SCI, who have smoked considerably or previously had lung problems, remain on ventilators. If your injury is in the thoracic spine, your ability to inhale is still weaker than if you didn't have an SCI, but it is better than that of someone with a cervical injury. Table 1.3 summarizes the muscles involved in breathing and the effect of SCI on those muscles.

Table 1.3. Effects of Spinal Cord Injury on the Muscles Involved in Breathing

SCI Level	Muscles Involved	Function of the Muscle	What happens if I have an SCI at this level?
C1-3	Sternocleidomastoid	Helps with inspiration	Can only breathe for a few hours after injury. Beyond that time will need a ventilator
C4	Diaphragm	Main muscle used for inspiration	May or may not need a ventilator either permanently or temporarily after SCI. Will have a very weak cough.
C5-C8	Scalenes	Helps with inspiration	May need a ventilator temporarily, but in most cases should be able to breathe on own. Will have a weak cough.
All thoracic	Intercostals	Control expiration/coughing	Cough will be somewhat weaker.

Coughing is our way of forcefully exhaling to remove mucous, phlegm, or other unwanted particles from the lungs. Both thoracic and cervical SCI weaken your ability to cough. We know from experience that people with SCI tend to cough up more phlegm. If there is difficulty clearing secretions and phlegm from our lungs, then the possibility of an infection, such as pneumonia, is more likely. Keeping upright (as opposed to lying down), keeping active, and sometimes asking for someone else to assist you with coughing are ways to help clear the lungs of unwanted material.

Other factors influence your ability to breathe in addition to the level of your SCI. These factors include whether you had a previous history of lung disease, whether you smoke or not, and your age. Respiratory problems after SCI can result from many causes. The most common cause is infection, such as pneumonia. Signs of respiratory problems include:

• Shortness of breath
• Rapid breathing
• Congestion or increasing lung secretions
• Morning headache
• Fever
• Abnormal drowsiness

What Can I Do to Have Healthy Lungs?

You can do several things to keep your lungs in the best shape possible. First and foremost, if you smoke, you should stop. Smoking causes more mucous and phlegm to develop, which are harder to clear from your lungs because of the muscle weakness associated with SCI. Smoking is also the major factor contributing to lung cancer. If you stop smoking, you can actually dramatically decrease your chance of getting lung cancer.

As stated above, when you are immobile, such as during periods of bedrest, mucous and phlegm tend to accumulate in your lungs. Portions of your lungs may collapse. Therefore, activity and exercise can help to keep your lungs healthy and prevent lung problems.

If you have a cervical or high thoracic level of SCI, or if you have other lung problems, you should strongly consider getting a pneumonia vaccination (called a "pneumovax") every five years and a flu vaccine yearly. Periodically, your SCI specialist should test your forced vital capacity (FVC). This simple test can be done in the outpatient department where you breathe into a hand-held device. These tests go a long way toward preventing much bigger problems.

WHY DO I HURT NOW?

Pain is another common problem after SCI. It contributes to both emotional and physical stress. There is a close relationship between **spasticity** (involuntary movement of one's arms and legs) and pain. Increased pain seems to trigger greater spasticity, which in turn can lead to painful postures and deformity.

Pain can be classified in different ways. One system classifies pain as mechanical, neuropathic, visceral, and "other" pain. Table 1.4 shows the types of pain, what causes them, and what you might do about the pain.

Table 1.4. Types of Pain and What to Do About Pain

Type of Pain	Causes	What The Pain Feels Like	What to Do
Mechanical pain	Injury to the muscles, bones, tendons or ligaments.	•Felt at or above the level of the SCI, though may be felt below the level of the injury in incomplete SCI •Feels like a dull ache or sharp pain	•Rest, bracing •Ice over areas that have normal feeling •Anti-inflammatory medications such as Ibuprofen •Narcotic medications • Surgery
Neuropathic pain	Damage to the central or peripheral nervous system, such as compression or pinching of a nerve	•Felt above, at, or below the level of SCI •Feels like burning, cold, shooting, stabbing, electricity, shock-like, tingling, numbness, squeezing/tightness, or hypersensitivity	•Difficult to treat •Appropriate medications such as Neurontin, Amytriptyline, Nortryptyline, or Klonopin •Implanted pump to deliver pain medicines •Epidural block •Surgery, such as rhizotomy
Visceral pain	Due to a problem with your internal organs (such as constipation or appendicitis)	•Felt above, at, or below the level of SCI, often in the abdomen (stomach area) •If you have a high level of SCI, may feel like any of the above	•Have a doctor evaluate •May require any of the above medications or surgery to correct the problem

To effectively treat your pain, you and your doctor need to determine the cause of the pain. Neuropathic pain is usually the most difficult pain to treat, and it may take several different types of treatments to decrease the pain.

Often, we can't totally eliminate neuropathic pain, but if we can decrease the intensity, it will help.

SEXUAL AND FERTILITY CHANGES

Despite the changes in your body, people with SCI can continue to lead sexually active lives. The physical aspects of sex may be different after SCI, but sexual intimacy is still possible. Below is an overview of sexual changes men and women may experience. Chapter 11 offers more detailed information about sexuality after SCI.

How Your Sexual Response Changes After Spinal Cord Injury

For men, major aspects of sexual change involve erection, ejaculation, and orgasm. Men's bodily systems are designed to create two types of erections. Reflex erections occur when the penis, scrotum, or the area around the genitals are stimulated (touched). Psychogenic erections occur when a man thinks or fantasizes about sex, or when sounds and smells trigger sexual excitement.

The level and type of SCI affect whether a man can have an erection and the "quality" of the erection. Men with higher levels of injury (high thoracic and cervical) tend to be more likely to be able to have a reflex erection compared with men who have very low injuries (below T12). The more incomplete the spinal cord injury is, the more likely an erection will occur. If your injury is below T12, reflex erections are less likely, but you may be able to have psychogenic erections from thinking or fantasizing about sex.

After a SCI, many men also find that their ability to ejaculate decreases. While most men can have an orgasm, which are described as similar, weaker, or different than before the injury, the ability to ejaculate depends on the level and completeness of the SCI.

Despite changes in their bodies, women with spinal cord injury can remain sexually active and have satisfying intimate relationships. Research has shown a similar pattern for women's vaginal lubrication as that for men's erection, such that women with complete injuries at or above the T12 level of the spinal cord are more likely to have reflex vaginal lubrication in response to touch. Some women with complete SCI also are able to have an orgasm with similar feelings and body reactions as women without spinal cord injury.

Will I Be Able to Have Children?

Infertility is a problem for most men with SCI. Infertility can result from an inability to ejaculate (called "anejaculation") and from poor sperm quality. While men with SCI produce a normal amount of sperm, many of the sperm do not move or "swim" well enough, making it less likely for them to travel as far as needed to reach and fertilize a woman's egg and achieve pregnancy.

Because of these issues, researchers have developed a variety of techniques to retrieve sperm and increase men's chances of fatherhood. These techniques include penile vibratory stimulation, in which vibration is applied to the head of the penis; electroejaculation, in which a probe is placed in the man's rectum and electrical stimulation is applied; and needle aspiration, in which sperm are removed from the testicles using a fine needle.

After healthy sperm are obtained, assisted reproductive techniques may help you and your partner become pregnant. These techniques include artificial insemination, in vitro fertilization (IVF), gamete intrafallopian transfer (GIFT), and intracytoplasmic sperm injection (ISCI). Chapter 11 describes sperm retrieval and assisted reproductive techniques in more detail.

Women with SCI do not have a change in fertility and are able to become pregnant. It may take a few months for you to begin having periods again after the injury, but after your periods return, pregnancy is a possibility. If parenthood is not your goal, then be sure to use birth control to prevent unintended pregnancies.

SOME COMPLICATIONS OF SPINAL CORD INJURY

Urinary Tract Infections

Recurrent urinary tract infections and upper tract complications are the most common medical complications seen in persons with SCI. These complications can impair your long-term health and survival. Associated problems include kidney stones, renal (kidney) insufficiency, kidney failure, hydronephrosis, and cancer.

Urinary tract infections with symptoms such as urinary incontinence, increased spasticity, fever, malaise, lower abdominal pain, and autonomic dysreflexia should be treated with antibiotics. Routine urinary system evaluations should be done every one to three years. Such evaluations can help detect problems and help maintain normal renal function. Diagnostic urinary studies include:

- A renal sonogram (ultrasound) to detect tumors, cysts, and stones in the urinary tract

- A renal scan to assess kidney function and blood supply in the kidneys
- An abdominal X-ray
- Cystoscopy to diagnose problems inside the bladder
- Urodynamic studies to provide information about the mechanics of void-ing urine
- A 24-hour creatinine clearance (a test involving collection of urine for a 24-hour period to check kidney function)
- Urinalysis (to look for chemical and cellular products)
- Urine culture to look for infection
- Urology consultation

Spasticity

Spasticity (uncontrolled, involuntary movement of one's arms and legs) is a common condition that arises with spinal cord injuries above the conus medullaris (the lower part of the spinal cord). The reflex muscle contractions that come with spasticity may be either flexor spasms (bending of your arms or legs toward your body) or they may be extensor spasms (rigid straighten-ing of your arms or legs away from your body).

You may experience spasticity when you stretch your muscles or when your skin is touched or irritated. You may also find that spasticity increases when you have an infection, pressure ulcer, constipation, urine retention, bladder stones, abdominal problems, or fracture. In addition, you may expe-rience spasticity if you wear tight clothing or if you come in contact with other irritating stimuli.

Although spasticity can cause problems, it does have some benefits. For example, spasticity can:

- Promote blood circulation in your limbs
- Alert you to a new or worsening medical condition, such as a pressure sore, in an area without sensation
- Help maintain your muscle bulk
- Help with bowel function by maintaining sphincter tone
- Assist you in obtaining a grip needed for to pick up objects
- Assist weak or paralyzed muscles in doing activities such as rolling in bed, transfers, and ambulation.

On the other hand, spasticity can negatively affect your quality of life. For example:

- Painful or recurrent intense spasms can interfere with your sleep, position-ing, wearing of splints, driving, sex life, and balance.

- Spasticity can interfere with your functional activities such as transfers, bed mobility, and walking.
- Abdominal spasms can impede your breathing.
- Sustained spasticity can decrease your range of motion and lead to joint contractures (tightness of tissue around joints and in muscle that limits movement and function). In turn, sustained spasticity can interfere with daily living skills like dressing and bathing.
- Sudden severe spasms may cause you to fall out of your wheelchair or off your bed, which may result in a bone fracture or skin breakdown.

Your doctor may consider treating spasticity if its disadvantages outweigh its advantages for you. Treatment may be needed if spasticity leads to skin breakdown or joint contracture; prevents or interferes with positioning, transfers, gait, or activities of daily living; causes pain; interferes with sleep or movement; or prevents the use of splints.

Treatment is aimed at improving function and relieving pain or discomfort. It may include:

- Sustained stretching of the extremities
- Special positioning to reduce spasticity and maintain proper body alignment
- Application of heat or cold
- Therapeutic exercise
- Splinting
- Electrical stimulation
- Oral medications

Autonomic Dysreflexia

Autonomic dysreflexia (AD), also called hyperreflexia, can be a serious complication of SCI. When you have an episode of AD, your blood pressure can rise to dangerous levels, possibly leading to stroke or death. Therefore, this condition should be considered a medical emergency. People with SCI at the T6 level or above are at greatest risk for AD. AD mainly arises because of an imbalance in the body systems that control your blood pressure. When an irritating stimulus is present, a reflex causes your blood vessels to constrict (become more narrow) and raise the blood pressure. With an uninjured spinal cord, the same stimulus would cause another set of reflexes to stop the blood vessels from constricting too much. However, when the spinal cord has been injured at the T6 level or above, the signals telling the blood vessels to relax cannot be sent through the spinal cord.

In addition, uncontrolled activity of the nerves at the T6 level can cause the blood from the gut to flow into the rest of the blood system. Blood pressure can then rise to a dangerous level.

Examples of irritating stimuli that may cause AD include:

- *Bladder problems* (the most common cause of AD). Such problems are caused by urinary tract infection, urinary retention, a blocked catheter, an overfilled urine collection bag, and not adhering to a **catheterization** program
- *Bowel problems.* Such problems include overdistention or irritation, constipation/impaction, distention during a bowel program (such as during digital stimulation), hemorrhoids or anal infections, and infection or irritation
- *Skin-related problems.* Such problems are caused by pressure from a shoe or chair, cut, bruise, or abrasion; a pressure sore; an ingrown toenail; a burn, including sunburn or a burn from hot water; and tight or restrictive clothing
- *Sexual activity.* Such activity may result in overstimulation during sexual activity or pelvic stimuli that would be painful if you had sensation in that area
- *Reproductive-related causes.* Such causes include menstrual cramps and labor and delivery
- *Other causes.* Such causes include **heterotopic ossification** or acute abdominal conditions such as gastric ulcer, colitis, or peritonitis

If you detect warning signs of AD, be sure to find and remove the cause. Get immediate medical attention if you cannot locate the cause. The warning signs are listed in Figure 1.5.

WHAT ARE MY CHANCES FOR RECOVERY?

Soon after your injury, you probably had many questions about your recovery: Am I going to walk again? Am I going to be able to urinate again? Will I be able to move my bowels normally again? Will I be able to be intimate with my partner? Because all spinal cord injuries are different, each person's recovery varies. No one can say for sure how much you will recover.

Most people get the greatest amount of recovery during the first six months after the injury, although you can still have small amounts of recovery up to two years post-SCI. People with incomplete SCIs are more likely than people with complete SCIs to regain some sensation and movement.

Even if your doctor predicts that you won't regain all of your preinjury abilities, medical rehabilitation can help you to function and live productively after your SCI. Your rehabilitation should begin soon after your injury.

Autonomic dysreflexia (AD) is a serious complication of spinal cord injury at the T6 level or above. AD needs immediate attention. With AD, your blood pressure can rise to dangerous levels, possibly leading to stroke or even death. Signs of AD include:

- Hypertension: blood pressure higher than 200/100
- A pounding headache
- A flushed (reddened) face
- Red blotches on the skin above the level of injury
- Sweating above the level of injury
- Nasal stuffiness
- Nausea
- A pulse slower than 60 beats per minute
- "Goose bumps" below the level of injury
- Cold, clammy skin below the level of injury

If you have these symptoms:

- Sit up if you are lying down.
- Look for and remove the cause, which may be a bladder, bowel, skin, or other problem.
- Contact your physician and go to the nearest hospital right away.

Figure 1.5. Warning Signs of Autonomic Dysreflexia

Your rehabilitation team will help you learn new skills and relearn old skills. They will show you how to adapt to your limitations and increase your physical abilities. Team members will also teach you ways to confront barriers in your environment and help you and your family to cope with your **disability**. At first, many people with SCI feel limited and frustrated because they cannot do everything they did before the injury. With persistence and the help of family, friends, doctors, and other rehabilitation experts, most people with SCI can regain some of their abilities and independence.

What Can I Do?

As you adapt to life after SCI, it's important to:

- *Become an educated consumer.* Spinal cord injury is a rare injury or disease, depending on the cause. Unless your health care provider specializes in, or has a special interest in, caring for people with SCI, it is likely that he or she will be unfamiliar with the nuances of the care of people with SCIs. So, just as you need to take control of your care during rehabilitation, you need to take control of your health, wellness, and function for the rest of your life. This means advocating for yourself and, at times, educating your health care provider about spinal cord injury.

- *Keep in contact with your SCI rehabilitation team.* Your rehabilitation team will share changes in treatment options, therapies, and new research with you. Also, as you've learned, SCI puts you at risk of more medical complications that may need closer monitoring.

Where Can I Learn More?

To learn more about the physical effects of SCI, you may wish to contact:

- Your physiatrist (rehabilitation doctor) or other members of your rehabilitation team
- The Spinal Cord Injury Information Network (www.spinalcord.uab.edu)
- The National Spinal Cord Injury Association (www.spinalcord.org)

Appendix C provides information about additional resources.

IMPORTANT POINTS TO REMEMBER

- The spinal cord is a soft, rope-like structure of nerves that runs from the base of the brain to the lower part of the back. Its purpose is to carry information between the brain and other parts of the body. Spinal cord damage caused by injury or disease often results in some type of paralysis (or weakness) and sensory loss (loss of feeling).
- Spinal cord injury can affect your bowel, bladder, circulatory system, breathing, sexual function, and fertility. It can also result in various kinds of pain.
- Medical rehabilitation can help rebuild muscles that are still functioning and help you relearn how to use them. If no movement remains below the level of the injury, then the focus of rehabilitation becomes strengthening intact muscles above the injury level and finding ways to compensate for those that are unable to move.

This chapter was supported in part by funding from the U.S. Department of Education, National Institute on Disability and Rehabilitation Research, Grant #H133B031114.

2
Adapting Your Activities of Daily Living

WILLIAM BUTLER
LISA DINAPOLI
LORI EISEN
CARA HOSSLER SMYTHE
LINDSEY KANSKI

"Writing, feeding myself, dressing, and walking the dog all required adaptation that was achieved by trial and error, research, and out-of-the-box thinking." –Jennifer

Your spinal cord is the major pathway connecting your brain to the rest of your body. When that pathway is damaged, any or all of the muscles below the level of injury can be affected, leading to an inability to use those parts of the body. During **rehabilitation** you will learn new ways to adapt your **activities of daily living** so that you can become as independent and functional as possible.

In this chapter, you will learn about:

- Factors that can affect activities of daily living
- What to expect, depending on your level of injury
- Options for self-care and mobility
- Useful equipment
- The importance of setting goals and actively participating in the rehabilitation process

FINDING NEW WAYS TO DO DAILY ACTIVITIES

Before your spinal cord injury, you most likely took for granted your ability to do routine tasks. Without thinking much about it, you could get out of bed, dress, brush your hair and teeth, use the toilet, eat, walk to the mailbox, and drive to work. Now, all of that has changed. Depending on the level and extent of your injury, you must now find new ways to accomplish at least some of these activities of daily living (ADLs).

While you are in the rehabilitation hospital, your team will help you learn to do routine tasks as easily and independently as possible, sometimes with the help of adaptive equipment. They will also help you rebuild your strength and endurance so you can perform ADLs on your own or with the help of a caregiver at home. Your doctor, therapists, rehabilitation nurse, and other members of the team will work closely with you to find the best solutions to meet your individual needs.

As you think about performing ADLs, keep in mind that several factors come into play. These factors include:

- Sensation
- Motor (muscle) control
- Balance
- Trunk stability
- Energy
- Spasticity

Sensation: Spinal cord injury can affect **sensation** in different ways. For example, you may no longer be able to feel pain in some parts of your body; therefore, you may not know how to move away from the source of pain. You might also be less able to sense where you are in space (proprioception). This may make it difficult to know where your leg is when you try to walk or where your arm is when you try to get dressed.

Motor control: Motor control is your ability to move parts of your body when you want them to move. As explained in Chapter 1, each muscle in the body uses a nerve connection that travels through the spinal cord to the brain in order to create movement. Without that connection, the muscles are unable to receive the information they need to work. How much your muscles are affected depends on the level and extent of your injury.

Balance: Balance is essential for functioning safely and minimizing the risk of injury resulting from falls. To achieve balance, you must have enough strength to hold a particular position. Your brain must also receive the sensory information needed to provide feedback on whether that position is being maintained. For example, if you have a cervical (neck) spinal cord injury, you may not have the trunk strength and sensation needed to sit safely at the edge of the bed when getting up in the morning. However, through rehabilitation, you can learn to use your arms and vision to find your balance point and hold yourself safely in that position.

Trunk stability: Damage to the spinal cord at or below the thoracic (chest) level may prevent voluntary movement and sensation not only in your legs, but also in your trunk. Voluntary control of your trunk is the foundation of stability for all movement. If you lack trunk stability, you will need to find ways to complete tasks while maintaining your balance.

Energy: Because of changes in your body's performance, self-care tasks such as bathing and dressing will require you to use more energy than needed before your injury. Depending on the level of your injury, you will have to make daily decisions about how to the use your strength and energy. Getting assistance with self-care tasks may give you more energy and time for other activities, such as home and child care or going to work.

Spasticity: Normally, some reflexes remain present after spinal cord injury. For example, when you touch something hot on a stove, a reflex reaction will move your hand away from the heat. There are also centers in the spinal cord capable of causing those same reactions, but the reactions can be out of proportion to the stimulus (such as extreme heat). These reactions are known as **spasms**. The presence of spasms is referred to as **spasticity**. In some cases, spasticity can be helpful. For example, if you have spasms in your leg muscles, they may help you to stand. More often than not, however, spasms can be painful. They can make it difficult to maintain certain positions, such as sitting in a wheelchair over the course of a day. Your rehabilitation team should work with you to find the right combination of medication and positioning options in order to control spasms and increase your independence.

WHAT WILL I BE ABLE TO DO?

The American Spinal Injury Association (ASIA) has developed a classification system for spinal cord injury, commonly referred to as the **ASIA Impairment Scale**. This scale, described in Chapter 1, is widely used by doctors to identify the level and extent of a spinal cord injury and to predict functional outcomes (what the person eventually should be able to do). Knowing the level and extent of the injury helps the health care team to create an individualized treatment and rehabilitation plan.

Table 2.1 lists the function a person with spinal cord injury is generally expected to have in doing self-care, bed mobility, and mobility tasks, according to the level of injury. As the table suggests, some people may be able to do some tasks independently, often with the help of adaptive equipment. Others will need assistance from a caregiver to do daily tasks.

Keep in mind that every injury is unique, making it difficult to predict precisely what a person will be able to do at the end of the rehabilitation process. Sometimes, what a person actually can do is often different from what he or she should do. Some people have other medical conditions such as heart disease, diabetes, pain, or even being overweight that limit their ability to achieve as high a level of independence as possible. At the same time, others are very motivated, work very hard, and exceed expectations. Therefore, while characteristics of your injury and your health play into how independent you will be, motivation, positive attitude, and hard work are critical to succeed. Each of these activity areas is described in more detail below.

Table 2.1. Expected Self-Care, Bed Mobility, and Mobility Function by Injury Level

Level of Injury	Self-Care	Bed Mobility and Transfers	Mobility
C1-C3	Caregiver required for all self-care. An environmental control unit (ECU) can be used to control light switches, phones, etc.	Complete assistance from a caregiver required.	Independent with a power wheelchair.
C4	Caregiver required for all self-care. A mouth stick can be used for typing, writing, etc.	Complete assistance from a caregiver required.	Independent with a power wheelchair.
C5	Caregiver needed for some assistance and adaptive equipment for self-care.	Some assistance from a caregiver required.	Power wheelchair with possible limited use of manual wheelchair.
C6	Minimal assistance from caregiver for self-care.	Some to no assistance from a caregiver needed.	Manual wheelchair with possibility of power wheelchair use for longer distances.
C7	Independent self-care with use of adaptive equipment.	Independent transfer with possibility of assistance to manage legs only.	Manual wheelchair with possibility of power wheelchair use for longer distances.
C8-T7	Independent self-care without adaptive equipment.	Independent transfer with possibility of assistance to manage legs only.	Manual wheelchair.
T7-L5	Independent self-care without adaptive equipment.	Independent	Manual wheelchair.

SELF-CARE SKILLS

Since your injury, seemingly simple self-care activities such as brushing your teeth, showering, and dressing may present new challenges and difficulties. To complete daily tasks, you will need to learn new skills, find new ways to "get the job done," and use specially designed adaptive equipment. The level of difficulty for doing daily living tasks depends on the level of injury. Some people will be able to make up for lost use of a limb by using adaptive equipment or finding different methods of completing tasks. Other people will need assistance from a trained caregiver.

Upper-Body Bathing, Dressing, and Grooming

Upper-body dressing, bathing, and grooming demand more energy during large movements made by the body, such as moving your whole arm, than doing small movements, such as moving your finger. How well you complete these tasks depends on your ability to get to needed grooming and bathing utensils, water, and clothing. If your trunk control and balance are impaired, you will find it harder to change positions, lean forward, and move from your bed to your wheelchair. You might also find it difficult to do tasks that require reaching overhead.

In the rehabilitation hospital, you will first learn to dress and bathe while sitting with back support (in a hospital bed with your head raised or in a chair). As you regain trunk control and sitting balance, you will be more able to do upper-body dressing and bathing in an unsupported sitting position (such as on the edge of the bed). Table 2.2 describes positions your **rehabilitation team** may teach you for performing self-care tasks.

Lower-Body Bathing and Dressing

As with upper-body care, lower-body care is more efficient if you have good trunk control and sitting balance. If you can control your trunk muscles, you'll be able to manage your legs and reach for items more easily because your trunk acts as a stable platform from which your limbs are controlled. If you have limited trunk control, you must divide your energy and attention between maintaining sitting balance and getting into a position that gives you enough leverage for leg management. If you have poor trunk control and sitting balance, you may find that lower-body dressing and bathing are most easily accomplished in bed. This gives you the options of lying in bed and/or sitting with your trunk supported to complete self-care tasks including bathing, dressing, and grooming (brushing your hair, teeth, washing your face, shaving and/or applying make-up).

Table 2.2. Positions for Performing Self-Care Tasks

Supported Sitting
Sit with your legs outstretched on the bed with the back of the bed at less than 90 degrees upright sitting. Begin to lean forward to wash your back and put on a shirt. You will also begin to address leg management skills to progress in sequence.
Unsupported Sitting – In Bed
Slowly lowering the back of the bed, you begin using your arms for balance and support. Your legs are put in a folded or "frog legs" position to minimize overstretching of the leg, trunk, and long back muscles that assist in upright sitting. You will then progress to shifting your weight forward and maintaining sitting balance without the use of your arms. This makes it easier to wash and try your back and to get shirts off and on.
Unsupported Sitting – Edge of Bed
From this position, you will explore your ability to begin shifting your weight beyond your body's center of gravity to extend your reach and prepare to do lateral transfers. This position also makes it easier to bathe and dress your upper extremities, with the assistance of a long-handled sponge and a reacher to give you greater reach.

You may use the raised head of a hospital bed to offer back support in sitting. If you don't have the use of a hospital bed, you may lean against a wall next to your bed and/or use pillows behind your back for support. You might also use a device called a bed ladder to help you get into a sitting position.

By adjusting your legs while seated, you will be able to reach your lower legs and feet to complete self-care tasks. Some individuals may not be able to easily or effectively position their legs because of spasms, tight muscles, weakness, or lack of sitting balance. They can use adaptive equipment to assist with bathing and dressing, but they will probably need help from a caregiver to complete these tasks fully.

Bathing and dressing in a wheelchair require more energy. These tasks are more easily mastered by individuals with good trunk control and sitting balance. However, being able to perform lower-body dressing and bathing at the wheelchair level will give you more independence with bowel and bladder care in community settings. It will also reduce stress on your arms by reducing the number of transfers needed to complete your daily care routine independently. Bathing in the wheelchair also gives you easier access to clean water and the ability to set up (that is, independently get needed items) for cleaning and grooming. Getting to this level of function is a key to living without the need for daily assistance or the daily presence of caregivers.

Dressing your upper body in a wheelchair requires that you have the strength and balance needed to lean forward or turn to the side away from the back of the chair to provide clearance to allow clothing adjustment. Dressing your lower body again requires enough arm strength and flexibility to manipulate your legs into positions that allow you to clear the seat of the wheelchair to adjust clothing.

While providing protection from injury (especially to those with little or no sensation in their feet), shoes should not be fit or tied tightly. Shoes should be one-half to one size larger than your normal shoe size. The larger size makes it easier to get your shoes on and helps prevent interruption of circulation. This larger size will also account for any swelling that may result from less active movement in your legs. Socks, pant waists, and outer clothing material in general should not be tight in consideration of circulation. Pants should not be made of slippery material as this makes maintaining sitting positions difficult. Silk briefs may be worn beneath pants to help decrease the possibility of skin shearing (see "Skin Care" section below), which may occur during changes of body position. To further assist with skin care, you should avoid clothing with buttons, rivets, or thick seams on the buttock and thigh areas. Such clothing may increase the amount of pressure on your skin.

SKIN CARE

The loss of mobility and sensation that often accompanies spinal cord injury increases the possibility of skin damage. This skin damage is referred to as **pressure sores**, decubitus ulcers, or skin breakdown. Pressure sores develop because of an injury to the skin or excessive pressure, which decreases the blood flow to the skin leading to breakdown. Pressure sores develop most easily in areas where only a thin layer of skin is covering bone, but any area of skin can be affected. Normally, sensation acts as a warning system, signaling you to move or shift your weight to let blood flow to return to an area before damage occurs. Because you cannot feel discomfort or pain after spinal cord injury, you cannot depend on your sensation to cue you to move. In addition to pressure, shearing, moisture, extremes of temperature, improper nutrition and alcohol and/or tobacco use can increase your risk of developing a pressure sore.

Pressure: The most common cause of skin damage for people with spinal cord injury is pressure. Sitting or lying in one position for a long period of time can decrease the blood supply to the areas that are supporting the body's weight, resulting in a wound known as a pressure sore or pressure ulcer. A pressure ulcer may first look like a dark area that does not blanch (turn white) when you press on it.

Shearing: Skin damage can also be caused by skin **shearing**. For example, movement while getting into or out of bed and movement while doing transfers that allows an area of the body to drag across a surface can result in a burn or shear injury. Similar to a rug burn, this type of injury results from the skin being pulled in one direction by the bed or transfer surface while the body moves in the opposite direction. You can avoid shear injuries by lifting your body off the transfer surface rather than sliding across it.

Moisture: Moisture from perspiration, incontinence, or inadequate drying after bathing can cause your skin to become soft and easily torn. Use of talcum powder or antiperspirants can protect the skin from natural body moisture. Also, be sure to thoroughly dry all areas of the body, especially skin folds, your groin area, and between your toes. In addition, make sure to attend to bowel and bladder "accidents" immediately because waste material contains acids. These acids, combined with moisture, can quickly break down skin and increase the chance of infection if a wound develops.

Extreme temperature: Extreme hot and cold can also lead to significant skin damage, but you may be unaware of such temperatures because of impaired sensation. For example, you could be burned by placing hot items on your lap or accidentally coming too close to space heaters, radiators, stoves, or fires. In addition, during the winter months, people with spinal cord injury who live in cold climates may be at risk of frostbite. Often, people with burns or frostbite are unaware of the problem until a wound is seen. By then, though, there may already be extensive skin damage. Therefore, it is important to take special care to avoid skin problems when you may be exposed to extreme temperatures.

Nutrition: Proper nutrition and hydration are also important in preventing skin breakdown and in healing when a wound has occurred. Eating a properly balanced diet provides the vitamins, proteins, and other materials essential for healthy, elastic skin. Drinking plenty of fluids also can improve skin health. Poor fluid intake can result in brittle skin that tears or rapidly breaks down with prolonged pressure.

Alcohol and tobacco: Alcohol and tobacco can affect the condition of your skin as well. Excessive alcohol use increases stress on your bladder function and increases the possibility of incontinence, which can lead to skin breakdown. In addition, the nicotine found in many tobacco products causes the smaller blood pathways in the body to constrict, resulting in decreased circulation of blood and other essential fluids to the skin. Finally, the use of drugs for recreational purposes increases the risk of poor decision-making and incidents that affect skin health.

Tips for Pressure Ulcer Prevention

An important point to remember is that nearly every pressure sore is preventable. Although pressure sores are major problems after spinal cord injury, you can take steps to prevent them. Review the pressure ulcer prevention recommendations below periodically to make sure that you are doing everything you can to avoid skin breakdown.

Change Your Body Position Frequently

In upright sitting, 75 percent of your body's weight is concentrated on your buttocks. To relieve this pressure, shift your position so that weight is taken off this area and blood flow is allowed to return. Such shifting may be accomplished by taking the following steps:

- In a power wheelchair with a tilt-in-space feature or with the assistance of a caregiver in a manual wheelchair, tilt backwards while maintaining your body's 90 degree (upright sitting) position until you feel your weight shift onto your back and shoulders. Maintain this position for 1 minute every 15 minutes while you are sitting in the chair.
- Lean to one side, lifting your hip/buttock off the seat. If you have decreased active movement in your trunk, you may need to push off from the armrest on the opposite side or take an armrest off and lean onto a piece of stable furniture, such as a couch or heavy chair. Hold this position for one minute, then repeat on the opposite side.
- Lean forward in your chair until you can slide your hand underneath your buttocks. This may again require the use of a piece of furniture or a wall to assist with moving back into an upright sitting position.

Maintain Proper Body Posture

When sitting, maintain a 90-degree angle between your trunk and hips. Your lower back should make contact with the back of your chair or bed. Sitting in a "slouched" position puts more pressure on the bony lower back area and is a major risk for skin breakdown.

Place pillows under and/or between your legs when lying in bed to reduce pressure. For example, if lying on your side, place a pillow between your knees to stop these two bony surfaces from rubbing together and breaking down due to pressure. Pillows can be placed under your calves to prop your heels off of the bed. Keep in mind that the pillows reduce, but don't eliminate, pressure. Your position needs to change every two hours.

Avoid Sliding Over Surfaces

Sliding over surfaces causes friction and will damage skin by rubbing a raw or open area. Although it is impossible to completely avoid some friction by movement or shearing, you and your caregivers should pay close attention during transfers and to positioning in bed or in your chair to provide clearance of your skin and the surface on which you are moving. Clothing will reduce, but will not eliminate, this problem. Any red or scraped areas noticed during daily skin inspections are the beginning signs of serious skin damage and require a change in the way you are moving your body.

Inspect Your Skin Twice a Day

You should inspect or direct the inspection of your skin every morning as you bathe and dress for the day and every evening /night as you undress for bed. Any changes in the condition of your skin should be identified by description, measurement, and cause of damage. Inspecting your skin less than twice a day will make identifying the cause more difficult (by having to assess a 24-hour period of time versus a 12-hour period of time). Such delay allows more time for damage before resolving the problem.

Remember to direct others or to personally look for any areas of skin that are darker than your natural skin tone, red areas, bruises, cuts, scrapes, or swollen areas. These indicate potentially serious skin damage that should be immediately addressed and monitored. Breaks in the skin surface should be discussed with your physician and/or SCI treatment team.

Know the Causes of Skin Breakdown

Some of the causes of skin breakdown or damage include pressure, shearing (rubbing or scraping), damage from extremes in temperature due to decreased sensation, moisture, delayed cleaning of bowel or bladder accidents and poor nutritional intake. Also remember that the use of tobacco, alcohol and drugs (prescription and recreational) constrict blood pathways and may slow or stop the healing process when skin damage occurs.

FUNCTIONAL MOBILITY—GETTING FROM PLACE TO PLACE

Your **mobility** (ability to move from one place to another) likely has been affected by your spinal cord injury. You may no longer be able to get into and out of bed, get into or out of a car, or walk as you once did. With some persistence and patience, however, in the future you may be able to do these tasks with the help of **assistive equipment**, allowing you to be as independent as possible. Your rehabilitation team will help you learn the mobility skills you'll need at home and in the community, and they will introduce you to equipment that can make mobility possible. This section discusses four areas of mobility—bed mobility, transfers, wheelchair mobility, and ambulation (walking).

Bed Mobility

Bed mobility refers to all of the movements that occur when you get into and out of bed, as well as with changing positions in bed. These movements include rolling, coming to a sitting position, coming to a lying position, and scooting up or down in bed. In addition, certain positions must be assumed for specific activities of daily living or to achieve pressure relief. For example, you may have difficulty or be unable to move your arms, trunk, and legs, depending upon the level of your spinal cord injury. Moving in bed becomes more difficult, and it may require special techniques or equipment.

An important part of bed mobility is managing your legs. If you are unable to use your muscles to move your legs, you must rely on your hands or arms to lift, push, or pull your legs into the position needed to complete a move in bed. Most bed mobility requires assistance from a therapist or caregiver until you reach your highest level of independence.

Transfers

A transfer is the process of moving safely from one surface to another, such as from a bed to a wheelchair or from a wheelchair to a car. Transfers can be done in many ways, depending on your level of injury, body type, range of motion, muscle tone, skill level, and muscle strengths and weaknesses. Your rehabilitation team will help you learn to do transfers that are most appropriate for your abilities. For example:

• If you can stand up, you may be able to do a "stand pivot transfer," which involves standing up from the initial sitting surface, pivoting on your feet, and sitting down on the other surface.
• If you are unable to stand fully, you may be able to do a "squat pivot transfer," which involves pivoting from the initial sitting surface to the other surface while in a squatting position.
• If you are unable to hold your weight through your legs for the duration of a pivot, you may be able to do "sliding board transfer," which involves sliding your buttocks across a smooth board that serves as a bridge between the initial sitting surface and another surface.

- If you are strong enough to "pop" your buttocks over the gap between sit-ting surfaces without a sliding board, you may be able to do a "popover" or "lateral scoot transfer."
- If you are unable to do a popover, lateral scoot, or sliding board transfer, then a mechanical lift may be used to lift and transport you from one sur-face to another.

All transfers, except those using a mechanical lift, typically require assis-tance from a therapist or caregiver until you reach your greatest level of independence.

Wheelchair Mobility

When you were admitted to the rehabilitation hospital, you probably were assigned a wheelchair to use during your stay. If you have full use of your arms, you likely were given a manual wheelchair. If you have impaired arm strength, you likely were given a power wheelchair. If necessary, one of your therapists can modify the chair or get a different one if the one you were assigned is not comfortable, does not allow you to use good posture, or is too difficult to propel. Be sure to talk with your rehabilitation team if you have any problems with your wheelchair during your hospital stay.

Wheelchair skills will be taught throughout your rehabilitation stay. All manual wheelchair users will be introduced to basic skills. If appropriate, advanced wheelchair skills will be taught either while you are an inpatient or further along in therapy. You will not be expected to master all of these advanced skills for before you go home, but you should leave with a solid understanding of how to get around safely, both at home and in your com-munity.

First and foremost in therapy, you will be introduced to simple propul-sion (pushing) on level, even surfaces. Next, you will have many opportu-nities to practice the propulsion skills gained. Later, you will learn to pro-pel over different surfaces found in the community. These surfaces might include grass, sidewalks, gravel, and carpet. Early on, you will also learn skills such as turning and getting through closed doorways across the lips of elevators. As you develop your wheelchair skills, you will also be increas-ing your muscular and cardiovascular endurance, enabling you to do other activities of daily living while using your wheelchair.

Advanced wheelchair skills should be attempted only after you learn and practice beginning skills. Advanced skills include:

- Popping "wheelies"
- Going over curbs

- Going up and down ramps
- Falling out of the wheelchair
- Getting back into the wheelchair from the ground

Those with more complex injuries or other limiting factors may never be able to do all of these advanced skills independently. Everyone should understand these advanced skills, however, because you may need to instruct your caregiver in helping you to do them.

If you will use a power wheelchair, you must also learn new skills and understand your particular chair and its controls. For example, you will need to:

- Know if you have a tilt system (an electronic, automatic way to complete a pressure relief whereby the wheelchair tilts, reclines or both) and, if so, how to operate it
- Know which operating mode is most appropriate for a specific setting
- Be able to drive in reverse
- Maneuver around objects and within small spaces
- Parallel park next to your bed so you can transfer into bed independently
- Be able to engage and disengage the motor
- Know how to remove and charge the battery

Using a wheelchair as a primary form of mobility requires you to plan more carefully, even for brief trips into community settings. Challenges in accessing sidewalks, buildings, and public transportation arise daily and exist even in areas considered to be accessible to those who are handicapped or wheelchair-bound.

Persons with **paraplegia** are most often able to use manual or self-propelled wheelchairs for transportation. These chairs can be taken apart and/or folded to fit into the back or trunk of a standard car. Because of limitations with arm and trunk function, persons with tetraplegia often need to use power wheelchairs to access their environments. Because of their size and weight, these chairs are difficult to transport. Standard conversion vans can be modified with ramps or lifts that provide access for the chair. (Some automotive manufacturers offer financial assistance for choosing their companies.)

Public and private agencies provide transportation for users of both manual and power wheelchairs. However, riders are encouraged to plan an extra hour or more for both pickup and dropoff times because of potential delays. Contact your local department of public transportation or spinal cord injury program to obtain information about these services.

Wheelchair users have numerous rights concerning air travel, including the right to remain in your personal wheelchair up to the gateway of the aircraft. The U.S. Department of Transportation has a toll-free hotline for air travelers with disabilities. It provides education to assist with travel planning. This number can also be used at the airport to provide assistance with any disability-related air travel problems. This number is 1-800-778-4838 (voice) or 1-800-455-9880 (TTY).

Ambulation (Walking)

Ambulation is another word for walking. For a person with spinal cord injury, walking can be achieved with or without braces and assistive equipment, such as a walker, cane, or crutches. Your ability to walk depends on the level of the injury, whether the injury is complete or incomplete, your body size, and if you have any other medical problems (see Chapter 1).

Walking requires certain skills, strengths, and range of motion in the joints. If you are unable to move all or some of the muscles in your legs, braces can be used to provide support to your trunk, hips, knees, ankles, and feet. To begin to walk, you must be able to stand up and then keep your balance while in a standing position. You must then move one or both legs forward for a step. In order to do this, you must have the strength to move your legs forward, or the strength in your trunk to swing your legs forward like a pendulum. In either case, walking with or without braces and assistive equipment is often very tiring for a person with spinal cord injury.

Walking training often begins with standing and then progresses to walking over smooth, level ground. This process typically begins while using parallel bars with assistance from a physical therapist. The appropriate assistive device (such as crutches) will be selected, and walking training with that device will begin. After you master walking over smooth, level ground, you will learn to walk over rough, uneven ground and to use ramps and stairs.

Often, people with spinal cord injury, who attempt walking, find that using a wheelchair is a more practical, faster, and more energy efficient way to move around. Wheelchair use often becomes the choice of convenience for achieving the most independence.

MEAL PREPARATION

Although you may have assistance from others, you may also want to prepare meals on your own. This section gives some general tips for preparing meals safely and efficiently.

If you use a wheelchair:

- Try to collect items in one trip. A bag can be useful for transporting several smaller items at one time
- To move items around in your kitchen, drag them along countertops or position yourself between counters to pass items back and forth
- Put heavier items such as milk cartons on easy-to-reach shelves in the refrigerator and plates in easy-to-reach cabinets. Some people prefer to leave plates and cups on the countertop instead of up in a cabinet
- Use a reacher to take lightweight items, such as bags of chips of cereal boxes, from hard-to-reach shelves (whether they are low or high). Do not use your reacher to access heavy items or glass items
- Use bottled drinks and sealed containers to minimize the risk of spills when moving drinks or food items from one room to another
- Ask for help from family members and friends

Take these very important precautions when preparing meals:

- If you have impaired or no sensation in your hands or arms, avoid burns and skin problems by being aware of how you handle food or containers that are very hot or very cold
- If you have impaired or no sensation in your trunk or legs, do not place very hot or very cold items directly on your lap. Use a thick tray as a barrier between the items and your skin. Clothing alone is not thick enough to prevent burns.
- If you have back precautions from your doctor or are required to wear a TLSO (back brace), avoid bending forward, down low, or twisting to access items when preparing meals.

The following adaptations/home modifications can be useful for preparing meals:

- Lower countertops to ease access
- Add a freestanding sink that you can roll your wheelchair under
- Add an angled mirror over the stovetop so you can see the food cooking in the pots
- Use a stovetop that has front panel controls instead of back panel controls
- Add automatic faucet controls or lever controls instead of twisting controls if you have impaired hand dexterity

The following are pieces of adaptive equipment may be useful if you have impaired hand dexterity and strength:

- Universal cuffs to hold utensils
- Built-up grip utensils
- Adaptive cutting boards to secure food and rocker knives to make cutting food easier
- Nonslip mats to secure plates or bowls to keep them from moving when eating or preparing food
- Adaptive cups with lids
- Scoop dishes or bowls

Every person's self-feeding and meal preparation needs are different, depending on the level of the spinal cord injury and the home environment. Consult your occupational therapist to learn what works best for you in your kitchen and dining room.

TOILETING

If your spinal cord injury has impacted your ability to control your bowels and/or bladder, you and your **rehabilitation team** (including your doctor, nurse, and occupational therapist) will work together to set up an appropriate bowel and bladder program. As you are learning your bowel and bladder programs, it is important to remember that you will need to know how to perform them at home and in the community. It is very important to keep your bowel and bladder program equipment clean and dry and to perform toileting activities in good lighting.

For the bladder program, males and females will often learn to use catheters. "Cathing" usually needs to be completed several times a day. It is most convenient to complete it in a seated position in your wheelchair, especially when you are in the community. For females, an adapted mirror can be placed between the legs to help guide the catheter into the urinary opening. For males, a bungee cord or hook can be used to hold the pants away from the body when cathing.

For the bowel program, males and females will use digital stimulation and may use a suppository inserter. Suppositories can be inserted side lying in bed or seated on a commode. However, it is very important to complete passing of your bowels in an upright/seated position on the commode to allow gravity to help with the process of voiding.

Be sure to keep cleaning supplies on hand. Clean gloves, soapy washcloths to clean, wet washcloths to rinse, wipes to clean, and towels are all recommended items to use after completing your bowel and bladder programs. Be sure to keep your buttocks and perineal (genital) area both clean and dry to prevent skin breakdown. As mentioned above, acid from urine and bowel movements and moisture from not being completely dry can lead to skin breakdown. A person with impaired or absent sen-sation below waist level will not be able to accurately feel clean and dry skin without checking it several times with a dry and clean cloth.

Adaptive Bathroom Equipment

Adaptive bathroom equipment you may find useful for completing your bowel and bladder programs includes:

- Grab bars
- Padded and raised drop-arm commode
- Padded raised toilet seat
- Raised commode/shower chair
- Padded transfer tub bench

Your occupational therapist will help you choose the most appropriate type of bathroom equipment, depending on your level of spinal cord injury, to maximize your safety and independence with toileting tasks. The equip-ment will help you complete your bowel and bladder program at home in an upright position. It will also allow for ease and shortened time spent completing toileting tasks.

People with impaired or no sensation should use padded equipment to help prevent skin breakdown from pressure sores. Also, when sitting on any piece of bathroom for extended periods of time, be sure to shift your weight/perform a pressure relief to prevent pressure sores from developing. Raised bathroom equipment will make transfers to and from the wheel-chair much easier than trying to get on and off a low toilet. Placing a raised commode over a regular toilet will allow you to flush waste immediately rather then having to empty a commode bucket at wheelchair level. Some people have to use the commode outside the bathroom if their wheelchair cannot fit through the bathroom door.

Having a cut-out on one side of the seat of a commode chair allows eas-ier access to the buttocks and perineal areas. The cutout can be in the front or back or on either side of the chair depending on your preference.

MORE ABOUT ADAPTIVE EQUIPMENT

During your rehabilitation stay, you'll learn about many kinds of adaptive equipment that will help you become as independent and functional as possible. This equipment includes not only your wheelchair, but also wheelchair "accessories" including a backrest and cushion, splints, and environmental control units. These items are briefly described below.

Wheelchairs, Seatbacks, and Cushions

As stated above, you will be given a wheelchair for use during your rehabilitation hospital stay. Different types of wheelchairs are available and, if
necessary, your primary therapist may alter or exchange the original for a
more appropriate chair.

Most spinal cord injury patients also need a wheelchair when they go
home. At some point during your rehabilitation stay, your physical or
occupational therapist will measure you for a chair and, with other members of your team, will help you decide what type of chair is most appropriate for long-term use. You might have the opportunity to try out different types of wheelchairs, which will help you to choose a suitable model.
You and your rehabilitation team will order the wheelchair, as well as the
most appropriate cushion and backrest. Chapter 9 offers more information
about choosing wheelchairs and other mobility devices.

The wheelchair you are assigned and order will have a seat cushion and
most likely a specialized backrest. The cushion's main purpose is to prevent
skin breakdown and help improve posture. There are many different types
of cushions with a range of materials such as gel, air, and various types and
densities of foam. If necessary, your therapist and a rehabilitation engineer
can do "pressure mapping" to determine what the best cushion is for you
prior to ordering. Pressure mapping allows us to see on a computer screen
what parts of the cushion are bearing the most and least weight when you
are sitting. This information can then tell your rehabilitation team where
more padding or support is needed.

The backrest's main purpose is to ensure good posture to maximize your
respiratory function and prevent spinal deformities. Depending on your
needs, different types of backrests can be used. Backrests range in height,
material, and amount of support given. Side supports are also available
depending on how much trunk control you have. You will work with your
therapists to determine which backrest suits you best.

Splints

Splints are temporary-use devices made to position or protect body parts,
usually at a joint. Splints can increase your function and/or decrease
changes in the structure of your hands that may result from muscle weakness, lack of active movement, or changes in the soft tissue of your hands.
For example, a tenodisis splint may be used by tetraplegics who are able to
extend or lift their wrists. This movement allows the thumb to move
against the side of the index finger of the hand, forming a modified pinch,
which allows one to pick up objects. This type of splint is fashioned to

enhance the thumb to finger movement and allow a stronger grip.

Individuals who do not have functional control of their wrists and hands may use a support splint that holds the wrist in a neutral position. The addition of sleeves or Velcro® can help with the use of utensils such as forks, spoons, and brushes for eating and grooming.

Not everyone with spinal cord injury needs splints. The need for splints is determined on a case-by-case basis. If you need a splint, it will be ordered or made by your occupational therapy practitioner.

Environmental Control Units

As noted throughout this chapter, adaptive equipment can help you become as independent as possible in doing activities of daily living. For a person with tetraplegia, equipment choices include environment control units (ECU), which are computer-based technology that allow greater control over one's indoor environment. ECUs let the person control lights, telephones, entertainment systems, and other equipment.

If you are thinking about obtaining an ECU, it is important to consider both the cost of these systems and your level of comfort with computers and technology. Some people may find it easy to use these systems while others may not. Your occupational therapist, working in conjunction with a rehabilitation engineer, can help you explore your ECU options. Chapter 9 offers more details about ECU options.

SETTING GOALS

The rehabilitation process begins as soon as you enter the hospital and continues long after you leave. That process is successful when a team of individuals, including you, your family, therapists, doctor, rehabilitation nurse, case manager, social worker, and psychologist all work together.

Part of the recovery plan includes setting personal goals and monitoring the progress you make over time. The long-term goal in every situation is to help you resume as much independence as you had in your previous lifestyle. Smaller goals can be stepping stones toward that end result. The first step in this process is to identify problems and concerns specific to the situation. Then, by problem-solving with your family and rehabilitation team, a goal can be set to address problems one step at a time.

When goals are created, it is important to consider your usual environments such as home, school, and work, as well as your lifestyle, level of injury, prior health status, and available support system. Complete a home accessibility questionnaire to give the rehabilitation team important information, such as the layout of your home, size of doorways, and number of steps. In addition, it is important to discuss with your rehabilitation team any concerns about transportation, continuing leisure activities, and returning to work or school so they can help to solve any problems associated with your return to those activities.

This chapter has presented some general information about adapting your daily activities. Remember, though, that every person is different. You will likely develop your own strategies with the help of the rehabilitation team. Although this may seem intimidating at first, your rehabilitation progress will depend largely on your input and active involvement into planning. After all, you are the person who knows you best.

What Can I Do?

As you learn to adapt your activities of daily living after spinal cord injury, it's important to:

- *Work with your rehabilitation team.* Work with your occupational therapist and other members of your rehabilitation team to learn ways to accomplish the activities you need to do everyday—from bathing and dressing to driving.
- *Talk with your peers.* Other people with spinal cord injury might offer useful tips and tricks for doing daily activities. Before adopting advice about altering your routines or equipment, check with a rehabilitation professional to be sure the advice is safe and helpful.
- *Learn about technology.* Assistive devices and other technology can boost your ability to do activities of daily living. Chapter 9 offers more information about helpful technology.
- *Ask questions.* If you have questions about technology or how to do daily activities, or if you have problems accomplishing your daily goals, talk with members of your rehabilitation team.

Where Can I Learn More?

To learn more about adapting your activities of daily living, you may wish to contact:

- Your occupational therapist or the occupational therapy department at your rehabilitation hospital
- Your physician
- ABLEDATA, a source of objective information about assistive technology products and rehabilitation equipment (www.abledata.com)
- The American Occupational Therapy Association, which offers con-

sumer information and a directory of occupational therapy professionals (visit www.aota.org).

Appendix C provides information about additional resources.

IMPORTANT POINTS TO REMEMBER

- People with spinal cord injury often must find new ways to do activities of daily living (ADLs), such as dressing, bathing, grooming, using the bathroom, eating, and getting from one place to another. Your ability to do ADLs depends in part on the level of your spinal cord injury and on the amount of sensation, motor control, balance, trunk stability, energy, and spasticity you have.
- Your rehabilitation team can show you new ways to accomplish ADLs and tell you about adaptive equipment that can help you be as independent and functional as possible at home and in the community.
- Your rehabilitation team can also help you find creative ways to solve problems and reach your goals, both small and large.

3

Beyond the Body: Adjusting to Psychological and Emotional Changes

SAMUEL A. GORDON

"When I became a person in a 'tragic' situation, dealing with a spinal cord injury and dependent on a wheelchair, I just learned to live my life the best way that I could and to the best of my abilities. Now my message to all people, whether in a 'tragic' situation or not, is 'You can do it, too!'" —Tim

From early in our lives, most of us believe that we'll live actively and independently through at least our sixties. We envision ourselves being able to walk, run, bathe and dress ourselves, and perform all activities of daily living—from work and home management to play and other leisure activities—with full use of our arms and legs. In addition, many of us regularly exercise to ensure that we will be able to do these activities well beyond our retirement years. Unfortunately, for some of us, an unexpected injury or illness, such as spinal cord injury (SCI), changes our view of our physical future.

The chapter provides some basic information to help you and your family as you progress through the journey of adjustment and adaptation to life after spinal cord injury. It addresses some of the psychological challenges you and your family may experience after SCI. In particular, this chapter discusses:

- Common psychological and emotional reactions to spinal cord injury
- Psychological approaches to SCI adaptation
- The importance of positive social support

- The effects of SCI on relationships
- Spiritual issues
- When to ask for help and where to find it

YOU'RE NOT ALONE—
COMMON PSYCHOLOGICAL AND EMOTIONAL REACTIONS

The physical changes caused by SCI can be emotionally devastating, even for the most psychologically well-functioning individuals. The big challenge of adjusting to the change in your psychological sense of self and your relationships with the rest of society comes with the change in your view of your physical self. At first, you probably had a great deal of free time in the hospital and thought a lot about what happened to you. Maybe more importantly, you probably also thought about what would happen to you in the future. As the days passed, you received more and more information from professionals, family, friends, and other patients, or you found information on your own. All of this information and thinking may have made you ask questions like, "Will I ever be able to walk and/or hold things like I did before my injury or illness?"

Some experts have compared spinal cord injury survivors' reactions to the grief process of a person who has lost a loved one. After all, SCI, like death, involves a loss—that of the ability to move and/or feel certain parts of the body. Elisabeth Kubler-Ross (1997) has proposed that when a person loses a loved one, he or she goes through stages of emotional grief that include denial, anger, bargaining, depression, and eventual acceptance. A similar set of stages can be proposed for grieving the loss of one's physical abilities caused by SCI and other disabilities. Typical, although not universal, experiences include:

- Shock
- Depression
- Anger
- Anxiety
- Denial
- Hope
- Gratitude
- Integration of a new sense of self

As with death and dying, these stages do not occur in any fixed or predictable way. Not everyone experiences them. Instead, individuals have different emotional and psychological experiences at different times.

Shock

Shock may well have been your first response when realizing that you were no longer able to move your arms and/or legs. This is especially true for people who have experienced a traumatic event, such as an automobile or recreational accident, fall, or assault. Initially, you cannot believe that basic activities you have always taken for granted have been taken away. For most persons with SCI, the loss of the ability to walk causes the greatest shock. The shock may increase as you realize that you cannot get out of bed on your own. It may be even greater if you are unable to urinate or move your bowels without special devices, and greater still if you are unable to feed yourself. Although this shock subsides within weeks of the injury, the change in your thinking about how to live the rest of your life following SCI only really begins as the shock lessens.

Depression

Most persons with SCI experience some degree of sadness, but much of this sadness is within the normal range of social function. If you feel sad, it can help to express your feelings to others and to get encouragement from family, friends, the rehabilitation staff, and other patients who are going through similar physically disabling experiences. Nevertheless, sometimes SCI may cause more significant depressive reactions that require special attention.

Depression probably occurs more often than other emotional reactions after SCI, but not all SCI survivors become depressed. Significant psychiatric forms of depression (often called clinical depression) may require medication or intensive psychotherapy. In addition to sadness, excessive worry, and/or irritable mood, the following changes may be indicators of depression that needs medical attention:

- Sleep problems—either the inability to sleep or sleeping too much
- Appetite changes, especially for foods you normally like (that is, not just because it tastes like "hospital food")
- Lack of interest in pleasurable activities, especially those activities you enjoyed previously
- Feelings of helplessness, hopelessness, and worthlessness, which may be related to loss of physical capacities, or to a skewed sense of the social value of being able to be a good parent, spouse, or worker
- Social withdrawal, particularly when it results in isolation and inactivity
- Abuse of alcohol, illegal drugs, and/or prescription drugs
- Suicidal thoughts or actions, including decreased attention to self-care

actions needed to maintain good health (for example, bladder and bowel management programs)

You may experience some of these symptoms at some point during the early stages of your hospital stay, but most of these symptoms should go away or subside by the time active inpatient rehabilitation ends. However, any of these symptoms can benefit from professional attention. The first line of action should combine individual psychological counseling, support group counseling, rehabilitation team support, reassurance, education, and general involvement in a full day of rehabilitation therapies. In addition, antidepressant medications may be prescribed to help restore the positive mood, appetite, sleep pattern, and energy level needed for a healthy outlook on life. Depending on the severity of the symptoms, individual counseling may involve one to several sessions per week. In some cases, a psychiatrist may be consulted, particularly when complicated medication combinations are prescribed.

Anger

Anger often is seen as a sign of depression turned outward. It usually occurs as one faces serious physical limitations following SCI. For most people, it is extremely difficult to accept being dependent on others for activities that are very basic and/or intimate, such as getting out of bed or using the bathroom in private. The realization that you now need help with such activities can cause you to express anger specifically about your condition. You may also be angry at yourself or whomever you feel is responsible for your injury. You might also find yourself transferring this anger to life in general and perhaps directing it at the people who assist you with daily activities.

Many of the strategies recommended for depression (for example, individual and group counseling) are helpful in confronting anger. Your family members and other caregivers may find themselves on the receiving end of some of your anger, and they must also find strategies for dealing with your anger. You might suggest they use some of the strategies that are outlined in Figure 3.1.

Anxiety

Anxiety can begin at the onset of the injury and remain throughout the adjustment period, increasing at critical points in the rehabilitation process. Fortunately, most anxiety usually subsides to a manageable level as you recognize over time that the worst of the injury is over. Being in a supportive environment, such as a rehabilitation hospital, can help reduce your anxiety during your initial treatment. This reduction in anxiety should continue with the support of family and friends after you leave the hospital.

Nightmares about the injury, worry about new care or medical procedures, resistance to trying new activities, and discomfort about going out in public in a wheelchair are all common forms of anxiety. Your rehabilitation team should take the time to assure you and your family that each of these experiences is normal. The team members should also teach you skills to build your self-confidence in overcoming these worries. In some cases, anxiety can actually motivate you to learn information and techniques that will help you succeed, both in the hospital and after you have returned to the community.

Denial

Many people believe that SCI survivors, who do not display depressive or angry symptoms, are in denial. The issue of denial can also be seen when a person, who has little or no chance of recovering leg and/or arm movement, states assuredly that he or she will walk or grab things in the same way as before the injury. In these situations, professionals sometimes feel that expecting a great deal of recovery is unrealistic and therefore unhealthy. However, such a view may not always be accurate. In fact, in many cases, denial can be very helpful in avoiding deep depression that would require intensive professional intervention. In particular, during the initial hospital stay and the early phases of rehabilitation, denial can help provide the motivation needed to help you get out of bed every morning, work hard in therapy all day and therefore promote maximum recovery and independence, and thereby avoid medical complications that can set back the recovery process.

Nevertheless, denial can pose certain obstacles to your long-term rehabilitation. For example, a person who believes he or she will walk again may oppose the idea of learning skills needed to use a wheelchair in the home and community. Similarly, using a splint for feeding may seem a waste of time for someone who expects to regain the ability to hold utensils with his or her hands and fingers.

One approach sometimes used to overcome the obstacles posed by denial is to give the person hard facts about the irreparable damage done to the spinal cord and the permanency of the condition. However, such an approach may trigger the depressive symptoms discussed above that can lead to complete withdrawal from the rehabilitation process.

Rehabilitation professionals have increasingly adopted a more balanced approach to handling denial. This approach allows for the hope of long-term physical recovery while educating you about the benefits of learning skills for increased independence now. It lets you proceed with a greater sense of happiness and self-satisfaction while hoping for and, if feasible, working toward higher-level recovery of physical functioning. An important element of this approach is to encourage you to enjoy an increasingly independent life. In doing so, you might come to realize that, even if the hoped-for physical recovery does not take place, you can adapt and adjust to the disability, even if you never accept it as permanent. The important distinctions among adaptation, adjustment, and acceptance are addressed later in this chapter.

Hope

Although hope often is viewed as unrealistic and part of the denial process, most, if not all, persons with SCI hold onto hope at some level for most of their lives. Initially, you may expect or believe that something will change about the spinal cord damage that will result in healing and recovery of movement and/or feeling. However, this hope likely will evolve into a more subconscious wish that with time, medical advances, or a miraculous event some recovery will occur.

In any event, hope should not be challenged by others unless it prevents active involvement in physical and social activities needed to maintain good health and move on with life. In many cases, hope can motivate you to follow through with health promotion activities. With encouragement, you can be empowered to grow physically, mentally, and socially in ways that put you in a position to move on with life, regardless or whether the hoped-for recovery of movement or feeling occurs.

Gratitude

Particularly after a sudden near-fatal traumatic event, such as a car accident or gunshot wound, you may at some point, during and/or after your rehabilitation, feel the need to express an appreciation of having survived. You may also see the event as changing your life for the better or as preventing physical or social deterioration such as death or imprisonment. This appreciation is often associated with religious or other spiritual beliefs, but in general it represents a positive step toward psychological recovery. This step can increase your participation in rehabilitation, and ideally it can encourage you to make the best of the rest of your life.

You may feel gratitude for those you see as being critical to your success in overcoming the injury experience. These individuals may include doctors and other health care professionals who provided services at the scene of the injury, during hospitalization, and during the rehabilitation process. You may feel gratitude toward your family, friends, and other patients who have given you emotional support during difficult times. You may also feel gratitude toward family members or others who help with daily living activities, possibly for the rest of your life.

Some people with SCI may not find ways to express their thanks. Their gratitude may get lost in the anger, depression, and other emotions discussed above. However, it is important for loved ones to realize that gratitude truly exists, especially for those closest to the person with SCI and those who will provide long-term support and care.

Integration of a New Sense of Self

After SCI, physical changes usually are accompanied by changes in how the survivor views himself or herself. These self-image changes may include feelings that you are unattractive. These feelings may be most noticeable in your relations with the opposite sex (see Chapter 11). Changes in self-image may also affect your same-sex and other nonromantic relations, including your sense of respect and power.

The major challenge with these self-image changes is developing a healthy sense of yourself, despite being unable to do physical activities in the same way as before your SCI. Keep in mind that the most important parts of yourself are not tied to what you do physically, but how you relate to others socially and psychologically. This realization may take time. However, by working hard at the physical and social activities involved in rehabilitation, and by interacting positively with others within and outside of the hospital, you will come to realize that others will respect you. Although they may seem trite, saying such statements as, "Do unto to others as you would have them do unto you," and "Treat others as you want to be treated" are helpful to remember when trying to rebuild your positive sense of self.

MOVING ON—ADAPTING, ACCEPTING, AND ADJUSTING

Spinal cord injury rehabilitation can be considered from three different psychological approaches—adaptation, acceptance, and adjustment—each of which is discussed below.

Adaptation

Adaptation taps your physical, social, and psychological skills and resources to make the best out of the bad situation of being disabled. These skills may be learned during rehabilitation, or you may have had them before your injury. Adaptation may mean, for example, using a wheelchair to get around at home and get to work, recreational activities, shopping, and other quality-of-life activities. Your rehabilitation team likely has encouraged you to adapt your lifestyle activities to make you as independent and functional as possible. Your family and friends should also encourage you to adapt and, more importantly, to learn ways to adapt themselves. To do so, they must first learn how much help and support you need and then learn when and how to help.

Equally important, your family and friends must learn when and how not to help, letting you do what you can do for yourself. This process often starts before you are discharged from inpatient rehabilitation and the family training that sometimes takes place by your nurses, physical and occupational therapists. In such training, your family members may be taught how to help you transfer from your bed to your wheelchair, from your wheelchair to a car, etc. During this training, therapists may also inform family members when it is more appropriate to let you do things on your own (e.g., push your own wheelchair, do your own catheterizations).

After you are home, you may find that family members or friends who were not trained, or who still are not comfortable with your "abilities" as a person with SCI, may be too quick to lend a hand. In such situations, it is appropriate for you to say that you would much rather "Do it myself." These reactions are also important because as you grow stronger after leaving the hospital, there are things you can do for yourself, those that you were not able to do while you were in the hospital. When this becomes the case, try to tell overly helpful persons that by allowing you do to more things for yourself, they are helping promote your adaptation and independence. If needed, you might also enlist the help of rehabilitation therapists in assuring family and friends that it is adaptive, healthy, and safe for you to perform activities within your range of capabilities.

Acceptance

On the surface, accepting your spinal cord injury may appear to be a good thing. However, whether or not acceptance is desirable depends on how it affects your approach to life with SCI. In fact, one can consider acceptance and nonacceptance as being either positive or negative. The following framework of acceptance is one way psychologists view the idea of acceptance:

- *Positive acceptance* – The person approaches life after SCI thus, "I have a disability that is probably permanent, but I have as much to offer and have as much value as a person as I did before my SCI."
- *Negative acceptance* – The person approaches life after SCI thus, "I am disabled for life, and I do not have much value or much to offer because of my disability."
- *Positive non-acceptance* – The person approaches life after SCI thus, "I am not disabled for life but will work to improve myself, and I have value before and after I recover from my disability."
- *Negative non-acceptance* – The person approaches life after SCI thus, "I am not disabled for life. Therefore, I will wait until I am no longer disabled (for example, until I am walking again) to resume positive life activities and pursuits."

Within this framework, acceptance is not seen as good or bad. Rather, what one does with his or her type of acceptance is more important than the acceptance itself. As much as possible, your rehabilitation team and support system (such as your family and friends) should encourage you not to adopt either negative acceptance or non-acceptance because both can interfere with your ability to adopt a new, positive sense of self. In contrast, positive acceptance and non-acceptance can be critical in helping you to work toward a healthy lifestyle, physical mobility, and social/community reintegration—all of which are associated with life satisfaction after SCI (Putzke, Richards, Hickens & DeVivio, 2002).

Achieving positive acceptance or non-acceptance will be different for different people, but there are certain actions that may help you in this process. These include:

- Stay involved with others who, despite their SCI, are active in the community with healthy recreation, work, and other social activities.
- Spend time with persons who do not have SCI, but who respect and treat you as if your SCI really does not make a difference in enjoying life.
- Keep informed about the latest opportunities for persons with SCI – including research on ways to increase your physical capabilities, and opportunities for greater social integration. The internet, local and national SCI consumer organizations, and publications can be valuable information resources.
- Do not put your life goals on hold until you are able to walk again. Instead, take steps to pursue your social goals (such as your career, relationship, and housing goals), with the understanding that achieving your goals won't prevent you from walking, and—when or if you

walk again—achieving those goals will be all the more satisfying.

Adjustment

In some respects, adjustment is a form of "fine tuning," which is a life-long process for persons with SCI. When combined with adaptation and either positive acceptance of positive non-acceptance, adjustment is a key to living a happy life with SCI. Regardless of whether one has a spinal cord injury or not, life is filled with stressors and changes that challenge our coping capacities. However, for a person with SCI, every-day hassles most of us can overcome by taking one or two deep breaths can cause major stress. Such seemingly routine hassles include, for example, having to go to the bathroom in the middle of the night, spilling hot coffee on your lap while rushing to get to an appointment or work in the morning, missing a bus, finding that a building entrance is blocked or an elevator broken, encountering others who are inconsiderate of your personal space, attending to health and hygiene needs while in the community, having to shop for and make dinner, helping your children with homework, and getting ready for the next day.

These everyday stressors, combined with the natural changes that come with aging, require an ability to adjust time and time again to the challenges of life after SCI. This process is not easy. It may take months or years to implement fully. In fact, most persons with SCI don't really begin thinking about the true long-term impact of the injury until after the one-year anniversary of the injury. Fortunately, during that first year, the rehabilitation process will prepare you to take on most of the above challenges, and with a positive attitude, the subsequent years can become increasingly productive.

Beyond the first anniversary, it is still important for you to keep an eye on how you are doing with the life-long adjustment process. Often this process may involve feedback from others. Again, involvement with others is a helpful way to get this feedback. SCI support groups, geared for persons who have returned to the community, usually meet weekly to monthly, and they often allow persons to attend periodically as their time and needs permit. Attending such groups even once a year can be helpful in gaining a sense of how well you are doing adjusting to your SCI as the years go by. Meeting persons who are more recently injured, and others who have been injured longer ago than yourself, can provide valuable insight about how far you have come and how far you still want to go. It can also help you see some of the negative directions that you want to avoid.

In addition to support groups, more individualized feedback and self-assessment can occur during annual visits to your rehabilitation physician. Although it is important that even able-bodied persons go for their annual physical and may be screened for mental health issues, it is even more critical for persons with SCI to have such issues discussed during their annual doctor visits. If nothing else, basic questions such as, "How are you coping with daily activities?" can get you thinking about how easy or hard your life with has become with your SCI.

Finally, family members and friends can still be a readily available source of discussion about how well you have done over the years since your SCI. In fact, a healthy sign of your adjustment process is your willingness to start the adjustment discussion with individual members of your support system by asking questions such as, "How well do you think I'm doing living with my SCI?," or "Do you think there is something I could be doing to improve my life with my SCI that I'm not doing?" However, and with whomever you discuss such questions, the most critical point is to continue to do self-checks on your adjustment to, and coping with, your SCI throughout your life. The underlying motive should be maintaining a positive attitude about yourself and positive behaviors to keep yourself healthy.

THE IMPORTANCE OF SOCIAL SUPPORT

The support and encouragement you receive from loving, concerned family members and friends are critical in your adjustment to SCI. In contrast to the services rendered by health care professionals as part of their jobs, the support of persons, who knew you before your injury or who have become friends since your injury, can feel more sincere and genuine. Remember, too, that your loved ones often are struggling with feelings of their own and may need to make adjustments. If handled appropriately, these adjustments can lead to a process of mutual support. Figure 3.2 presents some simple steps that family members and friends can take to support you psychologically and emotionally.

Unfortunately, for some persons with SCI, the support from family and friends that many of us take for granted was not present in the past or has been lost since the injury. This lack of support may occur because you had limited close family and friends before your injury. (For example, A lack of support may happen if you are a "loner" or of single status and recently moved to a new town. Also, in some cases, friends and family members, who were close before your injury, are not able to deal with your current condition and may withdraw from regular contact with you.

In each of these cases, involvement in the local and national SCI support community is especially important. To find this type of support, you should probably start with the facility where you received your rehabilitation. Professionals from those facilities (especially your inpatient therapists, nurses, and doctors) can direct you to organizations, mentors, and other SCI sources that provide opportunities for bonding and promoting a healthy overall life after SCI. Most importantly, don't forget fellow SCI patients (and other patients) whom you met during your rehabilitation. They can give you valuable support and are likely to benefit from the support you can give them. This mutual peer support can be accomplished simply by talking about life (whether about disability or non-disability issues) and by doing things together to just enjoy life (such as movies and other healthy recreational activities).

Everyone involved in the life of a person with SCI should strive to maintain a balance between sympathetic understanding of the major challenges of coping with physical losses and assertive support for the inner strength that will allow the person to find happiness and achieve some degree of independence despite the losses. Achieving this balance may depend greatly on how well one understands the way relationships may change as a result of SCI. This topic is discussed below.

HOW SCI CHANGES FAMILY AND OTHER RELATIONSHIPS

One of the most important social changes that can occur after a spinal injury involves the various roles one plays in life. These various roles are particularly apparent among males, who comprise the majority of persons with SCI. For many men, the loss of physical capacities to run, lift, and use the bathroom normally is seen as a loss of the dominance and strength that defined their manhood and physical attractiveness. Women with SCI may also experience feelings of similar losses in their physical capacities and social role functions. For both men and women, these losses may result in conflicts in their relations with significant others (spouse, boyfriend, or girlfriend) and with their parents, children, and friends.

Communication is the key to resolving conflict and meeting the challenge of re-establishing mutually supportive relations. A first step in dealing with relationship changes is to keep in mind the common psychological and emotional reactions persons with SCI experience (see above). It is important to discuss these emotions, focusing on how the SCI is affecting you and those who are important in your life. Such a discussion can set the stage for future talks about role changes and healthy ways to attend to each other's needs. Remember that both you and your loved ones are adjusting and adapting to the injury. With this in mind, you can negotiate with your family and friends about how to perform various life activities, such as housekeeping, money management, transportation, taking your children to school, shopping, and running errands.

Romantic Relationships

Relations between romantic partners (for example, a boyfriend and girlfriend or husband and wife) are possibly the biggest social role challenges following SCI. It is not uncommon for depression and anger over the care needs of the person with SCI to cause significant conflict between couples. However, with your own and your partner's involvement in the rehabilitation process, greater mutual understanding can develop. This understanding in turn can help promote healthy communication. For example, you and your partner may choose to limit the types of care your partner provides so that you can separate your partner's caregiver and sexual partner roles. On the other hand, for some couples, complete involvement of the able-bodied partner produces a more intimate relationship. In either case, open communication can build a partnership that can endure the periods of anger and depression that are part of coping with the aftermath of SCI disability.

Paid Caregiver Relationships

In many cases, the caregiver role is assumed by a paid health assistant. This person may be called a **personal care assistant** or aide (PCA) if you are living in the community, or he or she may be a nurse and/or nursing assistant if you are living in a nursing home or other long-term care facility. Relationships with paid caregivers can pose significant challenges, particularly if you have more than one assistant. As the person receiving care, you will have to be patient, as each assistant will likely need time to develop a good understanding of your care needs and personal preferences. This patience will have to be balanced with assertiveness to ensure that the care you have contracted to receive is provided with respect and dignity, and that you are not taken advantage of or otherwise abused.

Keys to a successful paid caregiver relationship include making sure that you give respect in directing how your care is provided, and that you get respect from the person providing your care. If either of these key parts is lacking, you might enlist a third party to mediate a solution. The third party might be the agency through which the PCA was hired, or it might be a mental health professional (such as a psychologist or social worker), a relative, or a close friend who can help negotiate a solution. In more extreme cases in which you are being physically abused or threatened, it may be necessary to contact the state government agency responsible for protecting the health and welfare of disabled and elderly persons. (This agency is sometimes called Adult Protective Services.)

Parent and Child Relationships

Parental responsibilities can also be affected by SCI. For example, researchers have found that in families in which the mother has SCI, household and child-care tasks are more equally shared than in families with able-bodied mothers (Alexander, Hwang & Sipski, 2001). Achieving this type of equality is likely to produce a happy, successful marriage or partnership over decades. If the father has been injured, he is likely to feel more fulfilled if he increases the time spent providing social and educational guidance to make up for some of the physical activities he may no longer be able to do with or for his children.

In addition, parent-child relations may change significantly after SCI. Often, the mother or father of the person with SCI is forced to resume care of an adult child. This scenario is often filled with mixed emotions, with the parent readily providing care and assistance when needed, but often without meeting his or her own needs. At the same time, an independent adult child with SCI may feel both gratitude for the care provided by the parent and resentment for again being dependent on the parent. In contrast, if the parent has been injured, multiple challenges can arise. For example, roles may suddenly be reversed, with the adult child assuming a parent-type role in caring for and sometimes making decisions for the parent. In either situation, it is important for both the parent and the adult child to communicate openly and empathetically about their feelings and commitment to work together to foster a good quality of life, despite the SCI.

Finally, parents with SCI who have children between infancy and adolescence face special challenges. In this situation, it is important to remember that the physical contributions of parenthood are not as important as the social guidance and supportive encouragement of parenting. The SCI may force you to develop your verbal skills to ensure that your children know that you intend to maintain the loving authority and structure needed to guide them into successful adulthood. Chapter 13 provides further information about parenting after SCI.

SPIRITUAL ISSUES

At some point, most people with SCI ask why they suffered such a devastating injury. Many people also ask whether they deserved such a fate.

In turn, these questions can stimulate thoughts about the role of God, spirituality, and religious beliefs in the injury and disability process. Although it is difficult to explain why some people have spinal cord injuries and others do not, spirituality and religious beliefs can be extremely helpful in developing one's capacity to cope with the situation.

Studies suggest that religiousness and spirituality can improve the psychological well-being of persons with chronic illnesses or disabilities (Gordon, 1987). For example, marital relationships can be influenced by a spiritual foundation and by the strong values and commitment that are usually associated with religiousness (Rohrer, 2001). Also, seeing oneself as a burden is associated with less spiritual activity (Dyeson, 2000). In some cases, spirituality and religiousness may cause people to believe that prayer, church attendance, and faith will lead to healing of the spinal cord. In other cases, spiritual and religious beliefs and practices provide the emotional strength needed to cope with the hard work that comes with living with SCI. In either case, spirituality and religiousness, like SCI itself, is very individualized. You should incorporate those beliefs that will help you make the best out of a challenging situation.

One key to the successful use of spiritual and religious beliefs in coping mechanisms lies in your adoption of a "survival mentality" versus a "victim mentality." A person with a survival mentality looks to his or her spiritual and religious beliefs to generate a purpose in life, believing that God saved him or her for a reason. In contrast, a person with a victim mentality is more likely to focus on the question, "Why did God allow this to happen to me?" Throughout the recovery period, you and those who support you will benefit more from focusing on survival as a reason for living life in a positive and fulfilling manner, based on healthy spiritual and religious beliefs.

WHEN TO ASK FOR HELP AND WHERE TO FIND IT

Most of us who have worked with persons with SCI have learned one thing: successful rehabilitation requires input from many people—both professionals and non-professionals. Each of us must be humble enough to admit that we need the help of others in order to be as helpful as possible to the person with SCI. Similarly, you, your family, and your friends must admit that help from outside of your immediate support network is sometimes needed. Ideally, this willingness to seek help will be present by the time you complete your inpatient rehabilitation. In most cases, the earlier you ask questions, ask for information, and seek assistance, the better.

To promote your own psychological and emotional health, keep in mind some of the points mentioned above about common reactions to SCI. Emotional reactions, such as shock, depression, anger, anxiety, and fear, are common after SCI, but don't always need treatment. Sometimes, however, specialized help is needed. Pay particular attention to signs that any of the reactions described above is interfering significantly with your own or your loved one's quality of life. Shock, depression, anger, or anxiety that is constant and lasts more than two weeks after the injury is stabilized should cause you to seek outside help, especially if you have symptoms such as too much or too little sleep, poor or excessive appetite, and failure to perform normal activities of daily living (including grooming, hygiene, chores, work, and socially enjoyable activities).

If you find yourself (or your disabled loved one) making suicidal or aggressive threats or statements, or if you experience or see any behaviors that pose an immediate threat to life, call a professional as soon as possible. Contact a hospital emergency room, the police (call 911), your rehabilitation mental health specialist, or a local suicide hotline.

Fortunately, in most cases, emotional reactions are not of an immediate life-threatening nature and can be handled in a less dramatic fashion. When it becomes apparent that the distress is not getting better after two weeks, however, it is appropriate to contact resources in your community that can help you resolve the psychological problems that you or your loved one may be experiencing. Depending on where you live, it may be possible to start with your SCI rehabilitation facility. Your rehabilitation physician may be able to refer you to mental health specialists trained in helping persons to overcome the emotional challenges associated with SCI. Alternatively, you may choose to ask for help from clergy at a place of worship or another religious institution. As mentioned above, it is also helpful to join support groups and organizations that seek to advance the lives of persons with SCI and other disabilities.

Whichever type of assistance you choose, keep in mind that seeking help is not a sign of weakness. Rather, seeking help is a sign of knowledge and commitment to improve the quality of your life, despite the challenges posed by your SCI.

What Can I Do?

To help make your ease your psychological and emotional adjustment and rebuild a positive sense of self after spinal cord injury, you can:

- *Stay active.* Be sure you stay involved in positive family, community, career, school, volunteer, and community activities.
- *Trust yourself.* Listen to and acknowledge your concerns, feelings, interests, and goals, and take an active role in making decisions that will help you maintain control of your own future.
- *Remember that you're still important to others.* Keep in mind the many nonphysical and physical contributions you can make to your family, your friends, your community, and society in general.
- *Accept or decline help as needed.* Arrange for help and tell family members, friends, and co-workers when you need help, but be assertive in letting others know which tasks you prefer to do independently.
- *Get support.* In addition to getting support from family members, friends, and clergy, join a support group, stay in touch with other patients you met while in rehabilitation, locate a peer mentor (see Chapter 15), or connect with others with SCI via the Internet.
- *Ask for help when needed.* If you feel depressed or feel you need professional help adjusting psychologically or emotionally, talk with your doctor, a psychologist, a social worker, or a clergy member as soon as possible.
- *Become an advocate.* Learn about and stand up for your disability rights (for example, the rights to health care, employment, and education) and for the rights of others with disabilities.
- *Teach others.* Help raise others' disability awareness by talking with school children and adults in your community about your experience with SCI and disability.

Where Can I Learn More?

To learn more about adjusting to the psychological and emotional effects of spinal cord injury, or to locate a mental health professional, you may wish to contact:

- Your rehabilitation doctor, psychologist, or social worker
- A local SCI support group (locate a support group through the National Spinal Cord Injury Association (www.spinalcord.org)
- Clergy at your place of worship or another religious institution
- Your local Center for Independent Living (visit www.ilru.org for a directory of these centers)
- The Spinal Cord Injury Information Network (www.spinalcord.uab.edu)
- The American Association of Spinal Cord Injury Psychologists and Social Workers (www.aascipsw.org)

Appendix C provides information about additional resources

IMPORTANT POINTS TO REMEMBER

- Spinal cord injury can bring about many different psychological and emotional challenges. Reactions may be similar to the stages of grief and can include shock, depression, anger, anxiety, denial, hope, gratitude, and integration of a new sense of self.
- Rehabilitation can help a person adapt to, accept, and adjust to the injury's effects. Spiritual issues sometimes play a role in these processes.
- Relationships with family members, friends, and others may change. Good communication and an understanding attitude are important in maintaining positive, strong relations. Support groups and mental health professionals can also help people to confront the psychological and emotional challenges posed by spinal cord injury.

REFERENCES

Alexander CJ, Hwang K, Sipski M. Mothers with spinal injuries: Impact on family division of labor, family decision making, and rearing of children. Topics in Spinal Cord Injury Rehabilitation, 2001. 7(1): 25-36

Dyeson, TB. Burden self-image: A mediating variable of depressive symptoms among chronically ill care recipients. J of Gerontological Social Work, 2000; 33(1): 17-33

Elfstrom ML, Kreuter M., Ryden A, Persson LO, Sullivan M. Effects of coping on psychological outcome when controlling for background variables: A study of traumatically spinal cord lesioned persons. Spinal Cord, 2002; 40(8): 408-15

Gordon SA. Religiousness and psychological functioning in chronically ill/disabled adolescents and their mothers. Doctoral Dissertation University of Maryland, 1987

Kubler-Ross E. *On Death and Dying*, New York: Scribner 1997

Putzke JD, Richards JS, Hickens BL, DeVivio MJ. Predictors of life satisfaction: A spinal cord injury cohort study. Archives of PM&R, 2002; 83(4): 555-61

Rohrer, JR. Factors in the marital adjustment of couples after spinal cord injury of one of the partners. Thesis Information, Ed.D. University of Cincinnati, 2001

This chapter was supported in part through a grant from the U.S. Department of Education, National Institute on Disability and Rehabilitation Research, Grant #H133B031114.

---4---

Taking Charge of
Your Own Life

SUZANNE L. GROAH

*"You know best what your wishes and needs are. Nobody can take
that away from you." –Steven*

Having a SCI is a catastrophic
event that changes your life and presents you with challenges you never
thought you would have to face. Suddenly, you can't move your legs
and/or your arms. Tasks that were simple and taken for granted before
your injury, such as reaching for a glass of water, brushing your teeth, or
getting out of bed, are now hard, if not impossible. You have to relearn
ways of doing such tasks, which before had been done without even
thinking.

You can call on yourself and others to help you to deal with the SCI.
At first, you may need others to care for you and to help with your physical needs. Although others may supply all or part of the physical energy
to help you, all of that energy does not need to come entirely from others. You can still use whatever strength you have to contribute in whatever way you can. Whenever you ask someone else to help, you should
also be commanding and demanding of yourself to do your part of the
work. This kind of determination however, requires knowledge and
understanding of your new self, your environment, and anything else that
might affect you.

When you are in rehabilitation, your therapists, nurses, and others
help you by giving you instructions as to how to overcome some of the
effects of your SCI. For example, they will teach you how to get out of
bed, dress yourself, and stay healthy. The way you accomplish these activities is usually different than before your SCI. Along the way, you may
find that modifying what you were taught in rehabilitation actually works
better for you in the long run.

This chapter:
* Discusses the importance of taking charge of your own life
* Suggests a goal-planning and problem-solving process
* Shows how to use a goal-planning worksheet

HOW CAN I HELP MYSELF?

As you proceed with your SCI, it's healthy to periodically reevaluate the way you do certain things and how you take care of yourself. This periodic reevaluation helps to take care of changes that you were unaware of, changes that might become bigger problems in the future. In this chapter we will walk through a stepwise process of reevaluating aspects of your life and your care, asking yourself questions and developing a "plan of attack." This process will help you take charge of your life and prevent problems in the long run.

Part of this process may involve changing the way you think. You may need to reorganize the ways you go about planning your life. Things that you did without thinking in the past now require more thought—more planning and thinking ahead. Plans you will make involve several steps:

* Decide *what* you want to accomplish
* Decide *how* to do it
* Decide *when* to review your plan

Ask yourself these questions periodically (every month, 3 months, or even every 12 months) as you may need to change your plan. We have developed a Goal Planning Worksheet. Figure 4.1 shows an example of a blank Goal Planning Worksheet that we have used to help people identify and set goals with the help of their therapists, nurses, and doctors when going through initial rehabilitation after SCI.

Putting your thoughts into words often helps you to commit actions to your thoughts. You may find it helpful to talk with others as you go through this process. Get ideas from your friends and family, other people with spinal cord injury, and your health care provider(s). Once you have your problems, goals, and solutions identified, prioritize them so that #1 becomes the most important problem, goal, or solution, and #3 becomes the least important. Then, give yourself some time to accomplish the task at hand.

HOW TO USE THE WORKSHEET

The Goal Planning Worksheet can be adapted to a variety of topic areas in this book, from skin care to bowel management, from learning to pop-up a

Question 1: What are my current or future problems with my

_____ ?

Problem 1: _____[Date]

Problem 2: _____[Date]

Problem 3: _____[Date]

Question 2: What are my goals? When do I want to reach these goals?

Goal A: _____[Date]

Goal B: _____[Date]

Goal C: _____[Date]

Question 3: What methods will I use to accomplish these goals?

Solution A: _____[Date]

Solution B: _____[Date]

Solution C: _____[Date]

Figure 4.1. Goal Planning Worksheet

curb to intimacy issues. Although the questions are the same, the answers to the questions about problems, goals, and methods used in keeping your skin healthy are different from those you might face in reestablishing intimacy and sexual life, managing your bladder or bowels, or getting back to work.

LET'S GO THROUGH IT TOGETHER

Let's start with the Planning Worksheet used for skin problems. First a little primer on pressure sores after SCI. Pressure sores—also called pressure ulcers and decubitus ulcers—are serious, but often preventable complications of SCI. Pressure sores usually appear over more bony surfaces, such as the tail bone, hips, and heels. Pressure sores are caused by too much or prolonged pressure or friction on the skin, which cuts off the blood supply. When the blood supply is cut off, there can be damage to the nearby tissue. The damage starts in the deep muscle and advances outward toward the skin. Although a pressure sore may seem small on the surface of your skin, it can be more extensive underneath the skin. Even some redness that doesn't go away should be dealt with very quickly and seriously. Once you see redness, a blister, or even breakdown on the outer surface of the skin, you can be sure that the inner surface is even more damaged!

Since you've had your SCI, you may lack the sensation needed to know when there is too much pressure or friction on their skin. Your body doesn't warn you that it is time to move or to relieve pressure from the skin. Other factors that can make things worse include poor nutrition, infection, urine or bowel incontinence, and lack of exercise and mobility.

Pressure sores are classified by the amount of redness on the skin and the depth of the skin damage. Knowing the stage of a pressure sore can help health care professionals plan for treatment. The four stages of pressure sores are:

• **Stage I:** A reddened or darkened area can be seen and does not turn white when pressure is applied.
• **Stage II:** A superficial break in the skin with an abrasion, blister, or shallow crater.
• **Stage III:** Tissue damage extending down to the layer that covers the muscle.
• **Stage IV:** Tissue damage extending down to the muscle, bone, or structures such as tendons and joint capsules. All of the tissue between the skin and these structures are destroyed.

Pressure sores can develop quickly and can be a serious complication of SCI. Therefore, it is important to try to prevent them and get early treatment when needed. Proper positioning equipment, good nutrition, and prompt attention to signs of a sore can help prevent serious problems. If advanced pressure sores develop, you may need to undergo surgery and long-term recovery.

So, let's say you've had a pressure sore that required prolonged bed rest or even surgery. After it's healed, it is a good time to make a Skin Care Planning Worksheet. Let's do it together starting with the problems.....

Question 1: What are, or could be, my problems that led to my SKIN breakdown?

Problem 1: Pressure
Problem 2: Wetness
Problem 3: I didn't monitor my skin, so I didn't know there was a problem until it was too late

Good. You've identified three problems in taking care of your skin that could really have contributed to skin breakdown. As an example, other problems might include skin infections, skin ulcers, skin sores, pain, inability to see the breakdown, or incontinence. Let's move on to your goals. For each problem, try to think of a solution that will solve the problem. Let's see what we came up with below....

Question 2: What are my SKIN goals? When do I want to reach these goals?

Goal A: Decrease the pressure and friction on my buttocks today!
Goal B: Keep my skin clean and dry_____1 week
Goal C: I (or someone else) need(s) to see all parts of my skin____2 weeks

Now, for the best (and hardest) part: how do you reach these goals? The answer is by thinking, reading, educating yourself, and talking to others. Don't be afraid to ask other peoples' opinions, including your health care provider. Now, let's finish the worksheet and come up with some solutions to your skin problem.

Question 3: What solutions will I use to accomplish these SKIN goals?

Solution A1: Perform pressure relief every 15 minutes for a minute while sitting
Solution A2: Avoid lying in a semi-reclined position
Solution B1: Clean my skin carefully every day
Solution B2: If sweaty, change clothes into something dry and clean
Solution C1: Regularly inspect my skin twice daily
Solution C2: Use a mirror to see all parts of my skin

As you've surely noticed, we actually came up with two solutions for each problem. See how many solutions you can develop. Other examples of solutions might include:

• Keep moving
• Keep my skin from drying out too much
• Use proper shoes and stockings
• Have proper equipment, such as beds and sets
• Eat the right foods
• Drink enough fluid
• Stop smoking!

In this way you can make a big difference in your life by realizing that you have set what we call "goals," that you have accomplished them and have seen what works. Now you are ready to continue to reach even higher goals.

Let's review what we actually did here. We identified a big problem that's associated with spinal cord injury, and then we figured out the solution. Next, we developed ways to accomplish our solution.

An important thing to remember as you work with the Goal Planning Worksheet is to pace yourself. Initially, you may want to accomplish all of your goals at once. For example, your long-term goal may be "to do pressure relief every 15 minutes." If you were only doing a pressure relief every hour before your skin breakdown occurred, changing your life and lifestyle to every 15 minutes might be pretty difficult. So, you may want to come up with some shorter-term goal that may be related to your longer-term goal. In other words, take baby steps! For instance, decide that you are going to do pressure relief every 45 minutes for the first week, then every 30 minutes the next week. In the third week, you will have accomplished your long-term goal of every 15 minutes.

In identifying a short-term goal, make that goal clear enough so that you can measure the results of your progress. We call that being specific, describing not only *what* you want to see happen but *how much* or *how well*, *where or when*. For example, the goal of "doing pressure relief every 15 minutes" tells you more clearly the result you are looking for by answering not only what you want to do (pressure relief) but how frequently you will do it (every 15 minutes).

REVIEW YOUR RESULTS

The next question to be asked is what result have you had. In answering this new question, it is important to build on the work you did earlier to be clear about your goals. If you have a clear specific goal, you can measure the results. Sometimes the results are more than we expected and sometimes less. Even with fewer results, it is still useful to list the results. The purpose of this question is to have a better basis for hope for the future now that some progress has occurred. Also, sometimes progress is so slow that we don't realize that we are actually making progress and meeting our goals.

The experience of the extent to which results did occur within certain timelines can also now help in establishing the rate at which results may be expected in the future. The rate of progress, for example, in being able over a week to "do pressure reliefs every 45 minutes" can provide a rough estimate of the progress that can be expected during the next one-week interval.

By using this simple process of identifying problem areas, developing solutions, and setting goals to accomplish those solutions, you help yourself grow in a variety of areas throughout your life. This type of process can be used whether or not you have a SCI and for problem areas related or unrelated to SCI. You can also develop a worksheet and go through the process with a friend, family member, or significant other. Remember, many problems encountered throughout life are preventable, or at least can be minimized, by being knowledgeable about problems that occur with time, age, or SCI. You should always stay knowledgeable about your body and your functional capabilities. Arm yourself with knowledge, reevaluate yourself often, and don't be afraid to change the ways you used to do some things. By making certain changes, you will be improving yourself and/or your relationship with others.

IMPORTANT POINTS TO REMEMBER

• Periodically evaluating different aspects of your life and care can help prevent problems in the long run.
• A simple, step-by-step process like the one suggested in this chapter can help identify problems, find solutions, and achieve your goals.
• Once you've identified your goals and any problems, you can prioritize them. Then give yourself a reasonable amount of time to accomplish the task at hand.

5

Getting Ready to Go Home

ASHLEY M. HARMON

"I wouldn't say that any part of my journey has been easy. . . . In the months that followed my homecoming, I continued to coach baseball, learned to use my voice-activated computer software, and was taught how to drive my accessible van." –Robert

Your inpatient rehabilitation is a time of major adjustments and transitions in terms of your emotions, body, and lifestyle. Part of what you will do, or have begun to do, during your rehabilitation stay is to make plans to go home. Getting ready to go home may seem like something you would do at the end of your hospital stay, but the earlier you begin to plan for your transition to home, the more smoothly your return to home will be. In fact, this process should start as early as your admission to the rehabilitation hospital.

As difficult as it may be for you to focus on your departure from the hospital, your **case manager, social worker,** and other team members will need to discuss your living situation when you go home. They will ask you questions such as:

- Where you will live when you leave the hospital?
- Is your home wheelchair-accessible?
- How many steps are there to enter your home?
- How much assistance do you need to complete daily activities and tasks like dressing, bathing, making meals, getting in and out of bed, and using the bathroom?

The answers to these questions are important because they will help to plan for your **discharge**. This chapter discusses several key factors in making your post-hospital plans. These factors include:

- Planning for follow-up care
- Finding and hiring a **personal care assistant**
- Planning for transportation
- Identifying support groups
- Modifications to your home

A list of questions to ask when planning for your discharge from the rehabilitation hospital is also provided at the end of the chapter.

BEYOND THE HOSPITAL WALLS—PLANNING FOR FOLLOW-UP CARE

Your inpatient rehabilitation likely will last several weeks, if not months, but your rehabilitation should continue well beyond the time you leave the hospital. Your discharge from the hospital can be thought of as a transition to another level of care or rehabilitation. As discussed below, your continuing care should include physician follow-up and home or outpatient care.

At home, you may receive health care services, such as nursing care, **physical therapy, occupational therapy, speech therapy**, or **social work** services. In an outpatient rehabilitation setting, you may receive individual therapies, participate in a day treatment program, or receive physician care. You and your rehabilitation team, including your case manager or social worker, will plan for follow-up care based on your individual needs and your insurance benefits.

Physician Follow-Up

People with spinal cord injury (SCI) need different levels of follow-up care after discharge from inpatient rehabilitation. It is very important to follow up with your primary care physician within two to three weeks after being discharged from the rehabilitation hospital for ongoing medication management and to continue to address your medical care. To help your primary care doctor manage your care effectively, it is important for you to have a copy of your discharge summary and a summary of significant medical procedures that were performed during your stay (such as X-rays and MRIs). Some hospitals and facilities will forward the discharge information to the primary care physician, but ultimately it is the patient's responsibility to make sure that the doctor receives the appropriate information.

Your primary care physician can prescribe or renew prescriptions and provide ongoing treatment as needed. Be sure to tell your doctor about medications you're taking and discuss any concerns with him or her. If you were to have an earache or the flu, for example, it would be important for

your doctor to know the medications you're taking, so that any new treatment or medication will not cause problems or further discomfort.

It's also important to see medical specialists if recommended by your
doctor. For example, many patients with SCI will need to see a urologist
regularly to manage bladder issues. Also, if you had surgery, the surgeon
(most likely a neurosurgeon or orthopedic surgeon), will need to monitor
your healing progress and make any further recommendations post-reha-
bilitation. Your primary care physician can also refer you to other specialists as needed.

Home Health

After discharge from rehabilitation, people with SCI often return to their
homes or a family member's home. Many people continue to receive nursing care and therapy at home. **Home health care** providers are trained to
teach skills and provide ongoing treatment. They may recommend changes
and adaptations to improve your level of independence and safety and to
conserve your energy.

The types and amount of home health services provided depend in part
on your insurance and benefits. Many home care agencies follow the
Medicare guidelines for home health services. These guidelines say that a
person can receive home health care if he or she:

- Is under the care of a physician who can establish a plan of care
- Is "homebound" (has an injury or illness that restricts his or her ability
  to leave the home other than to attend medical appointments)
- Has an intermittent need for skilled nursing care, home health aides,
  physical therapy, occupational therapy, speech therapy, and/or social
  work services

Typically, the primary care physician is the doctor who renews home
health orders and works with the patient and the home health agency on
the plan of care. Home health services may include:

- Nursing care
- Therapy
- Social work services
- Case management services

Home health nursing services may be provided with the expectation that
a caregiver will be trained to provide services. These services might include
bowel and bladder management, wound care, PEG (feeding) tube care,

provision of intravenous medication, monitoring of vital signs, and more. Usually, the home nursing staff's goal is to teach the caregiver(s) to provide the care and then to follow up two or three times a week to answer questions and respond to concerns.

Therapy in the home provides an opportunity for you to put the skills you learned during your inpatient hospital stay to practical use. As therapists work with you at home, they may modify or adapt the skills they teach based on your needs and home environment. Physical therapy, occupational therapy, and speech therapy are all services that can be provided in the home. Services are typically provided two or three times a week for a short duration of time, with the expectation that you will transition to an outpatient setting for continued therapy services.

Social work and case management services can also be provided at home. The social worker can assist with community reentry and can identify resources in the community to increase your independence. For example, the social worker could help you identify transportation or grocery delivery services. Home health social work services are usually limited. You and your caregiver will need to follow up and complete forms on the resources provided by your social worker.

The case manager is responsible for communicating to your health insurance provider your progress and the functional changes you are making. He or she will also talk with you about any home health services that are not covered benefits (and therefore your financial responsibility).

Outpatient Services

Outpatient rehabilitation services may be prescribed if you need ongoing or periodic medical care and therapy. Depending on your needs and community resources, outpatient services can be received from different sources, including the rehabilitation hospital, hospital outpatient clinics and centers, private therapy services, and physicians' practices.

Patients who receive outpatient services typically receive therapy two or three times a week with the expectation that they will continue to practice the skills and exercises at home. The duration of outpatient therapy varies, depending on your level of participation and functional goals. Outpatient services may include, but are not limited to:

• Medical care
• Physical therapy
• Occupational therapy
• Speech therapy
• Hand therapy

- Aquatic therapy
- **Vocational rehabilitation**
- Social work
- **Psychology** services
- **Therapeutic recreation**
- **Orthotics** and prosthetics services

Some larger and more specialized outpatient rehabilitation providers, such as the National Rehabilitation Hospital, also offer seating and mobility, fertility, wound care, and other clinics. Depending on your needs, you might receive only one of these services, or you might receive a menu of services as your rehabilitation progresses.

Day Treatment

Day treatment programs are a type of outpatient program, that provide full-day, intensive services. These "interdisciplinary" programs are designed for people who can live at home but continue to need services three to five days a week. To enter a day treatment program, a person must have minimal nursing needs and must be able to take part in a physically intensive program that may include a variety of therapies each day.

After an initial evaluation, the day treatment team will design an individualized plan designed to help you achieve specific goals. The program may include a combination of individual therapies, group therapies, and community outings. These services will allow you to practice new skills and help you feel comfortable and confident in your transition from the hospital back to your community. As your abilities change, your treatment goals will also change, reflecting the dynamic process of rehabilitation.

GETTING HELP AT HOME—PERSONAL CARE ASSISTANCE

Many people with SCI (up to 40 percent) need extra help with daily activities after they go home. Often, family members provide the required assistance. Think about personal care assistance as early as possible. Discuss with your rehabilitation team members if and how much assistance you might need.

As you think about personal care assistance, think about what your daily needs will be within a 24-hour period. These needs may include assistance with activities of daily living (bathing, dressing, using the toilet, grooming, and eating), getting into and out of bed, preparing meals, and using transportation. Think about who can assist with each specific task. Some people are most comfortable with assistance from family members or friends. Others choose to hire personal care assistants or a combination of family, friends, and paid help.

Family Members as Caregivers

When making decisions about who will be your primary caregiver(s), you will need to think about who in your family is willing to assist, the time needed from the caregiver, and who is physically able to perform the more labor-intensive activities (such as **transfers**). You will also need to think about where you will get additional support if needed.

If you are thinking about having your spouse or another family member as your primary caregiver, consider how care giving may change your relationship with him or her. For example, intimate interactions with your spouse or partner may become less frequent or limited due to managing your daily care needs. Your family member also may be afraid or anxious about the physical or emotional changes stemming from your SCI. In addition, your family finances may change, which could add stress or anxiety at home. Together, you may need to answer questions such as:

- Which family member(s) are working and can they return to work?
- How will bills be paid?
- What financial obligations do both individuals have and how will they be met?

Remember that the caregiver's roles are often very demanding, both physically and emotionally. It's important to understand that the stresses felt from the caregiver's point of view will be different from the stresses the individual with the spinal cord injury may experience. Caregivers may feel overwhelmed or guilty about having to say "no" to you. They may feel resentful about not having time for themselves and their own activities. In contrast, you may be concerned with the physical aspects of your SCI, such as walking, bowel and bladder care, change in or lack of sexual function, and frustration when doing simple tasks. Both you and your caregiver will most likely worry about continuing health care, time constraints, financial means, and changes in your work or household roles.

Keep in mind that your caregiver's needs and concerns are as important as yours. He or she must find a balance between their needs and your needs. To alleviate burnout, resentment, and anger, make sure that you communicate openly and seek additional assistance if needed.

To ensure a successful relationship, you and your caregiver should try to maintain a healthy, balanced lifestyle by eating three meals a day, exercising, getting plenty of rest, and finding times to pursue enjoyable activities either together or apart. Good time management and organization are also essential to maintaining this balance. For instance, getting your finances in order will reduce stress that might jeopardize your relationship with your caregiver.

Getting a little extra assistance from other friends, family members, and caregivers can also help you and your caregiver maintain a positive out-look. Keep a list of tasks and chores you need help with, and pull it out when others ask what they can do to help. Shopping, making a meal, and doing afternoon child care once a week are good examples of how others can help alleviate some of the overall care.

Finally, finding friends and support in the community is essential to alleviate the stresses of being a caregiver. Caregivers who seek out friends to talk with or join support groups (see below) have a better chance of adjusting to their loved ones' SCI and their new roles.

Hiring a Personal Care Assistant

Most often, family members serve as primary caregivers for persons with SCI. In some instances, family members acting as caregivers may need to hire additional help. For example, a family member may be able to help with bathing and dressing but unable to help the person with transfers from the bed to the wheelchair, bedside commode toilet, etc. In such cases, a personal care assistant (PCA) could be hired to take care of the daily routine needs of a person with a disability. Hiring a PCA can:

- Keep the roles of the caregiver and family members separate
- Enable the person with SCI to live more independently
- Give other family members or caregivers the opportunity to return to work or to take care of other obligations

Your insurance and financial resources may determine if you can hire a PCA. Although unusual, some insurance policies have benefits covering personal care assistance. **Medicaid** policies vary from state to state, and some states' Medicaid programs offer PCA services or waiver programs that may provide additional services. Some long-term care policies have PCA benefits. Community resources, such as Vocational Rehabilitation Services, may provide a PCA if the services provided will enable the person with SCI to return to work. Also, contact your local **Center for Independent Living** and the National Spinal Cord Injury Association to identify SCI support services in your area. In other instances, individuals may have financial means to pay for a PCA's services. If you plan to pay for a PCA yourself, you will need to determine how many hours a week you can afford an attendant's services.

Hiring a PCA can be done two ways—either through a home health agency or privately. Home health agencies often offer PCA services that can be obtained in four-hour time increments. Agencies are often required to maintain certification and medical records for their staff members. It is important to understand the agency's billing process and to know if the agency will file claims with your health insurance plan (if applicable).

If you hire a PCA privately, be aware that it can be a lengthy process. It is important, however, to take enough time to find the right person. Many of the job duties are very personal and, although you will be the PCA's employer, you will also be dependent on him or her.

Start your search for a PCA by determining what your care needs will be and the number of hours required to complete each duty. Consider hiring several people to perform different job duties. For example, you may hire one PCA to do shopping and light housekeeping, another PCA to assist with activities of daily living (ADL) in the morning, a third PCA to assist with evening ADLs, and a fourth PCA to assist with activities throughout the day. This schedule could eliminate burnout and allow each PCA to have a standardized, simple, efficient routine.

Make a detailed list of the PCA job duties. (Figure 5.1) Determine what salary range you can afford to pay and decide whether you will offer any

---

- Bathing
- Dressing
- Housekeeping
- Medication
- Range of motion exercises
- Shopping
- Meal preparation
- Setup for meals
- Assistance with eating
- Toileting (bowel and bladder care)
- Transfers
- Wheelchair maintenance
- Miscellaneous tasks such as errands and those related to recreation activities

Figure 5.1. Duties That May Be Performed by a Personal Care Assistant

added perks, such as room and board, meals, or use of a car. If you need assistance in paying your PCA, contact your local Center for Independent Living or the National SCI Association to identify local SCI support services, and/or your health insurance provider. Be sure to keep accurate records about the amount and method of payments, and adhere to local, state, and federal level tax rules. Talk with a tax advisor or certified public accountant if you have questions about payment methods and taxes.

Next, write a brief but clear advertisement or announcement that will help you find a PCA. Place an advertisement in community newsletters, newsletters produced by places of worship, local employment offices, or human service agencies. Bulletin boards may also be seen by the type of person who would make a good PCA for you. Think about publications and places where you might connect with people who care about helping others. College students and medical students make good PCAs because of the flexibility of their schedules and nature of their studies. Mothers with children in school during the daytime also can have schedules that allow them to provide PCA services. An advertisement may look like one of the following:

AIDE Needed to Assist Male with a Disability: Duties include personal care, light home cleaning, errands and meal preparation. 4 hr/day, $7.00/hr. Call Bob at 555-1234.

OR

STUDENT OPPORTUNITY: Room and board, flexible hours in exchange for assisting disabled female. Please call 555-1234.

Develop a brief list of questions to ask applicants on the telephone to determine if you should have a face–to-face interview. Be very clear about the hours required. If you have any pets or assistance animals (such as a helper dog), inform the applicant during the telephone interview. If you invite the applicant for a more detailed interview, ask him or her to bring a list of references and/or a local security report from the local police department. Figure 5.2 lists some important qualities to look for when hiring a PCA.

During the face-to face interview, give the applicant a detailed list of job duties and explain the rules. For example, explain your policies on smoking, personal phone calls, specific room temperature, vacation time, and calling in sick. Review your schedule and the importance of the job duties. You also may need to educate the applicant about SCI. Explain that you are not sick but need assistance because of the limitations resulting from your SCI.

Some important interview questions to ask applicants include:

- Do you have any outside responsibilities (such as classes, other jobs, and family) that could interfere with your work as a PCA and your PCA schedule?
- What is your level of education?
- Do you have dependable transportation?
- Do you have a valid driver's license?
- Do you have any lifting limitations?
- Are you willing and able to cook if needed?
- Are you willing and able to do housework if needed?
- Do you have additional skills that might be helpful?
- What are your long-term goals?
- What are your social interests?

- Punctual
- Dependable
- Trustworthy and honest
- Able to follow instructions
- Thorough
- Comfortable with following an established routine
- Good communication and listening skills
- Sense of humor
- Patience

Figure 5.2 Important Qualities of a Personal Care Assistant

The interviewee's experience may vary from person to person. There is no right or wrong type of applicant. However, you need to feel comfortable with the person's current skill level and/or with training him or her to meet your needs. Small talk is okay as you are first meeting each other. It helps break the ice and identify common areas of interest that could make or break a working relationship.

You can purchase employment applications and background check forms at a local office supply store. Remember, the person you choose will be in your home, and you will need to feel comfortable with his or her presence. Be assertive about getting needed information and be decisive in defining the job duties. At this point you may want to provide a more detailed and specific checklist of the job duties needed to be performed. Figure 5.3 shows some items you might include in a checklist.

Once you have chosen the applicant you wish to hire as your PCA, extend a written offer and contract outlining the job duties, wages, any benefits, your policies, and grounds for termination. You might also want to establish a trial evaluation period, such as one month, to be sure the arrangement is a good "fit." Preparing and agreeing to a detailed written contract can make the working relationship easier because both parties will clearly understand the expectations. Sign the contract, ask the PCA to sign it, give a copy to him or her, and keep a copy for your records. Figure 5.4 lists items you might include in the written offer and contract.

Bathing Preparation:
- Select outfit and lay it out
- Run warm water (temp between 70 degrees Fahrenheit and 80 degrees Fahrenheit)
- Make sure three towels, soap, and facial washcloth are next to tub

Routine:
- Undress me and put nightgown in closet hamper
- Assist me with a sliding board transfer to wheelchair
- Roll wheelchair/me into restroom
- Assist me with sliding board transfer to tub bench
- Assist with bathing upper extremities, lower extremities, and perineal area

---

Figure 5.3. Examples of Items to Include in a Job Duty Checklist

You may find the process of hiring a PCA to be lengthy, but your efforts in identifying the right person and attention to detail will help ensure that both you and the PCA are satisfied with the arrangement. Once a PCA is hired, you can look forward to establishing a routine for your daily activities and pursuing other rewarding life interests.

GETTING HOME FROM THE HOSPITAL

Before your discharge from the rehabilitation hospital, you will want to figure out how you will get home. The day of discharge from rehabilitation can be busy, and you don't want to have to scramble to find transportation that day. Your rehabilitation team can help you decide the best way to get home based on your medical needs and the distance you will need to travel. Your case manager, your social worker, or the discharge planner can assist you with coordinating transportation—whether by car, van, plane, or train.

Your rehabilitation team can help you determine if you can ride in a vehicle in the seated and upright position or if you need to lie down on a stretcher. If you can ride in a vehicle in the seated position, you will need

- Duties (specific tasks you will need assistance with)
- Hours of work required
- Wages and payment schedule
- Tax withholding arrangements
- Arrangements for backup assistance if the PCA has an emergency that may prevent them from working on any given day.
- Policies for vacation and sick days
- Length of trial employment (evaluation) period.
- Length of time for services (such as six months or one year)
- Insurance benefits, if any
- Reimbursement of expenses for travel to and from work, meals, and other out-of-pocket costs
- Personal phone call policy

Figure 5.4. Items to Include in a Written Offer/Contract with a PCA

to know what kind of wheelchair (manual or power) you will use the day you are discharged from the hospital. In preparation for transportation on the day of discharge, following are a few sample questions:

- What is the driving distance from the hospital to my discharge destination?
- Can a family member provide transportation?
- If I have a manual wheelchair, will I be able to transfer into the passenger seat of a car? If yes, how much assistance will I need to transfer?
- Do I have a power wheelchair and what is the best way to transport it?
- Will I need to travel seated in my wheelchair in a wheelchair-accessible van?
- Will I need to use a transportation service offered in the community?

Cost can also be a factor in deciding how to get home from the hospital—and how to get around after you're living at home. Transportation benefits vary considerably from one insurance policy to another. Check with your insurance provider to determine what will be covered at the time of discharge. Some insurance plans cover the cost of transportation from one medical facility to another medical facility, but they do not pay for transportation from a medical facility to home.

Most cities have transportation services to accommodate people with disabilities. Contact your local public transportation provider, bus system, or subway or rail system to inquire about service in your area. You may also contact the National Spinal Cord Injury Association or your local department of motor vehicles. If you are a veteran and have a service-related injury, you could also check with your local U.S. Department of Veteran Affairs office to find out if you qualify for transportation services.

Many people with SCI travel by train and airplanes if their discharge destination is not within driving distance. Talk with your physician and rehabilitation team members to determine if you are medically stable to travel by these other means of transportation.

If your physician determines that you are medically stable to travel by means other than by car, contact the local train station or airlines to discuss the accommodations you will need. Again, the case manager, social worker, or discharge planner can work with you and assist with coordinating services.

Trains are equipped with wheelchair ramps and wheelchair lifts. Depending on the overall distance you will travel by train, you may need to arrange to have a handicapped- accessible sleeper car. This car will allow you to get out of your wheelchair, do pressure reliefs, and take care of your bowel and bladder management.

If traveling by airplane, you should sit in the bulkhead row or in the first-class section. When you make your reservation, be sure the ticket agent is aware that you have a disability and, therefore, that you are unable to sit in an emergency exit row. You may need to purchase more than one seat, depending on the overall duration of the flight and the possibility that you may need to lie down across several seats.

Upon arriving at the airport, the airline staff will assist you in getting onto the plane. This may involve transferring from your wheelchair into an airline chair that is narrow enough to use in the aisle. Keep your pressure-relieving cushion with you so you may sit on it in your airplane seat. To ensure that all the components of your wheelchair stay together, ask that all detachable parts be labeled and taped together. Also, be sure you have arranged transportation that can accommodate your needs when you arrive at your destination airport or train station.

ACCESSIBILITY OF YOUR HOME ENVIRONMENT

Your home is more than a building. It is your place to live and it reflects your personality, taste, and style. After a spinal cord injury, however, accessibility of your home becomes a top priority. A place that allows you to live as independently as possible can become your home. It is not uncommon for people with SCI to need home modifications, such as ramps or wider doorways, to accommodate the use of a wheelchair or other **durable medical equipment (DME)**.

Who would I like to have involved in planning for my discharge (for example, spouse, child, or a friend)?

Name: _____

Home telephone number: (___) _____

Work telephone number: (___) _____

Cell phone number: (___) _____

My *Follow-Up Care*
- Will I need any follow-up care (such as physical therapy, occupational therapy, psychology, nursing care, or laboratory services)?
- Do I need to come back to see my rehabilitation doctor after discharge?
- Which other doctors will I need to see after discharge?
- Will I need any home care services (such as nursing care or therapies)?
- Will I need outpatient therapy or day treatment?

My *Caregivers at Home*
- Who will provide my care at home (for example, a family member, home health care service, personal care assistant)?
- Can my family/caregiver receive care giving training at the hospital or elsewhere?
- When and where will this training be held?
- Is my family/caregiver ready for my discharge?

My *Home's Accessibility*
- Do I need to make changes to my home to make it accessible?
- Who can recommend changes?
- What changes will be needed?
- Who will make the changes?

Figure 5.5. Questions to Ask When Planning for Discharge from the Rehabilitation Hospital

(Figure 5.5 continued)

My *Equipment and Supplies*
- Will I need any durable medical equipment (such as a wheelchair, braces, or raised toilet)?
- Is the equipment covered by my health insurance?
- Will I need to pay a co-payment for the equipment?
- Do I need any special supplies for wound care, bladder, or bowel management (such as dressings, tape, saline solution, and catheters)?
- Where will I get the supplies?

My *Medications*
- What medications will I be taking when I leave the hospital?
- What are the medications used for?
- What side effects might the medications cause?
- Where can I get prescriptions filled?
- Will I need to pay a co-payment?

My *Discharge Day*
- What day will I be discharged?
- What time can I leave?
- Who will pick me up from the hospital and where will I meet him or her?
- Do I have any valuables stored with security or elsewhere in the hospital?
- What time and where can I pick up my valuables?
- Will I need assistance when I leave the hospital?
- What will I need help with?

—Jennifer Hendricks, LICSW, Care Coordination Manager, National Rehabilitation Hospital

If you are returning to your current home, a friend or family member's home, or considering other options, you will need to think about the accessibility. Other options could involve looking at a sub-acute facility or skilled nursing home, a group home, or a shelter. Most sub-acute facilities or skilled nursing homes are modified to accommodate someone with a disability who uses a wheelchair. Family or friends are encouraged to visit potential facilities to determine those that will meet your needs. They can talk with staff members and current residents, take a tour, and look around.

A tape measure can be helpful during this visit to measure the size of door-ways, bathrooms, etc., to ensure you are able to maneuver your wheelchair safely.

To help make a smooth transition from the hospital to home, be sure to talk with your rehabilitation team to review any potential barriers. The Home Accessibility Questionnaire is a tool used to guide you and the team in discussing your home. This form will allow the therapist and rehab team to make recommendations for modifications based on your abilities. Many variables come into play when planning for home modifi-cations. For example:

- How will you enter your home?
- Are there steps? If so, where? How many?
- Do you need a ramp? If yes, what kind of ramp? Is it portable or perma-nent?
- How many exists are available in case of an emergency?
- How wide are the doors and do they need to be widened?
- Which rooms do you need to access?

Modifications can range in cost and duration of completion. It's impor-tant to prioritize those modifications that need to be done before discharge and those that may be completed at a different time. For example, widen-ing a doorway could be very timely and expensive versus removing the door and adding a curtain for immediate privacy. Whether you own or rent your home, be sure to follow any rules or regulations set forth by the property owner, association, community, county, etc.

Home modifications can be costly, so take time to research programs in your community that may pay for a portion of the cost or all of the cost. To identify programs, consider inquiring with your local housing authority, city hall, county resources, banks, and Center for Independent Living. Additional resources could include the Medicaid Home and Community Based Waiver program, Veterans Administration programs, your state vocational rehabilitation program, Fannie Mae, the U.S. Department of Housing and Urban Development's (HUD) Title I and Section 203k pro-grams, and the U.S. Department of Agriculture's (USDA) Rural Community Development program (formerly the Farmers Home Administration). Explore all funding options and communicate clearly with everyone so you understand the requirements, rules and regulations, and avoid making cost and/or timely mistakes.

The Americans with Disabilities Act (ADA) and the Fair Housing Act Amendments (FHAA) have set guidelines for people with disabilities to receive *reasonable accommodations* and *reasonable modifications*. Although the guidelines are set, landlords and property owners and federal tenant-based programs are not required to pay for modifications, especially if they are deemed unreasonable. *Opening Doors,* a housing initiative newsletter, defines "reasonable accommodations" and "reasonable modifications" as follows:

- *Reasonable accommodation:* A change in the rules, policies, practices, and/or services of a housing unit or program in order to ensure people with disabilities are not excluded or have their rights unfairly compromised. For example, designating a handicap parking space closer to your unit would be a reasonable accommodation.
- *Reasonable modification:* Alteration of rental housing to meet the unique needs of a person with a disability. Under reasonable modification, an owner must allow a person with a disability to make certain physical modifications to a unit if needed to fully use and enjoy the housing unit. An example of a reasonable modification is installing a ramp or a roll-in shower.

Be sure to communicate clearly with all people involved when making any modifications. Your rehabilitation team will need to have some basic information regarding home modifications that will be made so they may recommend the appropriate DME. Remember, not all modifications need to be completed before your discharge from the hospital. Some modifications will need to occur after you are home and you have an opportunity to live in your home. As you live in your home, you will have a clearer picture of changes that need to be made to maximize your independence.

ON THE ROAD AGAIN—DRIVING AFTER A SPINAL CORD INJURY

Driving after a spinal cord injury can be very liberating. With today's technology, adaptations can be made to accommodate people with a variety of disabilities, including spinal cord injury. In a 1996 survey, more than 72 percent of people with SCI reported that they were able to return to driving, although most of them said they had had their vehicles modified in some way.

Before driving, contact your state's Department of Motor Vehicles and your car insurance carrier to notify them of your spinal cord injury. Ask about the rules and laws set up for driving with a disability. Depending on your state's laws, you may need a prescription from your physician indicating that you are medically stable to drive.

You will also need to identify and enroll in a driver rehabilitation training program. Contact the National Spinal Cord Injury Association, your rehabilitation hospital, the local Veteran Affairs office, or your state department of vocational rehabilitation for information about driver training programs. Ask about the cost of the program and if adapted vehicles are available for use during the driver training. Funding for driver training programs and vehicle accommodations depends on your needs, the type of vehicle, and the modifications needed. The evaluation and training process is usually completed by a certified driving rehabilitation specialist (CDRS), who can address your individual needs and recommend accommodations.

Once recommendations have been prescribed by the CDRS, contact an Adaptive Driving Alliance dealer or the National Mobility Equipment Dealers Association to discuss obtaining recommended vehicle modifications. Be sure to discuss all options—including leases, rentals, and purchase of used vehicles that have already been modified. Also be sure to inquire about rebates if you decide to purchase a new vehicle from a car dealership.

To learn more about driver training and vehicle modifications, see Chapter 9.

FINDING SUPPORT FROM OTHERS WITH SPINAL CORD INJURY

Spinal cord injury can be devastating to an individual and his or her family because life has changed drastically in an instant. Joining a support group can help you "work through" some of the issues you face and will help you and your family understand that you are not alone in confronting the challenges of living with SCI. A support group will give you an opportunity to exchange valuable information and experiences about living with SCI, and it can provide companionship, role models, community resources and more. It will also help you gather information about resources in your community and tips on how to simplify and modify your life after SCI. In other words, becoming part of a support group can answer questions and alleviate some of the anxiety associated with SCI.

Your social worker, psychologist, or other rehabilitation team members can help you identify an SCI support group in your area. Also, you might find a group by contacting other local hospitals, the National Spinal Cord Injury Association, or the National Family Caregivers Association. If you are unable to identify a support group that specifically focuses on SCI, consider attending another type of support group. For example, there are support groups for people with traumatic injuries, caregivers, people with disabilities in general, and people with drug addictions.

In addition to support groups, Internet chat rooms can be a way to exchange and share information about spinal cord injuries. Internet chat rooms connect people to news groups, bulletin boards, discussion groups, message boards, for topics related to SCI and related disabilities. The Spinal Cord Injury Information Network hosts a few SCI chat rooms. Additional chat rooms can be identified by doing a Web search.

CONCLUSION

Your medical rehabilitation doesn't end when you leave the hospital. Rather, your discharge from the hospital can be thought of as a transition to another level of care that may include primary care, home health care, rehabilitation outpatient services, and day treatment. Throughout your rehabilitation stay, you will have learned new skills and gained new knowledge that you can use at home and in the community to become as independent and active as possible. Your family and friends can help you make the transition, but you can also look to your health care providers, support groups, and community-based organizations for additional support. If one type of support doesn't meet your needs, don't hesitate to look for other resources locally, nationally, or on the Internet.

What Can I Do?

As you prepare for your discharge from the rehabilitation hospital:

- *Speak up.* Be sure to ask questions and get the answers you need. Figure 5.5 lists some important questions to ask as you get ready go home from the rehabilitation hospital.
- *Communicate openly.* Your discharge from the hospital involves many factors. Talk openly with your social worker, case manager, and discharge planner throughout your rehabilitation. Don't hesitate to discuss your concerns and interests so you can be guided in your planning process.
- *Plan ahead.* Before you leave the rehabilitation hospital, take steps to ensure that your discharge destination is accessible, that your caregivers are identified and trained, and that you have identified a safe mode of transportation.
- *Arrange for needed care.* Be sure you have a continued care plan, and that follow-up medical care and therapies are scheduled. It is imperative that you have a primary care physician identified and that you have follow-up appointments scheduled with any specialty doctors. Also, make sure you know which medications and medical supplies you will need. Get a copy of your discharge summary from the physician and the rehabilitation team members for a clear understanding of

your rehabilitation and the continued care plan.

• *Understand your insurance.* Develop a good understanding of your insurance policy, including which services and equipment will be paid for, and where you can continue to receive therapies (for example, either in your home or at an outpatient clinic).

Where Can I Learn More?

To learn more about making the transition from the rehabilitation hospital to home or another destination, you may wish to contact:

• Your case manager, discharge planner, or social worker at your rehabilitation hospital
• Your health insurance provider (to learn what services are covered)
• Your local Center for Independent Living (visit www.ilru.org for a directory of these centers)
• The local chapter of the National Spinal Cord Injury Association (www.spinalcord.org for a directory of chapters)
• Spinal Cord Injury Information Network (www.spinalcord.uab.edu)
• National Family Caregivers Association (www.thefamilycaregiver.org)
• National Association for Home Care (www.nahc.org)
• Opening Doors newsletter (www.c-c-d.org/intro_page.htm)

Appendix C provides information about additional resources.

IMPORTANT POINTS TO REMEMBER

• After an inpatient rehabilitation stay, returning home or to another living situation is an important change. The earlier planning for this transition begins, the smoother the transition will be. In fact, this planning process should start early in the rehabilitation program. The patient's case manager, discharge planner, or social worker can help with planning.
• Good planning for continued care, transportation, and home modifications are important parts of the hospital discharge process.
• Many people with SCI need assistance with daily activities at home. Such help may be provided by family members or paid personal care assistants. Hiring a personal care assistant can enable the person with SCI to live independently and relieve family members from the need to help with all daily care tasks.

REFERENCES

(1) National Endowment for Financial Education, Paralyzed Veterans of America, National Spinal Cord Injury Association. (2002). *On the Move: A Financial Guide for People with Spinal Cord Injury.*
(2) Opening Doors: A Housing Publication for the Disability Community. (June 2000). *Accessible Housing for People with Disabilities.* Issue 10. Available at: http://www.c-c-d.org/od-june00.htm#Language.
(3) Research and Training Center on Independent Living, University of Kansas (1987). *A Step-by Step Guide to Training and Managing Personal Attendants.*
(4) *Rehabilitation Nursing,* Vol29, No 2 (March/April 2004). Support Groups: Why Do People Attend.
(5) University of Alabama at Birmingham, Spain Rehabilitation Center (1998). Medical RRTC in Secondary Complications in SCI: Caregivers for SCI (fact sheet).
(6) University of Alabama at Birmingham, Spain Rehabilitation Center (1994). Medical RRTC in Secondary Complications in SCI: Personal Care Assistants (fact sheet).
(7) Family Caregiver Alliance, National Center on Caregiving (2001). Hiring In-Home Help (fact sheet).

6

Peer Mentoring: Tap the Experience of Others with Spinal Cord Injury

THILO KROLL

"Mentors are important. Knowing (my mentor) when I had my accident prompted me to set high expectations for myself as I had a similar injury. He was a constant source of answers to my frequent 'how do you?' questions." —Jennifer

The first few weeks of living with a spinal cord injury (SCI) may be very difficult. During those weeks, you'll need to learn new ways of doing things and many new skills. You'll receive much information, which sometimes can be overwhelming and hard to understand. Peer mentors—people who are willing to share their knowledge and firsthand experiences with spinal cord injury—can help you work through some of this information and the challenges you may encounter during your rehabilitation and after you leave the hospital. For example, peer mentors can answer questions, offer advice, provide support, and help you make transitions back to school or work.

This chapter discusses:

- The role of peer mentors
- What peer mentors can and cannot do
- Where and how to find peer mentors
- How to work effectively with peer mentors

WITH SO MUCH TO DEAL WITH, I NEED HELP!

During your hospital stay, you'll get treatment, advice, and support from doctors, nurses, therapists, and others. Everyone will try to ensure that when you leave the hospital you can be as independent as possible and that you'll be able to take good care of yourself. However, too little time may be available to get all the answers to your questions. Health care professionals do speak English, but sometimes it seems they forget how to communicate with their patients. *Wouldn't it be nice to have someone available who can explain the effects of your spinal cord injury to you in plain English?*

At first, it may be very hard to come to terms with your injury. You may feel angry or sad, upbeat or frustrated, and scared or challenged. It may seem like an emotional roller coaster. *Wouldn't it be nice to have someone to talk to—someone who has a more personal understanding of your situation?*

After you're able to get out and about in your wheelchair, you may still feel a bit insecure. For instance, when you transfer into and out of the wheelchair, you may still feel shaky. Once in the chair, you may ask yourself questions like "How do I deal with stairs?" "What do I do if my chair breaks down?" and "What do I do if I fall out of my chair?" *Wouldn't it be nice to know someone who could show you how to deal with these situations based on his or her own experience?*

Then there's all of the paperwork. You may be entitled to disability benefits, you may want to tap into state vocational rehabilitation services, or you may want to use **paratransit** services to help you get around after you leave the hospital. Doing so typically requires you to complete many forms. *Wouldn't it be nice to get some help with this paperwork?*

If you answered "yes" to any of the questions above, then you might benefit from the help of a peer mentor, that is, another person who has had a spinal cord injury (SCI) who is willing to help.

JUST WHAT ARE PEER MENTORS AND WHAT DO THEY DO?

The word "peer" simply means someone who is similar to you, be it in age, gender, race, education, or disability. For example, a peer could be a friend, a fellow student, a coworker, or someone with interests like yours. "Mentoring" simply means serving as a trusted counselor or teacher. When we talk about peer mentors in the context of SCI, we mean other people who have SCI and have faced some of the same experiences and challenges.

Peer mentors have learned from their own experiences. They are knowledgeable about resources and living with SCI. They may be employed or work as volunteers at rehabilitation hospitals or for community-based organizations such as **Centers for Independent Living**. Most serious and responsible peer mentor programs choose their peer mentors carefully and provide them with comprehensive training and supervision.

Peer mentors can be helpful in many ways. For example, they can identify

Help You Deal with Your Emotions . . .

Many people with SCI feel angry, frustrated, anxious, or depressed, or respond to their injuries in other ways. Peer mentors are good listeners and can provide emotional support when you need it. After all, they understand what you're going through because they've been there themselves. Peer mentors can talk about their own experiences during the first weeks or months after injury. They can also tell you how they learned to confront their feelings and how they dealt with their injury from an emotional and psychological standpoint.

Advise You About Relationships and Sex . . .

Although specific experiences differ from person to person, it sometimes helps to hear from other people how they have dealt with changes in their relationships with friends, family members, teachers, and employers, and how they developed new relationships. Peer mentors may also serve as social role models. Joining them for a day out may help you to understand and redefine your own relationships with the people around you.

Most SCI survivors also wonder whether it will be possible to have fulfilling sexual relationships in the future. Most peers who "know the ropes" will tell you, "Of course it's possible!" Peer mentors can share their own experiences and point you to additional information, support, and resources that can help you deal with sexuality issues.

. . . and Help You Get Back to School and Work

Going back to school or work is one of the critical steps in resuming life after SCI. It may take time to get to this step because you need to deal with so many other pressing issues first. When you're ready, though, peer mentors can help you find information, give advice on completing college or job applications, suggest ways to make your workplace accessible, identify vocational training resources, and connect you with **vocational rehabilitation** counselors at the hospital or in the community.

Peer mentors may also help you with using computer hardware and software. Computers and other technology not only make communication with others easier, but also open up a wealth of information available through the Internet. Peer mentors can help you make sense of this technology, show you how to make a computer more accessible, help you develop your computer skills, and show you how to submit college and job applications and resumes through the Internet.

Peer mentors may also direct you to **social workers** at the rehabilitation hospital or in your community who can provide assistance with health insurance, **Social Security**, and financial issues.

PEER MENTORS CAN DO A LOT, BUT . . .

Peer mentors typically are not doctors, nurses, therapists, or other health care professionals, nor are they professional counselors. They can provide support and advise you on the practical aspects of life after SCI, but it's important for you to understand what they cannot—or should not—do for you.

First, peer mentors should never be seen as substitutes for health care professionals because they cannot and should not diagnose problems or treat you. Peer mentors can support you in being proactive, in taking charge of your own health, and in developing self-management skills. When you have health-related problems or concerns, though, see your doctor or another health care professional!

Second, peer mentors can't solve your family, social, work, school, financial, physical, or other life problems for you. They're partners in your effort to develop a better understanding of your life with a spinal cord injury— nothing more and nothing less. If you feel you need more or a different kind of help, talk with your doctor, psychologist, or a trained counsellor.

Third, peer mentors can't make decisions for you. Their role is to tell you about their own experiences, their solutions, and their ways of doing things. Their approaches may not be best for you. You may also have different ideas for resolving problems and reaching your goals. It's important to determine what is best for you and what advice you wish to accept, and to develop strategies that will work for you within the context of your life.

Fourth, peer mentors shouldn't be your only source of information or advice. Be sure to double check the information with a knowledgeable professional before making important health or life decisions.

Fifth, peer mentors can't be substitutes for your family or friends. They can advise and support you, based on their own experiences, and they can suggest ways to maintain positive relationships with important others in your life. However, they shouldn't be your sole source of emotional support or friendship.

Finally, peer mentors aren't personal assistants. Don't expect them to run errands for you, help with personal care needs, or lend you money.

CHOOSING AND USING PEER MENTORS

It's important to choose your peer mentor carefully. Typically, a peer mentor would be assigned to you by the team that runs and supervises the peer men-

Table 6.1. Questions to Ask Peer Mentors	
If you need . . .	**You could ask a peer mentor . . .**
Information about the impact of SCI on your life	• What does this health issue mean for my life? • How will it affect me? • Now that I know about it, what can I do about it? • Where can I find more information about this topic? • Who should I talk to? • Are there ways to get this information other than booklets and brochures?
Help with preventing and dealing with medical complications	• How do I know if something is wrong? • What are the signs of a urinary tract infection, autonomic dysreflexia, or a pressure sore feel like or look like? • How can I prevent complications? • What can I do to maintain good health? • Where and when do I need to seek help? • Where can I find additional information about specific complications?
Advice about healthy, active living	• What types of exercises can I safely do to gain more strength or to keep fit? • What kind of sports can I do? • Where can I find a place that provides for my needs? • Where can I find an accessible gym?
Information about leisure activities	• How can I get back to the hobbies or recreation activities that I enjoyed before my injury? • What can I do to be active and to satisfy my interests? • Where can I find information about accessibility? • What can I do together with other people with and without SCI? • Where can I find people who share my interests?
Advice about getting around your community	• What do I need to think about when planning to visit a friend or go to the movies? • Where can I find information about accessible public transportation? • What do I do if my wheelchair breaks down? • Where can I find spare parts for my wheelchair?
Emotional support	• How can I deal with my frustrations? • How can I overcome my anxiety to become more active? • What can I do to enjoy my life more? • Where can I find psychological counseling and professional help?

(continued next page)

(Table 6.1 continued)

Advice about relationships and sexuality	• How and where will I be able to meet people? • How can I make it easier for people who do not have a SCI to approach me? • What can I do to plan ahead for meetings with other people? • Where can I find information about sexuality?
Help with your return to school or work	• Where can I find job-seeking help? • What accommodations can be made for me at school or in my workplace? • How do I let potential employers know that I have a disability? • What assistance services are available to me in the workplace or in school? • How can I talk effectively with other students and my teachers about my disability?

toring program. The decision about whom to assign may vary from situation to situation. The primary matching criterion is that the "mentee" is comfortable with her or his mentor. Several additional criteria, including injury level, age, gender, interests and hobbies, and geographic area, may be considered. Some individuals may feel less comfortable with a peer mentor of the other sex, others think they would benefit more if they had someone with an injury that is very similar to theirs, while for others common interests and activities are the driving force.

Despite their best efforts, you might find that your peer mentor is not a "good fit" for you. However, you may want to give the relationship some time to see how it develops. If, after a few meetings, you can't see eye to eye or you feel you won't benefit from the relationship, contact the program manager, who will connect you with another peer mentor.

A good match between your peer mentor's personality, skills, interests, strengths, and availability and your own personality and needs is important. However, the qualities discussed briefly below are important, too.

A Peer Mentor Should Be Reliable and Dependable . . .

Your peer mentor should be available to you consistently and reliably over an extended period of time. If you set up a meeting with your mentor, you want to feel confident that he or she will arrive or call you at the appointed time. (Likewise, you should arrive or call your peer mentor at the appointed time.) Keep in mind, however, that your peer mentor won't be available to you 24/7.

Trusted . . .

You may want to share thoughts and feelings with the peer mentor that you don't share with anyone else—not even your best friend or members of your family. Because your relationship with your peer mentor will be very personal, you must be able to trust him or her. You need to feel safe and comfortable talking with him or her about your experiences and concerns.

Knowledgeable . . .

The foundation of the peer mentoring concept is that another person has some knowledge that can be of benefit to you. Therefore, your peer mentor should have a good understanding of spinal cord injury and of the information and resources that are available to you.

Resourceful . . .

When you work with a peer mentor, you want to make sure that he or she is able connect you to important resources at the rehabilitation hospital, in the community, and on the Internet. You can't expect the peer mentor to be familiar with every Web site or organization, but he or she should be resourceful enough to help you find the information you need. Keep in mind, however, that it may take time for the peer mentor to locate resources or the person or organization to help you.

Sometimes, several peer mentors work together as a team because they know they are resourceful in different ways. One peer mentor may be particularly knowledgeable about preventing medical complications, while another is active in wheelchair sports, and a third may be experienced in applying for college or for employment. Your needs and questions drive the extent to which additional peer mentors will be involved.

. . . and Active

Finally, because one of the important roles of peer mentoring is to ease your return to the community, to education, or to work, you want to choose a peer mentor who is active and involved in activities that are of interest to you. He or she should not only be resourceful but also be able to think of ideas about what you can do together. For example, the peer mentor might go with you to the movies, a basketball game, driver training class, or a meeting at an employment agency.

Peer mentoring programs and how they operate vary, depending on the hospital or other organization that sponsors the program. Below is an example of the peer mentoring process.

At the National Rehabilitation Hospital (NRH), peer mentors typically accompany a member of the clinical rehabilitation team to see new inpatients. The clinical staff member may be a psychologist, social worker, or therapist. After their introduction, they spend a few minutes to explain their role and the idea of peer mentoring. They will leave their contact information and a short brochure with the patient. In some instances, they show a short video that provides a quick and easy introduction of the peer mentoring program. Peer mentors answer the patient's questions and will return after a few days to see if the patient is interested in joining the peer mentor program.

After the individual's discharge from inpatient rehabilitation, the peer mentor will call to arrange an in-person meeting. The first meeting usually focuses on the situation immediately after discharge. Topics such as accessibility of the immediate living environment, transfers to and from the wheelchair, personal assistance, and the prevention of medical complications are common during these first weeks.

NRH's peer mentors seek to establish a regular contact pattern with their "mentees." They make sure that they at least talk on the phone once a week. The peer mentors may suggest social outings and leisure activities and may monitor for medical complications. They provide information, demonstrate skills, and refer the mentee to health care professionals when necessary. Over time, their contact typically becomes less frequent, as the mentee with SCI broadens his or her own social network of friends. The peer mentors are important facilitators in this process. At the same time, they will remain a resource that may be used whenever needed.

Figure 6.1. The Peer Mentoring Process

Figure 6.1 describes the peer mentoring process used at the National Rehabilitation Hospital.

BUILDING YOUR RELATIONSHIP

Every peer mentoring relationship is different. Not all contacts between peer mentors and "mentees" are in person. In fact, most contacts occur by phone or e-mail. Whether you communicate in person, by phone or e-mail, weekly contact with your peer mentor will help you establish and maintain a positive, fruitful the relationship. Some people decide to communicate more by phone or e-mail after a few weeks of direct face-

---

Peer mentor:

Name _____

Phone number _____

E-mail address _____

Scheduled meeting date: _____

Overall goals for the meeting:

1. _____

2. _____

3. _____

What do I want the peer mentor to do?

   Provide me with information about: _____

   Provide advice about: _____

   Show me where I can find help with: _____

   Show me how to: _____

   Join me to in this activity: _____

What did the peer mentor tell me or show me?

What will I do with the information/advice from the peer mentor?

Will we meet or talk again about the same subject? If so when and where?

Figure 6.2. Peer Mentor Meeting Worksheet

to-face contact. Sometimes, it's not possible to meet in person because of distance or lack of transportation. Thankfully, the phone and e-mail offer good alternatives.

It's up to you to decide how to develop and make good use of the relationship. Remember, though, that you must be an active participant if you are to benefit from the relationship. At your first meeting, your peer mentor will introduce himself or herself and explain to you how he or she can help. Similarly, you should talk about yourself and what you feel your peer mentoring needs may be. Then, each time you meet or communicate, you might want to define ahead of time what you wish to accomplish. The Peer Mentoring Meeting Worksheet (Figure 6.2) can help you prepare for your meetings with your peer mentor.

There are no clear rules about how long a peer mentoring relationship should last. Only you and your mentor can decide this! After a few weeks or several months, you may feel you've learned everything you need to learn in order to live as independently as possible, and may no longer want to contact or meet with a peer mentor. A rule of thumb is that six months after your injury, you may want to try out on your own what you have learned. At that time, be sure to let your peer mentor and the program team know that you're ready to move on, and that you appreciate all that he or she has done. Some people decide, after a short break from the relationship, that they would like to get back in touch with the peer mentor, perhaps to share recent experiences or to ask for specific advice.

IT'S UP TO YOU!

When thinking about using peer mentors, remember that you need to decide for yourself whether you want the support of peer mentors. You are in charge. If you choose to work with a peer mentor, you must decide what kinds of support you need, how often you want to meet or communicate by phone or e-mail, and how much support you need.

Peer mentors can provide support in many different ways. Keep in mind that their roles are to help you to deal with your disability and to get you started on the right track to independent living. They can't substitute for your family and friends, and they can't provide the type of help you receive from your doctors and other professionals. They also can't live your life for you, make your decisions, or take on your responsibilities. However, peer mentors can be good role models, and they can show you skills and techniques to help you live a healthy, productive, fulfilling life.   —

What Can I Do?

To develop or maintain a positive, beneficial peer mentoring relationship, be sure to:

- *Take steps to get started.* Talk with the staff of your rehabilitation hospital's spinal cord injury program to find out if the hospital offers a peer mentoring program. If not, ask them if they know of any local programs, or contact other organizations to find out if they can connect you to a program (see "Where Can I Find Out More?" box above).
- *Communicate your needs and interests.* Let the peer mentoring program team and your peer mentor(s) know what you feel you need and what kind of support you feel would help.
- *Have realistic expectations.* Your peer mentor can provide lots of support and information, but don't expect him or her to solve all your problems, be available around-the-clock, lend you money, or take the place of your doctor or other trained professionals.
- *Set goals.* Set reasonable goals for what you want to gain from the relationship and each meeting.
- *Be flexible.* Remember that your peer mentor has other responsibilities, such as work, family, and social activities. You should expect him or her to be dependable, but remember that last-minute scheduling changes might arise.
- *Be respectful.* Treat your peer mentor respectfully and courteously—just as you would like to be treated. If you can't make it to an appointment or be available for a call, let him or her know ahead of time. Remember that many peer mentors work as volunteers in this role!

Where Can I Learn More?

Peer mentoring programs have become more common in recent years. To learn more or to find a program, you may wish to contact:

- The spinal cord injury program team, a psychologist, social work or nurse on the team, or a representative of spinal cord injury advocacy groups at your rehabilitation hospital
- The local chapter of the National Spinal Cord Injury Association (visit www.spinalcord.org for a directory of chapters)
- Your local Center for Independent Living (visit www.ilru.org for a directory of these centers)
- The peer-to-peer program at your local U.S. Department of Veterans Affairs hospital (visit www.va.gov for a directory of VA facilities)

IMPORTANT POINTS TO REMEMBER

- Peer mentors are people who are willing to share their knowledge and firsthand experiences with spinal cord injury. They can help you work through some of the challenges you may encounter during your rehabilitation and after you leave the hospital.
- Peer mentors can answer questions, offer advice, provide support, and help you make transitions back to school or work. For example, they can talk with you about the impact of spinal cord injury, help you prevent medical problems, help you find ways to get around, and provide emotional support.
- To find a peer mentor, contact the spinal cord injury program team at your rehabilitation hospital. You might also find a peer mentor by contacting local spinal cord injury advocacy organizations or your local Center for Independent Living.

This chapter was supported in part through a grant from the U.S. Department of Education, National Institute on Disability and Rehabilitation Research, Grant #H133B031114.

7

Understanding Your Health Plan and Income Support Options

GWYN C. JONES
KIANDA BELL

"After my injury, and after medical bills had nearly depleted all my assets, I qualified for Medicaid so that I could continue my therapy as an outpatient. . . . For years, it seemed my father spent more time wading through the mire of private and public healthcare systems on my behalf than he did working in his law practice." –Jennifer

Living well with a spinal cord injury can require a lot of rehabilitation, medical care, and special equipment. It also can require making changes to one's home and work space. These services can be very expensive. The right blend of health insurance coverage and regular income support can help you live well with your spinal cord injury. You may have private insurance through your own or a family member's employer. If you do, then your health insurance will cover many of the costs of your rehabilitation and medical services. If you don't have private health insurance, then your federal and state governments offer some income support and health insurance programs that may help you.

This chapter discusses:

- Types of private and government health insurance
- Sources of income support, including **Social Security Disability Income** and **Supplemental Security Income**
- How your **rehabilitation team** and others can help you find out about health insurance and income support

111

HOW DO HEALTH PLANS DIFFER?

Many people find their health insurance plans hard to understand. Knowing how to work with your health plan can help you get the services that you need to live a "health-full" life with spinal cord injury.

People get their health insurance from different sources. Your insurance might be:

- A private plan that you or a family member buys
- Private health insurance bought by an employer
- Public health insurance offered by your state or federal government

Health insurance plans offered by those three sources can be:

- Fee-for-service
- Managed care
- Blended fee-for-service and managed care

Each of these three types is described below. Table 7.1 lists some of the advantages and disadvantages of each type. Knowing which type of plan you have will help you work with your health care providers to get the kind of care you need.

Fee-for-Service (FFS) Plans

Until the 1990s, fee-for-service plans were the most common type of health care plan. Now, most health care consumers belong to managed care plans. Often, fee-for-service plans offer more freedom in choosing health care providers. You may also have to pay out more of your own money for your health care. Fee-for-service plans, also known as "indemnity" plans, allow you to choose any health care provider who will accept the "usual and customary" fees paid by the insurance plan for each covered service. "Usual and customary" fees are the payments that doctors and other health care providers agree to accept as full payment for health care services.

Fee-for-service coverage usually requires you to pay a monthly insurance bill. You must also meet a yearly dollar amount in payments before your health plan pays for most services. This amount is called a **deductible** and is stated in the policy. Many health plans will not pay for some services until you pay the yearly deductible. For example, you may have to pay $100 or $200 of your own money each year, before your health plan will begin to pay for your medical care. Once you meet your deductible, the insurance

Table 7.1. Health Insurance Types

Plan Type	Advantages	Disadvantages
Fee-for-Service (FFS)	• Freedom to choose any doctor who accepts your health plan • Typically, the plan pays 80% of the cost for covered services	• You pay a monthly premium • You pay a deductible • Typically, you pay 20% of all covered charges after paying your deductible • You may have to pay 100% of the cost of services that your plan does not cover
Managed Care (MC)	• You pay a lower monthly premium • You pay smaller fees for doctor visits, prescription drugs, and other services • You can get many health care services in one location • Prescription refills can be mailed to your home	• You have limited freedom in choosing your doctors • You must get approval ahead of time for hospital care and visits to specialists
Blended FFS + MC	• You may have more freedom to choose specialists	• You may have higher co-payments for doctor visits and other services • If you choose a doctor who does not belong to your plan, you may have to pay all of the costs for seeing that doctor

company usually pays 80 percent of covered charges. You pay the other 20 percent of the approved fee to your doctors or other providers.

In some cases, you might also have to pay the difference between the amount your doctor usually charges for a service and the approved amount. This is called "balance billing," and it can be very expensive for you. When you visit a new doctor, be sure to find out if that doctor accepts your health plan's approved fees as full payment for his or her services. Figure 7.1 presents an example of "balance billing."

Robert has a spinal cord injury. He has finished his rehabilitation hospital stay and is now living at home with his family. Robert has private health insurance coverage through his wife's employer. The health plan charges a yearly deductible of $100 for each family member covered in the plan. Robert has already met his deductible.

When Robert visits his primary care doctor for a persistent urinary tract infection, the doctor suggests that he see a specialist. He decides to see the specialist his friend from the rehabilitation hospital suggests. This doctor charges $200 for the visit. Robert's health insurance allows an approved fee of $125 for the visit. The insurance company pays $100 (80 percent of the allowed amount), and Robert must pay the other $25 (his 20 percent of the approved amount).

Unknown to Robert, the specialist doesn't accept the approved amount that his health plan allows. The specialist bills Robert for the remaining $75 of the total $200 fee. Unless he has a second health insurance plan that will cover his 20 percent co-payment and the "balance billing" charge of $75, Robert will have to pay a total of $100 of his own money for the specialty visit.

Figure 7.1. Balance Billing: Don't Get Caught!

Managed Care

Managed care plans account for a large share of health plans in both private and public insurance programs. In fact, managed care is the most common form of health care plan today.

Managed care plans may take many different forms. The most common types of these plans are the:

- Health maintenance organization
- Point-of-service plan
- Preferred provider organization

Health Maintenance Organizations

In a traditional **health maintenance organization (HMO)**, a primary care physician (PCP) oversees your primary and preventive health care. This doctor also makes referrals for specialty care that you might need. You may get many of your health care services at a central location. These services could include primary care doctor visits, laboratory tests, X-rays, and prescribed medications. Most managed care plans offer the convenience of receiving prescription medicine refills by mail. This service can save you money, time, energy, and the stress of arranging for accessible transportation to go to the drug store.

If you belong to an HMO, your choice of doctors and other health care providers will be more limited than it is in a fee-for-service plan or a blended health care plan. You will also be required to get approval ahead of time for specialty care, hospital care, and other services. On the other hand, you will usually pay smaller monthly premiums and lower co-payments for doctor visits, and prescription drugs. You will also pay lower co-payments or no fees for hospital stays, X-rays, laboratory tests, and other health services. Managed care plans differ on these benefits, so check your policy carefully.

Point-of Service Plans

If you have a **point-of-service (POS)** option with your HMO plan, you can receive care from specialists who have not joined your health plan network. For example, you may need to see a neurologist, physiatrist, or rehabilitation doctor who does not belong to your HMO network. Co-payments and rules concerning point-of-service care vary, so it is a good idea to speak with someone in your health plan offices before seeking care through a POS option.

Preferred Provider Organizations

If you participate in a **preferred provider organization (PPO)**, you will have more freedom of choice in selecting health care providers. However, you may have to make larger co-payments to doctors in the plan's network than you would make with an HMO plan. If you go "out-of-plan" (that is, to a provider who does not belong to the health plan network) for medical care, you will probably have to pay for all costs charged by the out-of-plan provider. Before seeking care from an out-of-plan provider, it is a good idea to talk with a health plan representative about your specific medical needs.

Blended Health Care Plans

"Blended" health care plans have characteristics of both fee-for-service and managed care plans. For example, a person in a blended plan may have more choices for specialists than in a managed care plan. However, if you choose a doctor who does not belong to your plan, you may have to pay all of the costs for seeing that doctor. You might also have higher co-payments for doctor visits and other services.

WHAT ABOUT GOVERNMENT HEALTH INSURANCE?

Many people with spinal cord injury cannot return to work right away after completing their hospital rehabilitation. They may be able to use one or both of the two large government health insurance programs available to qualified people with disabilities—**Medicare** and **Medicaid**.

Medicare

Medicare is the nation's largest health insurance program, serving more than 5 million working-age adults with disabilities and 34 million senior citizens. This program covers adults who have worked a certain number of years in jobs that are covered by Social Security. To be eligible for Medicare coverage, a disabled worker must have received Social Security Disability Insurance (SSDI) payments for at least 24 months. (See "Work and Other Income Choices" section below for more about SSDI.)

Medicare has two parts: Part A (hospital insurance) and Part B (medical insurance). Once you qualify for Medicare benefits, you pay no monthly bill for Part A Medicare. If you decide to sign up for Part B Medicare, Social Security will deduct a monthly premium for Part B from your Social Security check. You can choose Original Medicare (fee-for-service) or a Medicare managed care plan. People who choose a Medicare managed care plan must sign up for Part B Medicare.

The federal government offers free booklets about eligibility rules for people with disabilities and covered services for people who receive Medicare. These free booklets can be viewed, printed, or ordered online at www.medicare.gov/publications, and copies can be ordered by calling 1-800-MEDICARE (1-800-633-4227).

Medicaid

Medicaid is the nation's second largest public health insurance program. Federal and state governments jointly fund this program. Under current laws, each state operates its own Medicaid program and decides who will receive services. Generally, Medicaid insures low-income children and adults and persons who receive Supplemental Security Income (SSI) because of disability. Many states now require people who receive SSI benefits to join a Medicaid managed care program.

You can get more information about Medicaid eligibility rules from your state Medicaid office. This office is housed in the Department of Health and Human Services in many states. You can also find information about Medicaid on the **Centers for Medicare and Medicaid Services (CMS)** Website: http://www.cms.hhs.gov/medicaid/consumer.asp.

WHAT DOES MY HEALTH PLAN COVER?

Both fee-for-service and managed care plans usually cover:

- Doctors' services
- Hospital care
- X-ray and laboratory services
- Emergency care

Some plans also cover:

- **Home health care**
- **Durable medical equipment (DME)**
- Prescription drugs

Your amount of coverage and co-payments depends on the type of health care plan you have.

HOW CAN I GET OTHER SERVICES I NEED?

As you move from the rehabilitation setting back into your community, you will need more supports and services that may not be covered by your health insurance plan. These supports and services might include:

- Assistance with personal care, such as bathing, eating, and dressing
- Help with meal preparation and household chores
- Specially designed clothing
- Disability-accessible, affordable transportation
- Assistance with shopping for groceries and personal care supplies
- Changes to your home or apartment to improve access to your living space

Regardless of your health plan type, you can get the most benefit from your health plan by building a strong working relationship with your primary care doctor. You can also get services that you need by explaining your special situation to your health plan's customer service representative. Learn all that you can about spinal cord injury and educate your health care team and health plan officials about your individual needs.

To locate the services and equipment you need, explain to your health care providers how spinal cord injury affects you and your family in your daily life activities. Make them aware of your special needs and ask about equipment that can increase your freedom and independence. Also, talk with your health care providers about ways to improve your quality of life with spinal cord injury.

Your rehabilitation team can connect you to your local Center for Independent Living and rehabilitation services that can help you return to work. Centers for Independent Living are also good places to find personal care assistants. People who work at these centers usually know about organizations that provide special equipment that is not often covered by insurance. In addition, you may want to join a support group for people with spinal cord injury in your community. If you have a computer or can use one at your local library or **Center for Independent Living**, you can use the Internet to find equipment and services that will improve your quality of life. You might also join an online support group or subscribe to an online mailing list or listserv for people with spinal cord injury. To learn more, visit the National Spinal Cord Injury Association's Website, www.spinalcordinjury.net.

Some states operate programs to repair donated computer equipment and other special equipment, which they then give to people with disabilities. Your rehabilitation team can help you find the organization that serves your community.

WORK AND OTHER INCOME SUPPORT OPTIONS

While you're recovering from your spinal cord injury, you may need a regular source of money to help you pay your medical and living expenses. This section describes some options that you may want to consider.

Employment

For many people with spinal cord injury, employment improves independence and overall quality of life. Employment after spinal cord injury can provide you with income to meet the costs of your living expenses and health care that are not covered by insurance. Your employer might offer you private health insurance to pay for your medical care. Coverage and benefits differ, depending on your employment. Usually, your employer contracts with a health plan and pays a part of the monthly premium. In most cases, if you join your employer's health insurance plan, your employer will deduct your share of the monthly premium from your paycheck. When you join a work-sponsored health insurance plan, your monthly payments are usually much lower than they would be, if you bought private health insurance yourself.

SSDI, SSI, and More

In addition to employment, two options may be available to provide you with cash benefits and health insurance coverage. Social Security Disability Insurance and Supplemental Security Income are government-sponsored programs that provide people with disabilities with monthly cash benefits and health insurance coverage. The Social Security Administration (SSA) operates both programs. To apply for benefits, you must be a U.S. citizen or a legally documented immigrant. These programs have some similarities, but they also have some very important differences.

Social Security Disability Insurance

Social Security Disability Insurance (SSDI) is a federally sponsored source of income support and health care coverage for qualified workers who become medically disabled. Applicants may also be disabled adult children of workers who pay Social Security taxes on their earnings. Your eligibility for SSDI and the amount of your monthly benefits after SCI depend on:

- Your citizenship status
- The severity of your spinal cord injury
- Your work history
- Your education
- Your age
- The length of time you have paid social security taxes on your pre-injury earnings
- Your ability to perform "substantial gainful activity"

Workers who pay Social Security taxes on their earnings receive work credits for each year of employment. The number of credits you need to qualify for SSDI benefits depends on your age at the time of your spinal cord injury.

For both of its income support programs, the Social Security Administration defines disability in the same way. A person with a disability must meet these criteria:

- You cannot perform any "substantial gainful activity" (SGA) because of a disability.
- You have a mental or physical impairment that is confirmed by a doctor.

- Your disability is expected to last for a continuous period of at least 12 months.

For disabilities other than blindness, performing "substantial gainful activity" means that you earn more than a certain amount of money per month ($830 for the year 2005). The Social Security Administration uses this definition to decide if you qualify for SSDI benefits. The same definition applies to keeping your benefits over time.

Once your SSDI application is approved, you must wait five months to get your benefits. The Social Security Administration recommends that you apply for benefits as soon as possible after your injury. You can begin the application process by calling 1-800-772-1213. A Social Security representative can take your claim information for SSDI benefits over the phone. He or she can also tell you about documents that you will need to give to the Social Security Administration to support your application. These documents include:

- Your Social Security card
- Your birth certificate
- A summary of your work history, including addresses and phone numbers of your work supervisors
- Your medical records describing your spinal cord injury and the treatment you have received
- Your bank account information for direct deposit of your monthly benefits

Social Security officials can tell you over the phone about any other information that is needed for your application and direct you to your nearest Social Security office for more help. If Social Security officials decide that they need more medical examinations or tests to support your application, they will make the necessary appointments and pay for these extra services.

The Social Security Administration processes a large number of applications for both SSDI and SSI. Be sure to keep a written record of your contacts with Social Security officials during the application process. Keeping careful records will help you to track the status of your application and follow up on program requirements. Your records should include the following information for each contact that you make:

- The date of each contact
- The name of the person you talk with
- The subject of the conversation
- Any advise or requests that you receive
- The steps you take to meet these requests

You should also keep copies of any written reports and letters that you send to Social Security officials or receive from them.

Did you know . . .

After you qualify for SSDI, you must wait another 24 months to qualify for health care coverage under Medicare.

Once you complete your rehabilitation program and return to your community, you may choose to return to work at a former job or new employment. People with spinal cord injury who receive SSDI payments and return to work are entitled to a nine-month trial work period in which they continue to receive their full cash benefits and Medicare coverage. After successfully completing the trial work period, these people will continue to receive full benefits for a three-month grace period. Medicare coverage may continue for 36 months after the grace period ends, but you must pay Medicare premiums each month to the Social Security Administration for this extra coverage.

Supplemental Security Income

Supplemental Security Income (SSI) is a "need-based" program available to people with disabilities severe enough to keep them from performing "substantial gainful activity." If you don't have the required work history to qualify for SSDI, you might qualify for income support and health insurance coverage under the federal and state-sponsored SSI program. The Social Security Administration uses the same disability definition and substantial gainful activity criteria for deciding if you can receive SSI, but more rules also apply to SSI. In addition to your monthly income (both earned income and unearned income), the Social Security Administration wants to know about any resources, cash, property, and other valuable things that you may have.

Family resources are sometimes included in deciding SSI benefits, depending upon state regulations. Generally, your eligibility for SSI benefits and continued receipt of these benefits is based on the amount of "countable" income you have. Benefits change from state to state, depending on how "countable" income is measured, as well as the amount of extra money that your state adds to the base federal SSI benefit.

If you receive SSI benefits, you might also qualify for health insurance coverage under Medicaid. Medicaid benefits vary from state to state, depending upon funding, service priorities, and existing waiver programs for people with disabilities. Some states require people who receive SSI benefits to apply for Medicaid and SSI separately. Other states cover both programs with one application.

Special rules apply to working and receiving SSI benefits. Contact your state's Medicaid office or the Social Security Administration for more information on allowable Impairment-Related Work Expenses that can be deducted from your earnings, if you have SSI benefits and you return to work. Social Security officials can subtract these allowed expenses from your monthly earnings before they decide if you meet the criteria for performing substantial gainful activity.

The PASS Program

You may be able to save some of your monthly resources that would be considered "countable" income toward a Plan for Achieving Self-Sufficiency (PASS). Your state's PASS program allows you to set aside some of your income for specific items or services that will help you achieve independence. Your vocational (work) rehabilitation counselor or social worker can help you design your PASS plan if you decide to sign up for the program.

The Ticket-to-Work Program

The Ticket-to-Work and Self-Sufficiency Program is the centerpiece of a law signed by former President Clinton in 1999, under the Ticket-to-Work and Work Incentives Improvement Act of 1999 (TWWIIA). This national law was enacted to assist people with disabilities with the training and support they need to go to work by giving them more employment options. The Social Security Administration (SSA) and the Department of Health and Human Services (DHHS) operate the Ticket-to-Work Program. People with disabilities who receive Social Security benefits can choose employment, work-related rehabilitation services, and other support services from public and private providers. Beginning in 2001 and extending through the life of the Ticket-to-Work Program, SSA has asked service providers to become Employment Networks (EN). If you receive Social Security benefits and want to return to work or enter the work force for the first time, you may contact one or more Employment Networks or state vocational rehabilitation agencies. You can discuss services and employment possibilities that are right for you.

If you decide to join the Ticket-to-Work Program, you will work with an Employment Network to design an Individual Work Plan (IWP). This IWP outlines the services that you will receive to help you reach your employment goals.

You can find more information on the Ticket-to-Work program on the Social Security Administration's Website (www.socialsecurity.gov/work) or by calling toll-free 1-866-YOUR TICKET (1-866-968-7842).

YOUR REHABILITATION TEAM CAN HELP

For most people with spinal cord injury, rehabilitation is a lifelong process because the effects of the injury change over time. As you move from one setting to another, take on different roles and responsibilities, and grow older, you'll make constant changes to health care services and income support options to meet these challenges. After you return to your community, there are some things you can do to access the health insurance and available income supports that you need.

Rehabilitation professionals, especially your **discharge planner, social worker**, and **vocational rehabilitation specialist**, can help you learn about resources and services. It's also important to think about your own role as a member of your rehabilitation team. After all, you understand better than anyone else how you want to live and participate in your family and community life. You know which of the health insurance and income support options presented to you will best fit your goals, needs, and interests. The rehabilitation professionals who work with you in the hospital may move on, but you will always be a member of your rehabilitation team.

As you prepare to leave the hospital and reenter your community, your discharge planner and social worker can help you complete all of the paperwork for public income support programs and health insurance options, as well as any claim forms for your private insurance. They can give you contact information for local offices and people in your community to help you check on the status of your claims and applications. These team members may also help you locate resource people in your community who can give you immediate cash assistance and other temporary supports that you may need, while your insurance claims and income support program applications are being processed.

Your vocational (or work) rehabilitation specialist can help you think about part-time and full-time work options that will best fit with your job skills, training, and prior work experience. He or she can provide:

• Direct referrals to vocational rehabilitation counselors in your community
• Information on local job banks and Internet employment resources
• Information on career changes, retraining, and educational options
• Assistance with a variety of other services and resources to help you become successfully employed and keep your job

The partnership you form with the other members of your rehabilitation team can prepare you for a "health-full" life with spinal cord injury.

Where Can I Learn More?

You can learn more about your health insurance plan and income support options by contacting the following people or organizations, or by visiting the Websites listed.

- Your discharge planner, social worker, or vocational rehabilitation specialist at your rehabilitation hospital
- Your employer's human resources office
- A customer service representative at your health insurance plan
- Your local Center for Independent Living (visit www.ilru.org for a directory of these centers)
- Your local Social Security office or the Social Security Administration (www.socialsecurity.gov or toll-free 1-800-772-1213)
- The federal Centers for Medicare and Medicaid Services (http://cms.hhs.gov or toll-free 1-800-MEDICARE or 1-877-267-2323)
- The federal Ticket to Work Program (www.socialsecurity.gov/work or toll-free1-866-YOUR TICKET)

What Can I Do?

To get the most from your health insurance plan and income support options, you can:

- *Become knowledgeable about your health insurance plan.* Review your current health insurance plan and make a list of covered benefits that apply to your new situation.
- *Look for gaps.* Identify any gaps in your current health insurance coverage.
- *Understand your options.* Make a list of income supports and other resources available to you.
- *Write it down.* Write down or tape record ideas and questions about your health insurance coverage and income support options that you want to discuss with your rehabilitation team.
- *Keep track of your contacts.* Keep dated records of contacts with health insurance officials and community agency staff who help you with your health insurance claims and applications to income support programs.
- *Keep good records.* Keep records of names, addresses, phone numbers, and e-mail information for health insurance and income support staff. Store them in one place, so you can find them quickly and easily when you need them.

- *Keep copies.* Keep copies of all letters and other materials that you provide to support your service and program applications.

IMPORTANT POINTS TO REMEMBER

- Your health insurance coverage depends on the type of plan and policy you have. Your plan may be fee-for-service, managed care, or a combination of fee-for-service and managed care.
- You may have private or public (government) health insurance. Public health insurance includes Medicare and Medicaid.
- After a spinal cord injury, your income support options may include employment; Social Security Disability Insurance (SSDI) for qualified workers who become disabled; and Supplemental Security Income (SSI), a need-based program for people with severe disabilities.

The authors wish to thank Phillip W. Beatty, Ph.D., for his assistance with this chapter.

8

Getting Back to School or Work

THILO KROLL

MARION LEVINE

"I learned that others also had apprehensions, questions, and fears about my new sit-uation. I learned that 'we'—me and all the people around me—were learning from this experience, growing together. I learned I was not alone." –Tim

School and employment might not have been the first things you thought about after your spinal cord injury, but they are keys to independent, productive living. Making the transition back to school or work is a process that requires a lot of guidance, patience, and planning. During this process, you'll have to think about your personal and career goals, and you'll need to make important decisions about your future. You'll also want to gather information, to set and achieve goals, and to solve problems with as much information as possible. In addition, you'll need to understand how to advocate for yourself.

This chapter provides information about the vocational rehabili-tation process and resources available to people with spinal cord injury to help with the transition back to school or work. It discuss-es:

- Challenges and opportunities in returning to school or work
- The role of **vocational rehabilitation**
- Important laws protecting and affecting persons with disabilities

HOW CAN I GO BACK TO SCHOOL?

Many people become spinal cord injured when they're still young enough to be in school. If you are in this younger age group, you might not yet have completed high school. The idea of going back to school may fill you with unease and concern. You may ask yourself questions such as:

- How will I get to and from school, now that I'm using a wheelchair?
- Who will help me at school if I need assistance?
- What will my classmates and teachers think, and how will they respond to me sitting a wheelchair?
- Will I be able to complete school, and what will come after that?

Asking yourself these questions and many others is understandable; they need to be answered. However, it is very important not to become overwhelmed by questions. They will be answered in due time, and solutions can be found. Finding solutions that meet your needs requires some planning toward realistic goals on your part, as well as the concerted efforts of your family, teachers, classmates, and vocational rehabilitation professionals.

As you make plans, you will want to identify your educational and career interests. Your vocational rehabilitation counselor can help you define the steps you can take to achieve success and satisfaction in those areas of personal interest.

If you're returning to school, involve your teachers as early as possible. If possible, talk with them while you're still in the hospital. Also invite classmates to visit you while you're completing your rehabilitation program. Tell them what they can do to support you and what you expect of them. For example, you might need help with note-taking in class or getting around the building quickly between classes. An open dialog is the best way to avoid misunderstandings and unclear expectations. Often people who don't have much experience with disability are uncertain about whether they should offer assistance and, if so, how they can assist a person with a disability. They might be concerned about making mistakes or hurting your feelings.

Only you can tell others how they can help you. People will rely on you to tell them what you need or don't need and instruct them about how they can support you. At times, well-meaning teachers and classmates will make decisions for you without knowing what kind of assistance you need Other people in your environment may have very good intentions, but they may lack experience with disability. Teachers and other students must learn from you about your needs and how they can make things work for you. The assistance you ask for might include making a classroom more accessible, tape-recording class sessions, granting you extra time to complete certain tasks, or planning field trips well ahead of time and in such a way that you can fully participate.

The Individuals with Disabilities Education Act (IDEA), passed in 1995, guides schools in delivering special education and related services to students with disabilities. This federal law gives children and youth with disabilities the right to request accommodations and services. The law was passed after the ADA with the same intention of equalizing opportunities for people with disabilities. You can visit the website for the National Dissemination Center for Children with Disabilities (http:www.nichcy.org/pubs/outprint/nd15txt.htm) or the Employment Center at the NRHhealthtown.org website for more information.

What about college?

All colleges, including community colleges, four-year colleges, and trade schools are required by law to provide modifications for students with disabilities. Universities and colleges usually have a disability support services office where you can find out about campus facilities, support, and activities for students with disabilities. You must take the initiative to contact this office and get special assistance if needed. Special assistance services can include, for example, tutoring, reading, note-taking, and support related to the use of assistive computer equipment and wheelchairs.

You might also find it necessary to adapt classroom environments and schedules. Making arrangements that meet your individual needs can be achieved by planning ahead and working with a vocational rehabilitation professional or the disability support services office. For example, you will want to:

- Make sure your place in the classroom is wheelchair-accessible and that you are able to follow all teaching activities.
- Make sure there are wheelchair-accessible bathrooms on the same floors as your classrooms.
- Talk to your instructors or professors to arrange classes in buildings and rooms that are wheelchair-accessible.
- Make sure you have **assistive equipment**, such as computers with voice-recognition programs, available to help you complete assignments.

HOW CAN I RETURN TO WORK?

Returning to work can mean many different things. For example, it can mean that you return to your old job where only minor accommodations are needed. These changes might include rearranging your desktop space or ergonomic reorganization of your entire workspace. Your return to work might also mean that your employer will make more extensive changes to your work environment, and perhaps buy special equipment to enable you to function independently at work. In some cases, you might need to take on different job responsibilities or a new type of job if you want to stay with your employer. For other people, returning to work means finding a new career path different from the kind of work done before the spinal cord injury.

Most people with spinal cord injury need time before they are ready to return to work. During the relatively short inpatient rehabilitation stay, your schedule no doubt was (or is) filled with many retraining and rehabilitation activities, with a focus on regaining your function and strength. Although you might receive vocational rehabilitation services while you're an inpatient, you might also be referred to your state vocational rehabilitation agency or a private agency when you're ready. Such referral means that you are cleared by your doctor to return to work.

The vocational rehabilitation staff at your rehabilitation hospital can provide information that will connect you with the staff at your state vocational rehabilitation agency and with potential employers. They can also provide advice on how to set new career goals. The section below discusses the role of vocational rehabilitation and getting ready to return to work.

WHAT CAN VOCATIONAL REHAB DO FOR ME?

Vocational rehabilitation (VR) helps people with disabilities return to school and work by defining feasible educational and employment goals and by helping the person work toward those goals. In general, VR offers vocational counseling and guidance as well as job search and placement assistance. VR professionals are specially trained to help people with disabilities become self-sufficient. They can be found working in different places, such as state VR agencies, private agencies, and rehabilitation facilities. Depending on where they work, their focus varies. Vocational rehabilitation professionals can help you by:

- Assessing the impact of the injury on the individual
- Determining work abilities
- Identifying personal education or employment interests and goals
- Identifying strategies to meet these goals
- Recommending vocational training
- Offering advice about **assistive technology** and **adaptive equipment**
- Providing training and referrals to resources that make the return to school and employment possible
- Providing other services that support achievement of education and employment

Every state and U.S. territory provides vocational rehabilitation services for people with disabilities through the state VR agency. These agencies provide evaluation, training, job placement, and follow-up services; the long-range goal is to return to work and/or independent living. These services take a case management approach, making referrals to appropriate resources. Professionals at these state agencies work with individuals, who after discharge from inpatient care, are at the maximum of their expected medical improvement with a reasonable expectation that they can return to work.

Vocational rehabilitation professionals working for private agencies often focus on workers' compensation cases; return to work is the main goal. Rehabilitation facility-based VR counselors offer job skills testing, counseling, guidance in the development of personal abilities, and services to help people with disabilities return to school or work.

Please note that you can't receive financial assistance for car or computer equipment adaptations, or for ergonomic modifications to your home unless these needs are directly related to work. Figure 8.1 describes the professionals you might meet in different settings.

Who can benefit from vocational rehabilitation services?

Vocational rehabilitation services are available for different age groups. For example, families of high school students may obtain information and practical assistance from VR counselors about returning to school. The counselors may identify tutoring or special services that may help smooth the transition back to school. Vocational rehabilitation also supports students who wish to begin or return to college. For example, VR professionals can help establish contacts with disability student support services at universities and colleges. Finally, vocational rehabilitation professionals assist working-age adults in a number of ways. One of their

As you prepare to return to school or work, you might work with two types of vocational rehabilitation professionals: vocational or employment counselors, or rehabilitation counselors.

School counselors work in the school setting (elementary through postsecondary) to help individuals and families make educational and career decisions.

Vocational (employment) counselors can help individuals make career decisions. They are often employed at public vocational rehabilitation agencies such as state VR agencies or private or private nonprofit agencies. They might explore and evaluate your education, training, work history, interests, skills, and they will arrange or give aptitude and achievement tests. They also might help you to develop job search skills and assist you in locating, and applying for, job openings.

Rehabilitation counselors usually work in hospitals and other health care facilities, workers compensation agencies (private for-profit), or nonprofit agencies, or are self-employed. They can help people deal with the personal, social, and vocational effects of disability. Rehabilitation counselors might interview you and your family; evaluate school and medical reports; and confer and plan with your physician, psychologist, occupational therapist, and employer to determine your capabilities and skills. By listening to you, the client, they develop a rehabilitation program that might include training to help you develop job skills. They also work with you to increase your capacity to live independently.

Figure 8.1 Professionals Involved in Vocational Rehabilitation

primary goals in working with adults is to identify vocational interests, plan realistic vocational goals, and assess the individual's abilities and skills.

Vocational rehabilitation professionals can refer you for career skills training, assist with job placements, recommend worksite accommodations, and enhance employers' understanding of your needs. They also coordinate special services with technical schools and colleges if you need more training or education.

Am I eligible for vocational rehabilitation services?

People with disabilities typically wonder whether they are eligible for VR services. You may be a candidate for VR if you have a documented disability that has an impact on your ability to attend school or work. A person is considered eligible for state vocational rehabilitation services if he or she has a physical or mental impairment that constitutes, or results in, a "substantial impediment." This statement means that, compared with an average person in the general population, he or she is unable to perform, or is significantly limited in performing, an activity. Factors considered include the nature and severity of the disability, how long the impairment will last, and its permanent or long-term impact.

What is vocational evaluation?

At the beginning of the vocational rehabilitation process, your VR profes-sional might suggest a vocational evaluation to help define your goals and abilities. This evaluation includes interest and aptitude tests and voca-tional counseling to determine job interests and abilities. It also considers your interests and achievements before your injury, specifically in the areas of education and work, and your current interests and functional abilities. The VR professional probably will ask you to complete a number of stan-dard tests. For example, academic achievement tests may be given to assess your basic reading, math, and spelling skills; a career interest test may be given; and other tests may be given to assess your functional and skill lev-els. These are not tests of intelligence or aptitude; they are simply used as a tool to understand better who you are and how best to design a VR plan to meet your needs.

After you have completed all of the tests, the VR professional will write a brief report about your test results, your interest areas, and his or her observations. He or she will also recommend steps you will need to take to achieve particular education and employment goals.

GETTING READY TO RETURN TO WORK

Going back to work involves making plans to return to your previous job or employer, or finding new employment. After evaluating your interests, goals, needs, and skills, vocational rehabilitation professionals can help you identify and apply for jobs. They can also help you work with your employer to make accommodations so you can return to productive work.

Applying for Jobs

When you're ready to return to work, your vocational rehabilitation counselor can assist you in the job application process. He or she can help you:

- Set a job goal
- Write your resume
- Conduct a job search
- Prepare to "network" with other people who may be able you find you a job
- Complete application forms
- Assess your own and employers' expectations
- Gather career and disability information

Making Changes That Let You Work

In many situations, even minor adjustments to a work environment can make the difference between being employed and being unemployed. Technology can also dramatically increase your employment opportunities. Just as able-bodied people take advantage of technology, people with disabilities today can use technology such as cellular phones with headsets, computers with voice-recognition and dictation software, and dictaphones to work productively. Using technology, people with disabilities can also work from home.

It's important that you examine your assistance and accommodation needs carefully. Vocational rehabilitation professionals, occupational therapists, and rehabilitation engineers can advise you about assistive technology and how to structure your work environment so that it works for you. They can analyze your job functions and tasks, and reasonable accommodations at your workplace. In addition, they can help you think about related issues, such as how you will get to and from work and your need for personal assistance in the workplace. Your VR counselor can assist you in this process and can help you convey your needs to potential employers.

For people with spinal cord injury, several types of accommodations can help improve opportunities to succeed in the workplace. These types include: accessible workplace facilities, modified workstations, assistive technology, modified work schedules, and job restructuring.

Accessible Workplace Facilities

Accessible workplace facilities will be needed if you use a wheelchair or have difficulty walking or climbing stairs. These accommodations need not be expensive. They can include:

- Designating extra-wide parking spaces near the workplace
- Designing an accessible route from the parking lot into the building
- Installing ramps to building entrances
- Leaving floors bare or installing low-pile carpeting
- Removing obstructions in hallways and walkways
- Making doorways wide enough for wheelchairs
- Installing automatic door openers or lever doorknobs
- Installing elevators with wheelchair level controls
- Providing wheelchair-accessible restrooms, lunchrooms, break rooms, and training areas
- Making copiers, fax machines, and other office equipment accessible

Modified Workstations

Modifying your workstation can help you work more efficiently and productively. Your vocational rehabilitation counselor can work with an occupational therapist or rehabilitation engineer, who can advise you about needed modifications. Some modifications might require buying new items, but sometimes only small changes to existing furniture or equipment are needed. Examples of workstation changes include:

- Rearranging files or shelves so you can reach them
- Relocating your desk or table to make it accessible
- Situating your desk in a way that allows face-to-face communication
- Raising your desk on wood blocks to accommodate your wheelchair
- Using a desktop turntable organizer to keep items within reach

Assistive Technology

As mentioned above, assistive technology can help you perform work functions and to work more productively. Examples of assistive technology you might use at work include:

- Typing splints or mouth sticks
- Specialty keyboards
- Large trackballs or joy-stick style mice
- Speech recognition technology
- Voice-activated computer software
- Voice-activated speaker phones, large button telephones, automatic dialing systems, and telephone headsets
- Page turners and book holders

Chapter 9 provides further information about assistive technology.

Modified Work Schedules

In today's work world, many people with and without disabilities have modified work schedules to accommodate their individual needs. Changing your work schedule can make a big difference in your ability to get to and from work and in your efficiency throughout the day. Work schedule changes can include:

- Working on a flexible schedule (flex-time)
- Sharing a job with another person
- Working at home
- Telecommuting, which allows you to use Internet technology to work at home on some days, including those times when transportation is unavailable
- Scheduling short, frequent rest breaks to avoid fatigue
- Working part-time

Job Restructuring

Job restructuring is another type of accommodation for people with spinal cord injury. When a job is restructured, nonessential functions are changed or reassigned to another employee in exchange for a task that you can do more easily. Such accommodations might include: to:

- Replacing frequent travel with teleconferencing and using e-mail
- Using a computer instead of writing by hand
- Rescheduling morning tasks to the afternoon or vice versa

Should I tell prospective employers about my disability?

One of the most frequently asked questions is whether the disabling condition should be disclosed, and if so, when and how. The resume is generally not the place to disclose disability issues. Some people choose to state in job applications that they qualify for the Affirmative Action Program under Section 503 of the Rehabilitation Act (see below), or they let the employer know that they are members of a wheelchair sports team.

Keep in mind that in your communication with potential employers you should emphasize your strengths and skills, not your weaknesses. Employers expect that the job applicant can perform the essential functions of the job. Their understanding of spinal cord injury and disability may be very narrow and limited, and they may only focus on the limitations of the disability. Therefore, you need to be able to advocate for yourself and convince them that you can perform the job for which you are applying. Barriers can be overcome if accommodations are made to your workspace. You have the responsibility of communicating that you will be successful in the job.

WHAT ABOUT MY LEGAL RIGHTS?

As you make plans to return to school or work, it's important to know about laws that protect you and give you rights or support you as a person with a disability. Brief descriptions of these laws are presented below. Table 8.1 summarizes the laws. For more information, talk with your vocational rehabilitation professional.

Americans with Disabilities Act of 1990

The Americans with Disabilities Act (ADA) of 1990 was signed into law to "establish a clear and comprehensive prohibition of discrimination on the basis of disability" and to ensure access and participation in society for persons with disabilities. Title I of the ADA prohibits employers with 15 or more employees from discriminating against qualified individuals. It also requires employers to reasonably accommodate the disabilities of qualified applicants or employees, including the modification of work stations and equipment unless undue hardship for the employer would result. Title I regulations also cover pre-employment screening, hiring, benefits, promotions, layoffs, and termination. The Equal Employment Opportunity Commission (www.eeoc.gov) is the enforcing agency for Title I of the ADA. The other ADA titles cover state and local government activities (Title II), public transportation (Title II), public accommodations (Title III), and telecommunications relay services (Title IV).

Rehabilitation Act of 1973

The Rehabilitation Act of 1973 was the first "rights" legislation to prohibit discrimination against people with disabilities. This law applies to federal programs, employers receiving federal funds (such as colleges participating in federal student loan programs), federal employment, and employment practices of businesses with federal contracts. The standards for determining employment discrimination under the Rehabilitation Act are the same as those used in Title I of the Americans with Disabilities Act. Title V of the Rehabilitation Act includes the following sections requiring that "reasonable accommodations" be provided:

Section 501

Section 501 requires affirmative action and prohibits employment discrimination by federal agencies. To obtain more information or to file a complaint, applicants or employees should contact the specific agency's Equal Employment Opportunity Office.

Section 503

Section 503 requires affirmative action and prohibits employment discrimination by federal government contractors and subcontractors with contracts of more than $10,000. This section applies to employers such as colleges and universities, training programs, and private defense and research companies that have such contracts. For more information or to file a complaint, contact the Office of Federal Contract Compliance Programs in the U.S. Department of Labor at (202) 219-9423 (voice/relay).

Section 504

Section 504 prohibits qualified individuals with disabilities from being excluded from, denied access to, or being subjected to discrimination under any program or activity that either receives federal financial assistance or is conducted by any executive agency or the U.S. Postal Service.

Parts of Section 504 regulations apply to individual federal agencies' programs and to agencies that provide financial assistance to or regulate entities that receive federal funding. Reasonable accommodations for employees, access to participation in all programs, facilitated communication for people with hearing or vision disabilities, and accessible construction and alterations must be provided.

Section 504 has promoted the development of disability support services in colleges and universities. It has also spurred the federal government to write disability employment policies. The "Handbook of Reasonable Accommodations," prepared by the U.S. Office of Personnel

Management, was the first such attempt to define the types of reasonable accommodations for people with disabilities, but focused primarily on modifications for people with physical or sensory disabilities.

Section 504 does not require that special education programming be developed for students with disabilities. However, it does require institutions to be prepared to make appropriate academic adjustments and reasonable modifications to policies and practices to allow for full participation of students with disabilities.

Architectural Barriers Act of 1968

The Architectural Barriers Act (ABA) of 1968 requires access to facilities designed, built, altered, or leased with federal funds. Passed by Congress in 1968, it was one of the first efforts to ensure access to the built environment. The Access Board, an independent federal agency devoted to accessibility for people with disabilities, was established under Section 502 of the Rehabilitation Act to enforce the ABA, which it does through the investigation of complaints. The Access Board develops and maintains accessibility guidelines under this law. These guidelines serve as the basis for the standards used to enforce the law, the Uniform Federal Accessibility Standards (UFAS). Four federal agencies—the Department of Defense, the Department of Housing and Urban Development, the General Services Administration, and the U.S. Postal Service—are responsible for the standards.

Federal agencies are responsible for ensuring compliance with the UFAS when funding the design, construction, alteration, or leasing of facilities. Some departments also require compliance with the ADA Accessibility Guidelines (which otherwise do not apply to the federal sector) in addition to UFAS.

If you are concerned about the accessibility of a facility that may have received federal funds, you may file a complaint with the Access Board. For further information, visit: www.accessboard.gov/indexes/enforceindex.htm.

Family and Medical Leave Act

The Family and Medical Leave Act (FMLA) provides certain employees with up to 12 weeks of unpaid, job-protected leave per year. It also requires that group health benefits be maintained during the leave. The FMLA is designed to help employees balance their work and family responsibilities by taking reasonable unpaid leave for certain family and medical reasons. It also seeks to accommodate the legitimate interests of employers, and promotes equal employment opportunity for men and women.

The Family and Medical Leave Act:

- Covers only certain employers
- Affects only those employees who are eligible for the protections of the law
- Involves entitlement to leave
- Maintains health benefits during leave
- Restores an employee's job after leave
- Sets requirements for notice and certification of the need for leave
- Protects employees who request or take leave
- Includes certain employer record-keeping requirements

Therefore, under the FMLA, an employee has more flexibility with maintaining employment under certain circumstances and their job must be kept open for them by their employers.

Workforce Investment Act of 1998

The Workforce Investment Act (WIA) of 1998 set in motion the first major reform of our country's job training system in more than 15 years. The new national workforce preparation and employment system is designed to meet both the needs of the nation's businesses and the needs of job seekers and those who want to further their careers.

WIA is designed to revitalize federal job training programs to provide a customer-focused system that offers individuals access to career tools and information while helping employers find skilled workers. It embodies seven key principles: streamlining services through the unified, coordinated One-Stop service delivery system; empowering individuals; making services universally accessible; increasing accountability; creating a strong role for local workforce investment boards and the private sector; increasing state and local flexibility; and improving youth programs. Title I of the legislation is based on the following elements:

- Training and employment programs must be designed and managed at the local level where the needs of businesses and individuals are best understood.

- Customers must be able to conveniently access the employment, education, training, and information services they need at a single location in their neighborhoods.
- Customers should have choices in deciding the training program that best fits their needs and the organizations that will provide that service. They should have control over their own career development.
- Customers have a right to information about how well training providers succeed in preparing people for jobs. Therefore, training providers must make available information about their success rates.
- Businesses provide information, leadership, and play an active role in ensuring that the system prepares people for current and future jobs.

Under WIA, nearly 1,000 "One-Stop Career Centers" have opened to provide information about, and access to, a wide array of job training, education, and employment services available to the public. The organizations that operate the centers are selected by the local workforce investment boards through a competitive process. At these centers, you can:

- Obtain information about employment-related services, including information about local education and training service providers
- Get help filing claims for unemployment insurance and evaluating eligibility for job training and education programs or student financial aid
- Obtain assistance with job searches and job placement, and receive career counseling
- Learn about job vacancies
- Access up-to-date labor market information which identifies skills necessary for in-demand jobs, and provides information about local, regional and national employment trends

Ticket to Work and Work Incentive Improvement Act of 1999

The Ticket to Work and Work Incentive Improvement Act (TWWI-IA) of 1999 is designed to modernize the employment services system for persons with disabilities and makes it possible for millions of Americans with disabilities to join the workforce without fear of losing their health insurance coverage. TWWIIA includes two key measures, described below.

First, the law created the Ticket to Work and Self-Sufficiency Program, through which recipients of **Social Security Disability Insurance (SSDI)** and **Supplemental Security Income (SSI)** are able to obtain job-related training and placement assistance from a Social Security Administration-approved provider of their choice. Individuals can receive a "ticket," which they may present to an approved Employment Network for services.

Second, TWWIIA expanded health care coverage so that individuals with disabilities can work without fear of losing their Medicare and Medicaid benefits, which in the past was one of the major barriers to employment for individuals with disabilities who wanted to work but had no alternative means of health care coverage.

Individuals with Disabilities Education Act

The Individuals with Disabilities Education Act (IDEA) is the nation's special education law. It originally was enacted in 1975 as the landmark Education for All Handicapped Children Act to help states and localities protect the rights of, meet the individual needs of, and improve results for infants, toddlers, children, and youth with disabilities and their families. The law was amended in 1997 and again in 2004.

The IDEA Amendments of 1997 (known as IDEA '97) were the first major revision to the Act in more than 23 years and represented a major milestone in the education of children with disabilities. They retained and strengthened the basic rights and protections under IDEA, including the right to a free, appropriate public education for all children with disabilities in the least restrictive environment appropriate to their individual needs. IDEA '97 also required public school systems to develop an appropriate Individualized Education Program (IEP) that outlines specific special education and related services for each child. The Individuals with Disabilities Education Improvement Act of 2004 (IDEA) aligned IDEA closely to the No Child Left Behind Act of 2001 (see below), helping to ensure equity, accountability and excellence in education for children with disabilities.

No Child Left Behind Act

The No Child Left Behind (NCLB) Act of 2001 is intended to improve student achievement. Under NCLB, each state must measure every public school student's progress in reading and math in grades 3 through 8 and at least once during grades 10 through 12. By the 2007-08 school year, assessments (or testing) in science will also be underway. These assessments must be aligned with state academic content and achievement standards. They will provide parents with objective data on where their child stands academically.

NCLB also requires states and school districts to give parents easy-to-read, detailed "report cards" on schools and districts, telling them which schools are succeeding and why. These report cards include student achievement data, broken out by race, ethnicity, gender, English language proficiency, migrant status, disability status, and low-income status. They also include important information about the professional qualifications of teachers. With these provisions, the No Child Left Behind Act ensures that parents have important, timely information about the schools their children attend—whether they are performing well or not for all children, regardless of their background.

BE A SELF-ADVOCATE!

As with therapy and other medical rehabilitation services, vocational rehabilitation requires your active input and participation. Vocational rehabilitation professionals can give you a lot of support and connect you to helpful resources, but you must actively take part in the process. In addition, like your therapists, vocational rehabilitation professionals can provide you with information, advice, and training, but they cannot make decisions for you. You are the ultimate decision-maker, planner, goal setter, and goal achiever!

As you work toward your goals, you must take responsibility for getting what you need to be successful at school or work. You must be clear about your goals, ask for help, be persistent, and not get discouraged. It might take a while before you get to where you hope to be, but the better you understand your own goals and the resources available to you, the closer you will be to meeting these goals.

Table 8.1. Laws Related to School and Work for Persons with Disabilities

Law	Coverage/Provisions
Americans with Disabilities Act (ADA) of 1990	Prohibits discrimination on the basis of disability in employment, state and local governments, public accommodations, commercial facilities, transportation, telecommunications. Title I of the ADA: • Requires employers with 15 or more employees to provide qualified individuals with disabilities an equal opportunity to benefit from the full range of employment-related opportunities available to others. • Restricts questions that can be asked about an applicant's disability before a job offer is made, and requires that employers make reasonable accommodation to the known physical or mental limitations of otherwise qualified individuals with disabilities, unless it results in undue hardship.
Rehabilitation Act of 1973, as amended	Prohibits discrimination on the basis of disability in programs conducted by federal agencies, programs receiving federal financial assistance, federal employment, and employment of federal contractors. Standards for determining employment discrimination are the same as those used in Title I of the ADA. • Section 501 requires affirmative action and nondiscrimination in employment by federal agencies of the Executive Branch. • Section 503 requires affirmative action and nondiscrimination in employment by federal government contractors and subcontractors with contracts of more than $10,000. • Section 504 prohibits exclusion of, denial of benefits to, and discrimination against qualified individuals in any program or activity that receives federal financial assistance or is conducted by any Executive agency or the U.S. Postal Service.

(Table 8.1 continued)

Law	Coverage/Provisions
Architectural Barriers Act of 1968	• Requires that buildings and facilities designed, constructed, or altered with federal funds, or leased by a federal agency, comply with federal standards for physical accessibility. • Requirements limited to architectural standards in federal buildings and facilities operated by the U.S. Postal Service.
Family and Medical Leave Act of 1993	• Provides a means for eligible employees to take up to 12 weeks of job protected, unpaid leave from their jobs in certain circumstances, including those times when the employee or an immediate family member has a serious health condition, or at the birth of a child. • Applies generally to private employers with 50 or more employees, as well as all public agencies (state and local government), including schools, regardless of the number of employees. Also covers most federal employees.
Workforce Investment Act of 1998	• Reforms federal job training programs and creates a new, comprehensive workforce investment system that is intended to be customer focused and to help U.S. companies find skilled workers. • Includes several key principles: streamlines services through the creation of the One-Stop delivery system, empowers individuals, promotes universal access, increases accountability, provides for State and local flexibility, and improves youth programs. • Section 188 prohibits discrimination regarding participation, benefits, and employment because of race, color, religion, sex (except as otherwise permitted under Title IX of the Education Amendments of 1972), national origin, age, disability, or political affiliation or belief.

(Table 8.1 continued)

Law	Coverage/Provisions
Ticket to Work and Work Incentive Improvement Act (TWWIIA) of 1999	• Modernizes the employment services system for persons with disabilities. • Creates the Ticket to Work and Self-Sufficiency Program, through which recipients of Social Security Disability Insurance (SSDI) and Supplemental Security Income (SSI) can obtain training and placement assistance from approved providers. • Expands health care coverage so that individuals with disabilities can work without fear of losing their Medicare and Medicaid benefits.
Individuals with Disabilities Education Act (IDEA)	• Requires public schools to make available to all eligible children with disabilities a free appropriate public education in the least restrictive environment appropriate to their individual needs. • Requires public school systems to develop an appropriate Individualized Education Programs (IEP) outlining specific special education and related services for each child.
No Child Left Behind Act of 2001	• Designed to improve student achievement and reform America's schools by overhauling federal efforts to support elementary and secondary education in the United States. • Founded on four major principals: accountability for results, an emphasis on doing what works based on scientific research, expanded parental options, and expanded local control and flexibility.

What Can I Do?

Vocational rehabilitation can help you explore your options and make decisions about getting back to school or work. You can take the following steps to start the process:

• *Get a referral.* Ask your doctor to refer you to a vocational rehabilitation (VR) professional if you have questions about returning to school or work.

- *Find out about services.* Learn about the VR counseling services available at your rehabilitation hospital, through the local office of your state VR agency, at a local One Stop Career Center, or elsewhere in your community.
- *Make lists.* Write down 5 to 10 questions you have about education and employment issues, and list what you think you will need to get back to school or work (for example, driving, transportation, and more education and training).
- *Set a date.* Schedule a meeting with a VR counselor.
- *Take notes.* Make sure a relative, friend, or assistant accompanies you to the meeting with the VR counselor to assist you with taking notes. If this isn't possible, ask the VR counselor to provide answers to your questions in a format that is convenient for you to use.
- *Be an active participant.* Play an active role in developing your Individualized Written Rehabilitation Plan (IWRP*) that details the next steps and a timeframe to obtain additional information, initiate training activities, and formulate support needs that can be addressed by the VR counselor.
- *Come to agreement.* Discuss the IWRP with your counselor and come to an agreement about what to do next.
- *Follow up.* Keep in touch with your VR counselor about the progress you've made to turn the plan into action.

> * IWRP is an individualized written rehabilitation plan and is an agreement between the state vocational rehabilitation agency's VR counselor and the client as to how the client's goals will be met. For example, if someone requires a wheelchair lift to get in and out of a car in order to get to a job, this can be included as a goal in the IWRP. It is similar to the IEP written by schools and is meant to define goals and what is needed to implement those goals with eventual return to work.

Where Can I Learn More?

To learn more about returning to school or work, vocational rehabilitation, or your rights, you may wish to use the following resources:

- Vocational rehabilitation professionals at your rehabilitation hospital
- Your state vocational rehabilitation agency (visit www.jan.wvu.edu/sbses/vocrehab/htm for state agency contact information)
- Your school principal or other staff

- Your college or university's disability support services office
- Your local One-Stop Career Center (visit www.doleta.gov/usworkforce/onestop/onestopmap.cfm to find a center near you)
- The Job Accommodation Network (JAN) (www.jan.wvu.edu)
- National Dissemination System for Children with Disabilities (visit http://www.nichcy.org/index.html)
- Council for Disability Rights (www.disabilityrights.org)
- NRHhealthtown Employment Center (www.nrhhealthtown.org)

Appendix C provides information about additional resources.

IMPORTANT POINTS TO REMEMBER

- The idea of returning to school or work after a spinal cord injury may seem daunting at first, but with professional guidance, patience, planning, and accommodations, it is possible.
- Vocational rehabilitation helps people with disabilities return to school or work by offering counseling, guidance, and job search and placement assistance. Vocational rehabilitation professionals work at rehabilitation facilities, for state vocational rehabilitation agencies, and for private agencies.
- Many federal laws protect the rights of persons with disabilities and support individuals' efforts to return to school or work. These laws include the Americans with Disabilities Act, the Rehabilitation Act, and the Individuals with Disabilities Education Act, among others.

This chapter was supported in part through a grant from the U.S. Department of Education, National Institute on Disability and Rehabilitation Research, Grant #H133B031114.

9

Putting Technology to Work

JENNIFER HENDRICKS
JOHN NOISEUX
MARIANNE OURSLER
NEEPA SHAH

"My home and office environments are filled with remote controls, adaptive gadgets, and software and hardware that allow me to be as productive as or more productive than anyone else." –Jennifer

Throughout your rehabilitation experience, you have been learning or will learn to do things in new ways. Sometimes these new ways will include using a device as simple as a dressing stick or a built-up handle on an eating utensil. They may also involve more complicated devices, such as wheelchairs, driving aids, and technology that help you control things in your environment or interact with a computer. Taken together, these devices are called assistive technology. This chapter explores some of the assistive technology that will enable you to get around, control your environment, and be connected and productive in new ways. In this chapter, you will learn about:

• Technology that can assist with mobility, stair-climbing, driving, self-care, environmental control, and computer access
• Funding for assistive technology
• The importance of the **Americans with Disabilities Act of 1990**

MOBILITY DEVICES

This section introduces you to mobility devices that can help you move around independently following a spinal cord injury. The type of mobility device you will use depends on the level of your spinal cord injury and the movement you have in your arms and/or legs. Your rehabilitation team, including your doctor, physical therapist, occupational therapist, and case manager, will help you choose mobility devices that are best for you. When ordering a wheelchair or walking device, you and the rehabilitation team will try to choose the device that makes you as independent as possible. The mobility device will enable you to get around your home, school, and work settings so that you can continue doing many of the activities you did before your injury.

Wheelchairs

If you are unable to walk following your injury, a wheelchair can help you get where you need to go. The type of wheelchair ordered for you will depend on:

- The level of your injury
- How active your movement will be
- How accessible your home is
- The types of activities you will participate in after you leave the rehabilitation hospital
- The type of insurance you have and what your insurance will pay for

Your physical therapist, occupational therapist, case manager, equipment specialist, physician, and rehabilitation engineer may all be part of the "seating and mobility team" that helps you decide on the chair that best meets your needs. Before ordering a wheelchair, your physical or occupational therapist will measure you and choose a wheelchair size based on the measurements. There are three types of wheelchairs: manual wheelchairs, power wheelchairs, and scooters.

Manual Wheelchairs

Manual wheelchairs come in different sizes, shapes, and weights. Most manual wheelchairs have a variety of features to choose from, such as different styles of armrests and footrests. When selecting and ordering a manual wheelchair, you and your seating and mobility team will want to consider three goals: ability to propel the chair well, adequate adjustability of the wheelchair, and comfort in the wheelchair.

The first goal is to choose a wheelchair you can propel (move) well. If you will propel it using your arms, you will want to choose the lightest-weight wheelchair possible. If you will use your arms and legs to propel it, you will want a lightweight chair that allows you to touch the ground with your feet.

The second goal is to get a wheelchair that is highly adjustable. As your functional status changes, you will want the wheelchair to be able to change as well. For example, when you are first injured, your ability to balance yourself while sitting in the wheelchair may be impaired. By using a wheelchair feature called an adjustable axle plate, the rear wheels can be positioned to make you and the chair feel very stable. As your balance improves, the position of the wheels can be changed on the axle plate to make the chair easier to push.

The third goal is to get a chair that is comfortable. There are two different types of wheelchair frames: rigid and folding. The type you choose should depend on which chair is most comfortable for you. The chair should be easy for you or your family to get in and out of a car or van. Your physical or occupational therapist will talk with you about the pros and cons of both types of frames and will help you decide.

Power Wheelchairs

If you do not regain full use of your hands or arms after your injury, your rehabilitation team may suggest that you use a power wheelchair. A power wheelchair enables you to get around many different places quickly and efficiently. Just as there are many different types of manual wheelchairs, there are also many different types of power wheelchairs.

Power wheelchairs fall into three main categories: rear-wheel, mid-wheel, and front-wheel drive. The main difference among these categories is the way in which they drive and steer. During your rehabilitation stay, you should have an opportunity to drive several different chairs to see and feel the differences. Ask your rehabilitation team to explain how the chairs differ and why one might be better for you than another.

Power wheelchairs can be operated in a variety of ways. If you are not able to use your hands to drive the chair, you can use your head, chin, or breath to operate it. In recent years, equipment companies have developed many systems to operate power wheelchairs. Most of the driving systems are interchangeable. You may learn to drive using one system, such as a head control, but as you gain greater strength in your arms, you may be able to switch to using your hands to operate a joystick. In the end, you should choose the system that you like and one that is the easiest and most reliable for you.

You should also think about whether you need to have a power-seating system put on your power wheelchair. These power systems include a tilt system, a recline system, and an elevating seat. The power tilt and recline systems will help you do pressure reliefs to help protect your skin. A power-elevating seat may be useful if you need to reach things from cabinets at home or at work.

Before ordering a power wheelchair, you and your family will need to consider several points. First, a power wheelchair cannot be folded and put into a car. You need to think about how you will get from one place to another with the wheelchair. People often transport their power wheelchairs in specially equipped vans, or they use public transportation. Second, because a power wheelchair will not go up and down stairs, you need to determine if you can get it into your house. You may need to have a ramp built to get the chair in and out of your house.

Scooters

You have probably seen TV advertisements for scooters. Many people like scooters because scooters are smaller and more streamlined than wheelchairs. In addition to smaller size, scooters have several other advantages, including the ability to be taken apart and put into a car for transport, and often at lower cost.

The biggest disadvantage of scooters, however, is their limited amount of options, and they are not very adjustable. They offer few or no options in seat size and drive controller. They can have a significantly larger turning radius than some wheelchairs, and often they cannot accommodate the special adapted seating needs of persons with spinal cord injury.

Walking Mobility Devices

Depending on your level of injury, you may or may not be able to walk again. However, if it is appropriate, your physical therapist will teach you to walk again and help you select walking mobility aids. These aids, which include walkers, canes, and crutches, can increase your stability and help prevent you from falling as you walk over different surfaces. Your therapist will help you choose the safest and most appropriate device for you.

Walkers are the most stable type of walking devices. These devices include standard walkers with four legs or rolling walkers with two legs and two legs with wheels. Most walkers can be adjusted according to the height of the user. A folding walker is the easiest to get in and out of a car.

Canes come in a variety of sizes and shapes. The most stable type of cane is one with a base and four legs at the bottom. Depending on the size of the base, the cane is called a "large-based quad cane" or a "small-based quad cane." A "straight cane" has a single point that touches the floor. Most canes can be adjusted according to the height of the user.

Some canes come in fancy colors and designs and are actually collectors' items.

Crutches are another alternative. "Axillary crutches" come up underneath your arms. "Lofstrand crutches" have a cuff that goes around your forearm. If you are learning how to walk with long leg braces (KAFOs), you will probably learn to use Lofstrand crutches.

If you do not regain full strength of all of your leg muscles, braces (orthotic devices) may increase your stability and make it easier to move your legs when you walk. Braces can be made to fit just around your foot and calf (AFO) or around your whole leg (KAFO). If you need to have a brace made, your physical therapist will consult an orthotist (a specialist in making orthotic devices).

STAIR-CLIMBING ALTERNATIVES

If you use a wheelchair, scooter, or walking aid, stairs can be a barrier in your home and elsewhere. You may need to find a way to overcome these barriers to get into and around your home. A number of alternatives to stairs are available. The most important factors in determining what modifications are possible include your needs and abilities, the amount of space in and around the staircase, the architectural layout, and funding.

Ramps

Where sufficient space is available and the elevation change is not too great, a ramp is a good, low-maintenance option for making a home accessible. The general rule of thumb for a ramp's slope is a 1-inch rise for each foot of horizontal run. For example, if there is a two-foot rise from the ground to the entrance, a ramp approximately 24 feet long is needed. In addition, a 5-foot square level turning area should be available at the top and bottom of the ramp.

Porch Lifts

Where space is limited or the height is too much for a ramp, a porch lift is a good option. A porch lift has a gate at the top and bottom, and a platform that travels vertically from the ground to the level of a porch or deck It should be remembered, however, that porch lifts do require some maintenance, and they are more expensive than ramps for heights less than several feet.

Stairglides

Inside the home, a number of options are available for travel between floors. Two options, stairglides and platform lifts, transport you up and down the stairs. To use a stairglide, you must have enough trunk stability to sit on a seat that is mounted on a rail along the stairs. The seat travels up the rail to the next floor. If you are using a wheelchair, you will transfer to the stairglide seat and locate a second wheelchair on the second floor. A family member or caregiver can also carry the manual chair up the stairs. This system has the advantage of being less expensive than the other options, particularly in cases where the staircase is straight.

Platform Lifts

A wheelchair platform lift is an option only in situations where the staircase is fairly wide (in most cases 34 inches or wider) and at least one wall along the stairs continues for several feet beyond the bottom of the stairs. A clear space at least 4 feet by 3 feet or more will be needed at the bottom of the stairs. Platform lifts allow you to remain in your chair while traveling between floors. However, space requirements at the bottom of the stairs and for the clear width of the stairs prevent many people from installing these lifts in their homes.

Residential elevators are also an option if you are using a wheelchair or mobility aid and will travel between floors. Residential elevators are much smaller than commercial elevators. They are more expensive than stairglides and platform lifts and require significant modifications in the home.

ADAPTED DRIVING TECHNOLOGY

If returning to driving is one of your goals, you are not alone. However, after a spinal cord injury, weakness, paralysis, sensation, balance, spasms, and skin integrity can all affect your ability to drive safely. These issues, as well as your strengths, are considered in adapted driver rehabilitation programs, which include training and adapted equipment to assist individuals with disabilities in returning to driving. Adapted driver rehabilitation may be able to assist you in becoming more independent in accessing your community, work, social, and recreation opportunities. This section offers information about the professionals involved in driver rehabilitation, the process of returning to driving, and the technology available to people with spinal cord injuries.

Adapted Driving Rehabilitation Programs

Individuals who may be qualified to provide driver rehabilitation services include, but are not limited to, occupational therapists, physical therapists, rehabilitation engineers, and driver training educators. Be sure to verify that the driver rehabilitation facility or professional that you choose is licensed by your state and has participated in a recognized accrediting process.

Your adapted driving rehabilitation program should address:

- Your abilities and limitations with strength, range of motion, endurance, vision, etc.
- Identification of appropriate types of vehicles.
- Safe driving strategies, including traffic safety skills.
- Use of adaptive driving equipment, including prescription, positioning, and instruction.
- Laws and regulations concerning standard and adaptive motor vehicles.
- Resources including mobility equipment dealers and other professionals involved in adaptive equipment and driver training

To begin the driver rehabilitation training process, you should first speak with your physician and get an order or prescription. Your physician must confirm that you are ready and safe to begin this process. It is important to realize that returning to driving after a spinal cord injury can involve a major time and financial commitment. Many insurance companies will not pay for this therapy, so check with them and your state's vocational rehabilitation agency to find out what will be covered.

You must also understand that you may not be cleared to drive even after participating in a driver rehabilitation training program. Your treatment team will make a recommendation, but the final decision lies with your physician. In addition, your motor vehicle administration (MVA) may require that you retake the driving portion of the driver's license examination and receive a new license. The license may authorize you to drive only with adaptive equipment in place.

It is important that you inform the MVA of any illness or injury requiring hospitalization before returning to driving. If you fail to do so, you may be putting yourself at risk. It is also advisable to report your status to your vehicle insurance company in order to protect yourself from denial of a claim. Regulations prohibit insurance companies from raising premiums on the basis of use of adaptive equipment unless the driver wants the equipment covered under comprehensive damage, loss, or theft coverage.

The Evaluation

Once you have decided to participate in the driver rehabilitation training program, you must start by making an appointment for a driving
evaluation. The evaluation consists of two parts. The first part is an in-
clinic evaluation at which the evaluator takes an in-depth medical and
driving history and learns about your goals for returning to the community. The evaluator will also assess factors involved in safe driving,
including:

- Range of motion
- Strength
- Coordination
- Balance
- Sensation
- Ability to transfer vision
- Cognition
- Perception
- Use of adaptive driving equipment
- Reaction time

During the first part of this in-clinic evaluation, you will receive initial recommendations for adaptive equipment and further therapies. The
second part of the evaluation is an on-road driving test using the appropriate adaptive equipment. The evaluator will assess factors such as those
assessed in the in-clinic evaluation, but in a more realistic driving environment. Training begins in a motor vehicle on a quiet driving range
where you will learn basic control skills and use of adaptive equipment.
After you master basic skills, your training will move to quiet public
roadways and then to city streets and highways as appropriate. Adaptive
equipment recommendations, if any, will be revised during the training
process, as needed.

Adapted Driving Equipment

Many devices are also available for adapted driving. Your driver rehabilitation specialist will be able to assist you in determining the most appropriate equipment. Work with him or her to choose equipment offered by
a manufacturer or vendor with a good track record and reputation for
safety and quality. Examples of driving equipment for accelerating, breaking, and steering are listed in Table 9.1.

One example of adapted driving equipment is hand controls. Hand
controls allow drivers to operate the accelerator and brake with their

hands. You will have your own style of hand controls that suits you and will allow the best access to safely operate the controls. If you steer with only one hand, a spinner knob is required. It is often used in conjunction with hand controls and is generally operated with the dominant hand while the hand controls are operated with the non-dominant hand. Other types of knobs or grips are listed below and may be appropriate depending on the amount of function and strength available in your hand. For those who have decreased strength in the shoulder or elbow, there are additional alternatives for steering (included below), such as reduced effort steering. A system that incorporates both steering and acceleration and braking is the Scott Driving system, which allows the driver to control all three functions with a single lever system.

Table 9.1. Adapted Driving Equipment

Adapted Equipment for Steering	Adapted Equipment for Acceleration and Braking

• Knobs and Grips
  ◦ Spinner knob
  ◦ Palm grip
  ◦ Single pin or post
  ◦ U grip
  ◦ Tripin or quad steering device
• Reduced effort steering
• Horizontal or reduced angle steering
• Joystick driving
• Digital or multiaxis steering
	• Hand Controls
	  ◦ Steering column-mounted
	  ◦ Floor-mounted
	  ◦ Electronic

Many alternatives are discussed above. It's important to discuss those items that may be appropriate for you with your therapist or rehabilitation driving specialist.

Last, modifications can be made to enhance access to the vehicle's ignition, parking brake, turn signals, horn, wipers, defroster, headlights, heater, etc. These modifications can increase the safety and comfort of the driver.

Loading and Unloading Yourself and Your Wheelchair

Two other keys to independent mobility are being able to get yourself in and out of your vehicle, and loading and unloading your mobility device (wheelchair or scooter). The level and completeness of your spinal cord injury will affect how you transfer in and out of a vehicle. Some people are able to do "pop-over" or "sliding board" lateral transfers. Others require more extensive assistance. Two power devices are available to assist you with transferring in and out of your vehicle. The first is a passenger seat that rotates and slides forward so you can enter the vehicle from an accessible position. The second is a power lift with a sling that is installed in the front passenger area of the car or minivan. Those needing to transfer into a pickup or sport utility vehicle can also use a power transfer board known as the EZ Rizer™. This device lowers to a height level with the wheelchair and then rises to the height of the driver's seat so a level transfer can be done.

Your ability to load and unload a wheelchair also depends on the level of your injury and how much upper body strength and balance you have. Some people with spinal cord injury are able to fold their wheelchairs and lift them into a car. Those who lack the strength, sitting balance, or mobility to do so may need to use a powered device. If you need a powered device, you may be able to use a switch-controlled, motorized wheelchair loader, which sits on the car roof and lifts the chair in and out of a storage compartment. This option only works with a folding frame wheelchair. For those with pickup trucks with extended cabs, there are several different options to assist you in loading your wheelchair either behind the driver's seat or in the bed of the pickup.

If you are using a power wheelchair, you may need to have a full-size or minivan modified to enable you to enter by ramp or lift while in your wheelchair or scooter. This option allows you to drive into the van with a wheelchair or scooter. Van modifications can include installing a side-entry or rear-entry lift or ramp, and a raised roof or dropped floor. Keep in mind that such modifications alter the structure of the vehicle and can affect its safety and reliability. Therefore, it is important to choose the right kind of van for modification and to be sure the modification is done correctly.

In addition to changes made for access to the vehicle, you will need to include wheelchair tie-downs and restraint systems for yourself and any other wheelchair user who will remain in a wheelchair while in the vehicle. In addition to using the vehicle's seat and chest belts (not the lap belt and chest strap that may be part of the wheelchair's seating system), a tie-down system is used to secure a wheelchair and the user inside a van. A tie-down system typically consists of a mechanical metal locking device or several belts anchoring the four corners of the wheelchair frame to the van floor.

Remember to consult with your occupational therapist and mobility equipment dealer before buying any equipment or altering your vehicle. They will be able to help you sort through the often confusing number of options and make sure you get equipment that meets your needs.

For more information and resources, contact the Association for Certified Driver Rehabilitation Specialists (ADED) (www.driver-ed.org). ADED can be reached at 318-257-5055 or 1-800-290-2344 (toll-free in the United States).

SELF-CARE AIDS

Many assistive technology devices are available for bathing, dressing, feeding, and other self-care tasks. "Low-tech" devices include dressing sticks, long-handled sponges, eating utensils with built-up handles, shower chairs, and bedside commodes. The use of some of these devices is discussed in Chapter 2. Many commonly available "off-the-shelf" devices also can be helpful for self-care. For example, electric toothbrushes (which can be used with a splint or cuff) can reduce the amount of arm movement required to brush your teeth, and electric razors can be safe alternatives to razor blades if you lack dexterity and fine movement.

Some of these commercially available devices may be used "as is." Sometimes, however, a small change made by you, a family member or friend, an occupational therapist, or a rehabilitation engineer can greatly increase the usability of an inexpensive appliance or device. For example, eating utensils, small tools, or a toothbrush can be modified with larger handles to make them easier to use with limited use of the fingers or with a splint, or u-cuff (a strap that fits around the hand and has a pocket to slip in eating utensils or small handles). The on/off switch on items like an electric razor or electric toothbrush can be adapted to make them larger and easier operate.

Other, more expensive and complex self-care aids can also be obtained if needed. For example, lifts to access a bathtub powered by the water pressure in your home, electric hospital style beds that assist you with independent bed position changes, and mechanical/robotic feeders that operate with a simple switch that can allow the user with very limited movement to feed himself or herself more independently.

ENVIRONMENTAL CONTROL TECHNOLOGY

Being able to control technology in your home or work environment is important for independence and safety. Even with a family member or care attendant nearby, it is still important for a person with a disability to be able to access the telephone. What if the family member or care attendant should need help? You may be the one that needs to call for assistance. A wide range of technology available today will let you control telephones, lights, fans, air conditioners, televisions, hospital beds, and more.

Remote Control Devices

Environmental control technology can be as simple as "universal remotes" used to operate infrared-controlled TVs, VCRs, and stereos. These inexpensive devices are available in local electronics and department stores and are commonly sold as replacement remote controls for TVs or VCRs. The universal models that control multiple devices will reduce your need to use several remote controls (which can be difficult to manipulate). Only one remote control device is needed. It can be held in your lap, on an armrest, or with Velcro® affixed to a wheelchair lap tray. Some of these remotes have large buttons, making them easier to use than those with small buttons.

More advanced universal remotes can control infrared-controlled TVs and VCRs, as well as items like lights and fans. These systems use "X-10" home-automation technology to control lights and fans by allowing you to turn them on and off. You simply plug the power cord of the device you want to control into a small control box and then plug the control box into an outlet. A starter kit with a universal remote and two control boxes can be purchased for under $50 at stores such as Radio Shack, some large hardware stores, and on Websites such as www.x10.com and www.smarthome.com. You can also add thermostat controls, window blind openers, controls for powered door openers, and even motion detector controls.

If multiple buttons will be difficult to use, you can use single-switch remote controls. These devices can be used to control a single feature of an appliance (on/off), completely control a single device (such as a TV or VCR), control multiple infrared devices (such as a TV and VCR), or multiple infrared and X-10 devices (such as a TV, VCR, lights, fan, and telephone). Single-switch remote controls typically allow you to plug in different types of switches so you can use the one that work bests for you.

Switches come in many designs. They can be activated when you blow into or sip on the end of a straw (a pneumatic switch), raise an eyebrow, press a large plate, or bump a plastic stem. When using switch control, it is important that a reliable switch site be identified. The switch should be located where you can repeatedly activate it when desired but not activate it accidentally. Your occupational therapist can help you identify the right type of switch and control site.

A single-switch remote, which controls more than one feature, will rely on scanning to allow the single switch to do multiple things. When you activate the single switch, the remote will scan through a list of options that will be highlighted or spoken one at a time. When the option you want is highlighted, you activate the switch again to, for example, to turn on a TV or turn off a light.

More complicated single-switch scanning systems let you control several devices, each with multiple features. (For example, TVs have on and off, volume control, and channel control, and VCRs have record, play, and rewind.) Single-switch scanning remotes are more expensive than the universal remotes discussed above, and they increase in cost as features are added.

All-in-One Systems

All-in-one environmental control systems also are available. These systems let you control infrared devices (such as TVs, VCRs, CD players, and cable boxes), X-10 devices (such as lights, fans, and door openers), telephones, and hospital beds using one or more switches or even your voice. Some of these systems are wireless and can be mounted onto a wheelchair for mobility. Others use cords and are designed for use primarily in one place. These systems can start at $4,000 to $5,000, depending on the options included.

Consult with an occupational therapist, rehabilitation engineer, and/or assistive technology specialist, to choose an environmental control system that best suits your needs and environment. These professionals can help you select appropriate features. For example, systems with multiple menus can be confusing, particularly for persons who are not generally comfortable with technology. Additionally, speech recognition should not be the primary means for controlling the device for a person who uses a ventilator or whose voice varies over the course of the day or from one position to another (for example, in bed to upright in a chair).

COMPUTER ACCESS

People use computers for many reasons. You may find them useful for paying bills, communicating with friends and family, keeping track of your schedule, storing addresses and phone numbers, writing reports for school and work, finding information on the Internet (from airline schedules to health information), and reading the newspaper. It is important to remember that a computer is a versatile tool—part calculator, typewriter, communication device, stereo, speakerphone, and game system. Using special technology to access a computer can be very helpful for persons with spinal cord injury who may have difficulty manipulating a pen, turn-ing pages of a newspaper, or getting out to the shopping mall.

Selecting a computer can be intimidating because of all the options in terms of manufacturers, operating systems (for example, Microsoft versus Macintosh), designs (laptops versus desktops), and software packages (such as word processing, spreadsheet, and photo editing software). Your specific needs, such as where and for what purpose you will use the com-puter, will help determine which system is best for you. An occupational therapist, rehabilitation engineer, assistive technology specialist, or vocational rehabilitation specialist can help you assess the many options available.

You may already be familiar with a computer keyboard and mouse. These two devices, along with the computer screen and speakers allow you to interact with the computer. If you have impaired arm and hand use, using the standard keyboard and mouse may be mildly difficult to impossible. However, many options are available to make the computers accessible to those who can type with a single finger, use a typing splint, or operate a mouth stick. Some of the simplest and least expensive options are already installed on computers when you buy them. For example, if you have difficulty pressing a key fast enough to avoid getting multiple keystrokes, the FilterKeys option will allow you to turn off or slow down the rate of repeated keystrokes.

If you type with one hand or finger, it can be difficult to perform oper-ations that require pressing two keys at the same time. The StickyKey feature allows you to press the keys one after the other but have the com-puter recognize them as being pressed at the same time. If you are having difficulty with the computer mouse but can access the keyboard, MouseKeys allows you to use the number pad keys (the set of number keys typically on the right side of the keyboard) to direct the pointer on the computer screen.

Another simple accommodation is the use of a keyguard placed over a standard or specialty keyboard. A keyguard is usually a metal or plastic sheet that rests directly above the keyboard keys. A hole aligned over each key helps your finger, typing splint, or mouthstick target just one key.

Many specialty keyboards are available as well. If you type with a sin-gle typing splint or a mouthstick, compact keyboards that include small-er keys arranged more closely together can reduce the amount of effort required to reach each of the keys. Large keyboards with oversized keys may be useful if you have difficulty hitting small keys.

Many mouse alternatives are also available. Large trackballs can be used if you have poor use of your fingers but good arm movement. Mouse alternatives also include joystick-style mice, multiple switches (one for up, down, left and right), and headpointer and eye-tracking technologies that use the movement of a reflective dot worn on the head, or eye movement, to move the mouse pointer. These mouse alternatives can also interact with software that puts an image of a keyboard on the screen to allow you to use the mouse to click keyboard keys. This arrangement lets you bypass the traditional keyboard nearly all together.

Speech recognition technology can also be used to access a computer. Although this technology is not perfect, it has improved greatly in recent years. It can be helpful to persons with clear speech and the ability to remember and consistently use a few spoken commands.

Special software and hardware also can allow computer access using just one switch to control the mouse and generate keystrokes. Because switch-access techniques tend to be slow, they and other computer access methods discussed above are sometimes combined with word prediction and abbreviation expansion software to increase typing rates. Word prediction software uses the first letter or letters typed to offer a list of words starting with that letter or letters. You then select the word from the list, and the word is automatically inserted, saving you from having to type the entire word. Abbreviation expansion software allows you to use just a few keystrokes to create frequently used blocks of text such as a full name or address.

These are just some of the many options available to make computers accessible. Talk with your occupational therapist, rehabilitation engineer, or helpful technology specialist to find out more about computer access and services, such as a computer access evaluation, that may be helpful for you.

FUNDING FOR HELPFUL TECHNOLOGY

Who will pay for assistive technology depends on your age; the state you live in; and what private, state, or federal sources of funding you are relying on to cover costs of your rehabilitation. Talk with your social worker or case manager at your rehabilitation hospital to determine which of the assistive technology devices that you need will be covered. He or she should also know whether and how to look for coverage for technology devices while you are an inpatient and an outpatient.

In general, if you are covered by Medicare (that is, if you are over 65 and have "paid into" the system over the years), then certain pieces of standard or "traditional" equipment will be covered. Durable medical equipment—wheelchairs, commodes, canes, walkers, and orthotic devices (braces)—are usually covered if you meet certain criteria set by

The Americans with Disabilities Act (ADA), passed by Congress in 1990, is a civil rights act for people with disabilities. It forbids discrimination in the workplace, housing, transportation, and other aspects of life. Before the ADA's passage, discrimination against persons with disabilities was illegal only in institutions receiving federal funding (such as schools with government grants) under the Rehabilitation Act of 1973.

The ADA has five sections or "titles." Title I prohibits discrimination based on disability by an employer against current employees who become disabled. It also prohibits discrimination in the application and hiring process. Under Title I, employers are required to provide "reasonable accommodation." Such accommodations are defined as any modification or adjustment to a job or the work environment that will enable an otherwise qualified applicant or employee to participate in the application process or to perform essential job functions without causing "undue hardship" for the employer.

Among other requirements, it means that an employer must accommodate, where possible, use of wheelchairs (for example, rearrange furniture, raise a desk, or modify restrooms) and use of other assistive technology (such as phone headsets, reduced-size keyboards, and customized settings for computer interfaces). The legal definition of "undue hardship" in the employer's case takes into account the size and resources of the company in determining the expense and complexity that constitutes a reasonable accommodation.

Titles II and III of the ADA address public and private accommodations. With respect to assistive technology and people with a spinal cord injury, the most important aspects of these sections of the law are their impact on new construction and mass transit systems. The ADA specifies that public facilities and programs must be accessible. The impact of this act can be seen in the proliferation of ramps and curb cuts, new public buses with wheelchair lifts, subway construction that includes elevators, and trains that have wheelchair spaces.

In addition, the ADA mandates that businesses providing services to the public must provide reasonable accommodation where it does not cause undue hardship. It also specifies guidelines for architectural accessibility for new construction (for example, wheelchair accessibility in hotels, movie theaters, shopping malls, and other public places).

The overall effect of the ADA has been to increase greatly the opportunities available for persons with disabilities to continue to enjoy the benefits of, and contribute to, their communities and society in general. If you are headed back to work, there is a reasonable chance that a current or potential employer, who finds you qualified, will be willing to make adjustments if the cost of accommodation is not too great.

Your state vocational rehabilitation service may help fund the workplace accommodations you need. You may also want to seek advice from the Job Accommodation Network (www.jan.wvu.edu; 1-800-526-7234) before making a pitch to an employer.

Figure 9.1. Assistive Technology and the Americans with Disabilities Act of 1990

Medicare. Other traditional low-tech equipment, such as reachers and long-handled sponges, is sometimes covered by Medicare.

If you are covered by Medicaid, the answer to the question of "Who will pay?" varies from state to state. If you have private insurance, coverage for technology varies widely. You will need to ask what is covered. Many private payers offer at least partial coverage for basic durable medical equipment. Chapter 7 discusses financial issues and insurance in greater detail.

Unfortunately, much of the technology discussed in this chapter is not covered by public and private insurance plans. In general, items are not covered because insurers continue to be governed by the notion of "medical necessity." They cover what is medically necessary, which often is narrowly defined. One might argue that independent access to the telephone is medically necessary for safety reasons. One might also argue that an inability to communicate reliably can cause depression, which can lead to failure to exercise, eat right, take medication, and other behaviors essential to good health. While sensible, such logic often makes no difference when it comes to funding for technology.

The bright side may be that the U.S. health care system is being reexamined, so changes in the future are possible. Disability advocates have been pushing for many years for coverage of technology based on functional need, rather than medical need. Keep an eye on the media for the latest news on this topic and ask your case manager or social worker to help interpret what you read.

If the technology you need is specifically related to employment, your state vocational rehabilitation agency may help pay for equipment that will get you back to work. This equipment might include items, such as a wheelchair porch lift at the home, so an individual can get to work. It also might include computer-access equipment or custom modifications to tools so you can do essential job tasks. Chapter 8 discusses vocational rehabilitation in more depth.

When it is clear that some system or device will not be paid for by your insurance plan or state vocational rehabilitation agency, you may want to turn to local civic organizations. Kiwanis, Rotary, Knights of Columbus, Lions, and Elks Clubs often take up worthy causes. They may be willing to raise funds for the environmental control system or computer adaptation that you need.

Your employer might also be required to provide assistive technology if it is deemed to be a "reasonable accommodation" (Figure 9.1). If you are in school, the school system should provide needed accommodations. Talk with your employer or school personnel, or with your hospital's vocational rehabilitation specialist, about your accommodation needs.

Chapter 8 also discusses getting what you need at school and work.

Funds for needed assistive technology also may be available through your rehabilitation hospital or other organizations in your community. Talk with your case manager or social worker and with other people with spinal cord injury to get their ideas about funding sources. You might also try searching the Web, using "spinal cord injury," "disability," "funding," and "support" as search terms.

CONCLUSION

We've covered a lot of ground in this chapter: how assistive technology can assist you in so many ways from how you can get around (mobility aids and adapted driving), how you can take care of yourself (aids to daily living), how you can control your environment (environmental control), and how you can access that tool, the computer, that is used for everything from staying in touch with family and friends, reading the news paper, and completing school and work projects. The goal in this chapter has been to give you just an introduction to assistive technology and some of the ways it can assist you in increasing your independence. We encourage you to speak with your rehabilitation team to find out more about what specific assistive technology may benefit you.

What Can I Do?

As you make decisions about assistive technology, it is important to:

- *Determine your needs.* Talk with your rehabilitation team, including your doctor, occupational therapist, physical therapist, rehabilitation engineer, vocational rehabilitation specialist, about your goals at home, at school or work, and in the community, and how technology might help you achieve those goals.
- *Educate yourself.* Learn as much as you can about different types of assistive technology, models that are available, and vendors. Your rehabilitation hospital may have technology available that you can look at and try out before making a decision.
- *Understand your insurance coverage.* Whether you have private insurance, Medicare, or Medicaid be sure to develop a good understanding of your insurance coverage, including which types of technology is covered and what portion of the cost is covered.
- *Consider different funding sources.* Talk with your case manager and other rehabilitation team members about where to find funding for the technology you need.

- *Work with your team.* Work closely with your rehabilitation team to select and order the technology that will benefit you. If you have questions about how to select, obtain, or use technology, be sure to ask questions and get the answers you need.

Where Can I Learn More?

To learn more about assistive technology, you may wish to consult the following resources:

- Your rehabilitation team
- Your health insurance provider, whether it is a private insurance plan, the federal Medicare program, or your state Medicaid program
- ABLEDATA, a source of objective information about assistive technology products and rehabilitation equipment (www.abledata.com)
- Your state vocational rehabilitation agency (visit www.jan.wvu.edu/sbses/vocrehab.htm for state agency contact information)
- The Job Accommodation Network (JAN) (www.jan.wvu.edu)
- The Association for Certified Driver Rehabilitation Specialists (www.driver-ed.org)
- The Adaptive Driving Alliance (www.adamobility.com)
- The Rehabilitation Engineering and Assistive Technology Society of North America ((to find a technology specialist near you) (visit www.resna.org and click on "ATP/ATS/RET Directory")

Appendix C provides information about additional resources.
your rehabilitation hospital.

IMPORTANT POINTS TO REMEMBER

• Assistive technology includes a range of assistive devices and technology—from simple dressing sticks to power wheelchairs and sophisticated environmental control units—that can enable you to get around, do self-care activities, control your environment, and use computers.

• Your rehabilitation team can help you choose appropriate technology to help you become as independent and functional as possible at home, at school or work, and in the community. Your team can also help you explore funding options.

• Depending on your age, state, and health insurance, some funding for assistive technology may be available. Medicare, Medicaid, your private insurance plan, your state vocational rehabilitation agency, your employer, local civic groups, or your rehabilitation hospital may help pay for needed technology.

The adapted driving section of this chapter was adapted from "Personal Transportation and Adapted Driver Rehabilitation" by Glen Digman, O.T.R./L., published by the American Occupational Therapy Association, Inc., 1996

—10—
Get Out and Play! Making Plans for Physical Activity and Recreation

JOAN PARCHEM JOYCE

"Get yourself together. Take care of yourself. Get out. Start doing things you did before. Get back into your hobbies. Don't sit around and mope." –Andrew

If someone asks us "What do you like to do?" most of us would not answer "work." Work is what we do to help us pay our bills and for our leisure activities! Everyone has different ideas about what "recreation" means. It can be reading, traveling to exotic places, playing sports, watching a ballgame or scary movie, sweating in aerobic classes, attending cooking classes, biking, sailing, being with friends, dancing, water skiing, painting, and more. The list is endless!

After a spinal cord injury, many people feel like they can't participate in recreational activities like they did in the past. That fact may be partially true, in part, but you still have many opportunities for recreation, maybe some you never considered before. Having a spinal cord injury may change the way you participate in activities, but it doesn't stop you from having fun. The changes may include using adaptive equipment, finding accessible facilities, and being creative. Many organizations and people can show you how!

This chapter shares ideas, skills, and information that can help you return to a satisfying leisure life. In this chapter, you'll learn about:

- **Therapeutic recreation** while in the rehabilitation hospital
- The benefits of physical activity and recreation
- Options for physical activity and recreation
- How to plan for recreation activities

DURING YOUR REHAB STAY

Leisure time is free time during which you can do what you want to do. Recreation is what you do during your leisure time. It's your decision how you will use your leisure time. You can spend it alone, with family and friends, or with people who have similar interests.

While you're in the rehabilitation hospital, most likely you will be introduced to recreational activities by a recreation therapist. You'll have the opportunity to try new leisure activities, adapt activities that you enjoyed before your injury, and learn where to participate in activities in your area. Recreation might be the last thing on your mind during your hospital stay. However, by participating in the activities offered, you'll be working on your therapy goals while having fun. You'll also gain experience doing everyday activities in a wheelchair or with walking aids.

In addition, as part of your recreation therapy, you'll also have the opportunity to take part in recreational activities that you can enjoy in the community. These activities might include going shopping, sightseeing, bowling, or to a movie. You might be nervous at first, but most patients return from these community outings more relaxed, reporting, "It's easier than I thought!" Experiencing the community for the first time in a wheelchair is easier with your therapists.

WHY SHOULD I GET ACTIVE?

Physical and recreational activities offer many physical and social health benefits. For example, these activities give us the chance to learn skills, relax, meet and socialize with people, and improve or maintain our physical health (Figure 10.1). Research suggests that for people with spinal cord injury, exercise can also prevent secondary conditions, such as diabetes, cardiovascular disease, **pressure sores**, **urinary tract infections**, and respiratory disease. In addition, exercise helps prevent deconditioning (getting out of shape) and obesity, and it provides mental health benefits.

You've heard all the experts say how important physical activity is for your health, but maybe going to the gym, lifting weights, or playing sports has never been your idea of fun. Are you aware that you can get many of the same benefits by participating in less strenuous recreational activities that you really enjoy? It's true! The Surgeon General has reported that just 30 minutes of moderate activity (added up over an entire day) most days of the week can help prevent disease. Actually, any increase in physical activity can help prevent medical problems and make you feel better! Think about shopping, traveling, visiting a museum, bowling, gardening, and walking the dog! All these activities get you moving and at the same time increase your conditioning.

The American Heart Association and other organizations stress the importance of daily physical activity. According to the American Heart Association, the benefits of daily physical activity include:

• Reducing the risk of heart disease by improving blood circulation
• Keeping weight under control
• Improving blood cholesterol levels
• Preventing and managing high blood pressure
• Preventing bone loss
• Boosting energy level
• Helping manage stress
• Releasing tension
• Improving the ability to fall asleep and sleep well
• Improving self-image
• Countering anxiety and depression
• Increasing enthusiasm and optimism
• Increasing muscle strength, giving greater capacity for other physical activities
• Providing a way to share an activity with family and friends

Figure 10.1. Benefits of Physical Activity

BUT I'M DISABLED—WHAT CAN I DO?

Many people with spinal cord injury find that they have a less active lifestyle after the injury than they did before the injury. They find themselves sitting around more, which leads to the body becoming deconditioned. In turn, this change in your physical well-being will lead to your becoming more dependent on others in your everyday activities, such as doing transfers and wheeling around. Inactivity also lead to less strength and endurance and will increase your risk of heart disease and other medical problems.

You can prevent all of these problems and benefit both your body and mind by developing a regular exercise program. According to the National Center for Physical Activity and Disability, the best types of exercise for persons with spinal cord injury are:

• Aerobic exercise, which builds and maintains cardiovascular health
• Strength training, which maintains the ability to perform activities of daily living
• Mobility and flexibility training, which improves range of motion and reduces spasticity

During your rehabilitation hospital stay, your therapists will work with you to develop an exercise program. When you leave the hospital, it will be important for you to continue your exercise program. Many individuals with spinal cord injury report getting out of the house less frequently after hospitalization, despite the fact that many people actually have more leisure time during the initial months following spinal cord injury because of not returning to work. So, although those first few months can be a difficult transition, recognize that you may actually have some extra leisure time on your hands. It's also important to find physical activities that you enjoy. If you don't enjoy a certain type of physical activity you've chosen, you probably won't stick with it for very long. Just look at all the exercise equipment for sale at yard sales!

Three good options for exercise include using a fitness center, getting involved in competitive or noncompetitive sports, and participating in outdoor sports. Each of these options is discussed below.

Use a Fitness Center

Fitness centers are a good option for exercise for many people, regardless of their physical abilities. These centers usually have weight equipment and stretching areas, and many have swimming pools and classes teaching aerobic conditioning, tai chi, yoga, and other types of exercise. Many fitness centers are now accessible for people in wheelchairs. If you already have a membership, call your club and ask about accessibility. Figure 10.2 suggests questions to ask about fitness centers.

> - Are the doors wide enough to go through with a wheelchair and do they have automatic door openers?
> - Are the locker rooms, restrooms, and shower area accessible?
> - Are there ramps or elevators outside and within the facility where needed?
> - Are there elevators inside the facility?
> - Are the spaces around the equipment wide enough to fit a wheelchair?
> - Is the equipment padded to protect your skin?
> - Have the center's fitness trainers worked with individuals with disabilities?
> - What are the trainers' certifications?

Figure 10.2. Questions to Ask About Fitness Centers

Don't assume that your fitness center is accessible, but don't assume that it's not! The chances are good that the center has had other members with disabilities and that the equipment and facilities are accessible.

Many hospitals and clinics also have exercise facilities with accessible fitness equipment. For example, if you are in the Washington, D.C., area, National Rehabilitation Hospital offers fitness memberships at its Irving Street facility. Check with the staff at your rehabilitation facility or other hospitals to find out if they have accessible fitness facilities that you can use.

Before joining a fitness center, take a tour and learn about the facility, programs, and staff. If you find that the facilities or equipment are not accessible, or if you need accommodations, talk with the staff. Most likely, they will be willing to listen and make reasonable changes to accommodate you and other members with disabilities. For example, a prospective member of a YMCA facility recently found that the shower chair in the locker room was not sturdy enough to hold his weight. After he talked with the membership coordinator, a more substantial shower chair was obtained and grab bars were installed. Just speak up and work with the staff if you need accommodations to help you use the center!

Take Up a Sport

Many communities have developed wheelchair sports programs for basketball, soccer, tennis, swimming, bocce ball, quad rugby, racing, track and field, softball, and sitting volleyball. Many of these programs offer introductory clinics, training for competitive teams, and opportunities to play the sport noncompetitively with friends and family.

As you look for sports opportunities, don't limit yourself to a sport that you participated in before your injury. One nationally ranked wheelchair racer was a wrestler before his injury. Another person, who had never played tennis before his injury, became a competitive tennis player. He attended a tennis clinic while he was in the rehabilitation hospital, and he was competing a year later.

Sports are also an excellent way to interact with friends and family. Often, the rules are similar to conventional ways of playing the sport. Wheelchair tennis is a great example. The only change in the rules is that the tennis player using a wheelchair gets two bounces of the ball if needed.

Many opportunities are available for learning about, and getting involved in, sports. Just getting out and throwing the ball around with a friend can be fun, but you can also look into getting more involved through wheelchair sports organizations. Going to wheelchair sports events and tournaments—from wheelchair racing to basketball to quad ruby—can give you a feel for what these sports are all about. You'll be amazed at the high level of competition seen at many of these events. Talk with your recreation therapist to learn more, or see the "Additional Reading and Resources" section at end of this book for list of wheelchair sports organizations.

Head for the Great Outdoors

Water skiing, snow skiing, sailing, kayaking, canoeing, hiking, mountain climbing, scuba diving, and other outdoor sports are all still possible despite your spinal cord injury. Many national organizations provide information about these activities and offer local opportunities to try out the adaptive equipment. These organizations are also a way to meet others with similar interests in your area.

For example, in the Washington, D.C., area, Baltimore Adapted Recreation and Sports offers year-round activities in snow skiing, water skiing, sailing, kayaking, and handcycling. For a small fee they provide instruction and the adapted equipment necessary to participate. Through such organizations, you can rent a handcycle and cycle with other club members or your family on local bike paths, or you can learn to snow ski in the winter, for instance. During the summer, local organizations also offer water skiing and sailing opportunities.

Appendix C (Reading and Additional Resources) of this book lists many of these organizations, and your recreation therapist can provide more ideas about how to get involved.

ACCESS IS GETTING BETTER

Since the **Americans with Disabilities Act (ADA)** became a law in 1990, opportunities for leisure activities for people with disabilities have multiplied! For example:

- Movie theaters now have accessible seats in the front, middle, and back. (Theaters removed three or more seats, so you can sit in your wheelchair next to the person with whom you have come.)
- Most performing arts theaters and concert venues also provide accessible wheelchair seating. In the Washington, D.C., area, the John F. Kennedy Center for the Performing Arts has a special price ticket program for people with disabilities.
- Bowling alleys have made their lanes accessible and provide a ramp to roll the ball on if needed! (People with good upper body control will not need this ramp.)
- Gardening is a relaxing activity that can also provide physical exercise. At your local garden shop, you can purchase long-handled tools so you can reach from your chair. Another idea is to raise your garden bed. Your local garden shop staff or a recreation therapist can tell you simple ways to raise the bed.
- Golfing is another activity that is still possible. Accessible golf carts can go

on the green, adapted golf clubs are available, and First Swing Golf clinics can provide basic instruction.

- Swimming is a great physical activity offering overall body toning. Many new swimming pools are being built with ramps so you can wheel in a water wheelchair right into the water. Others have lifts. Check with a local therapy program and see if they offer adapted aquatics lessons for your first time in the pool. Using adapted techniques and floats if needed, you can soon be swimming!

- Going shopping is also an option for exercise. Have you ever thought about how much energy you expend going from one end of the mall to the other? Many shopping malls now have walking programs and are open early to provide a safe, level, air-conditioned walking environment. It's a great way to build up your endurance. High schools and local parks also have tracks you can use.

As you can see, your opportunities for recreation really are endless! The key is to get moving. Think of all the things you enjoy doing and all the things you always wanted to do. Now you're ready to make a plan!

MAKE A PLAN

Even if you weren't recreation-oriented in the past, now is a great opportunity to get started! This section offers you the tools to start making a recreation plan that is realistic one that suits your personal needs and interests. There are three easy steps to get you thinking about what you want to do, where you can do it, and how you are going to do it! The steps are:

Step 1: Choose your activity
Step 2: Find out where you can do it
Step 3: Develop a plan with solutions

STEP 1: CHOOSE YOUR ACTIVITY

As you begin planning, let's get back to basics. Think about the reasons why you think you want to participate in physical activity or recreational activities. Is it because you want to get back to a sport you did before? Do you want to find new friends who share your interests? Do you need to get in shape? Remember that sometimes after an injury, a person's needs may be different than they were before the injury. For example, if you were very physically active at work before your injury, you may have participated in activities that were less physical after work. If you worked with crowds of people all day, in the evening you may have wanted time alone. Your situation may be differ-

---

The top two reasons I want to participate in recreation activities are to:

____ Be more physically active
____ Be around people and socialize
____ Reduce stress and relax
____ Feel a sense of achievement
____ Enjoy nature
____ Be adventurous

Another reason that's important to me:

Figure 10.3. Why do I want to participate in recreational activities?

ent now. Use the checklist in Figure 10.3 to assess the reasons you want to participate in recreational activities.

Consider All the Options

Now use the reasons you chose in Figure 10.3 to think about the types of activities you would like to do. Table 10.1 lists some options. It doesn't include all of your options, but it may give you some ideas. Remember to try any activity that sounds like fun to you! Finding activities that you can enjoy with family and friends is important!

Now that you've identified some activities you might enjoy, find out more about them. Talk with your recreation therapist, other people with disabilities, or representatives of adapted sports organizations to learn about an activity. Ask:

• What skills does it take to do the activity?
• Can I do the activity on my own or does it involve other people?
• What equipment will I need and how much will it cost?
• Can I find people in my community who will teach me to do the activity?
• Will I need to take a class or get certified to participate (for example in scuba diving)?
• Do I have to change anything about this activity to be able to participate? (If so, see the next section.)

Adapt It to Your Needs

Fortunately, we don't have to reinvent the wheel when it comes to adapting recreation activities to meet the needs of people with spinal cord injury! Many people have already done this and "know the ropes." Contact a recre-

If you checked:	You might want to:
Be more physically active	• Join a gym/exercise class • Join a sports team • Learn a new sport • Work out with an exercise video • Lift weights • Kayak, canoe, or sail • Hike • Handcycle on a bike trail
Be around people and socialize	• Join a club • Take a class (such as a computer, language, painting, or crafts class) • Plan a party • Join a sports team • Take a cruise • Attend a worship service • Be a volunteer
Reduce stress and relax	• Swim • Take a water exercise class • Learn or participate in yoga or tai chi • Garden • Go fishing • Kayak or canoe • See a movie or a play • Paint • Make crafts
Feel a sense of achievement	• Be a volunteer • Take a class • Learn a new craft • Complete a project
Enjoy nature	• Hike or backpack • Travel • Canoe, sail, or kayak • Camp • Scuba dive or snorkel • Ski • Ride horseback
Be adventurous	• Ski • Fly a plane • Mountain climb • Scuba dive • Travel to exotic places!

Table 10.1. What Can I Do?
Use the checklist in Figure 10.3 to assess the reasons you want to participate in recreational activities, then consider some of the activities listed below.

ation therapist in your area for help with finding out more about adapted activities. National and local organizations also can provide information and answer your questions. For example, the National Center on Physical Activity and Disability (www.ncpad.org) has compiled information about a variety of recreational activities and sports. If you have access to the Internet at home or at the library, your resources are virtually unlimited!

To participate in some activities, you may need adaptive equipment, such as a playing card holder, an adapted fishing rod, a handle grip for bowling, a sit ski, adapted computer equipment, or longer adapted gardening tools. Talk with your rehabilitation hospital's recreation therapists or rehabilitation engineers to find low-cost ways to adapt equipment.

Many sports have specific sports chairs for their competitions, but beginning players can participate in chairs provided by the team. When you're ready to make a commitment to a particular sport, you can buy a wheelchair specific to that sport.

Joining a sport team or organization will help you learn the rules of the sport. Most sports are adapted only where needed. As mentioned above, in wheelchair tennis, the only major rule change is that the person in the wheelchair can take two bounces when needed. In basketball, a big difference can be seen in is the dribbling rules. (You can hold the ball in your lap as you push twice.) Water skiing and snow skiing are done in a sitting position with a modified sit ski. Special organizations provide qualified instructions in their sports.

STEP 2: FIND PLACES WHERE YOU CAN DO IT

Now that you've identified a recreation activity you think you want to do, you'll need to figure out where you can do it. Figure 10.4 lists some of the many places you might find physical fitness and recreation activities in your community.

To find out about activities in your area:

- Get on the mailing lists of adapted sports organizations and your local parks and recreation department. These newsletters may spark your interest in something you never considered before.
- Look in the Yellow Pages to find places that offer recreational activities.
- Read your local newspaper, including activity listings.
- Ask friends and other people with disabilities where they go for recreational activities.
- Talk with recreation therapists and others at your rehabilitation hospital.
- Contact national organizations to find out if there are local chapters in your area.

- Search the Internet (using the activity name and your city or community name as search terms).

Questions to ask when you contact places that offer recreation activities in your community include:

- Where are you located?
- What recreational activities do you offer?
- Are your facilities and programs accessible to people in wheelchairs?
- What accommodations do you offer for people in wheelchairs?
- Do you have any adaptive equipment (such as a sports wheelchair) that I can use?
- Is the program open to everyone or is it only for persons with disabilities?

- Dance studios
- Community centers
- City or county recreation departments (contact the therapeutic recreation office for specific information on adapted recreation and accessible pools and facilities.)
- YMCAs and YWCAs
- Universities and community colleges
- Fitness clubs
- Shopping malls (may offer walking programs and/or aerobic classes)
- Yoga or tai chi clubs
- Bowling alleys
- Libraries (offer free Internet access, book groups, classes, and lectures)
- Craft stores (may offer classes and workshops)
- Theaters (some offer discounts on tickets)
- Museums (may offer tours, classes, lectures, and special events)
- Volunteer service organization
- Social clubs
- Hospitals and clinics (may offer lessons, workshops, and fitness centers)
- Senior centers
- Golf courses (many have at least one accessible golf cart that is allowed on the greens)
- Tennis clubs
- Garden clubs
- Horseback riding stables
- Religious groups and places of worship
- Travel groups
- Historic sites (may offer lectures and events)

Figure 10.4. Places That May Offer Recreational Activities in Your Community

- How much does it cost?
- What are the times and dates of program?
- How do I register?
- Can I be added to your mailing list?

STEP 3: IDENTIFY BARRIERS AND FIND SOLUTIONS

Have you ever heard yourself think or say, "I can't because . . .?" Most of us have said this at one time or another! Lots of factors can prevent us from continuing an activity or taking up a new activity—whether it's playing a sport with friends, working out regularly in the gym, going dancing, or doing a craft. We can all come up with physical, psychological, and other reasons not to do something, but sometimes we just need to find workable solutions to motivate us to get involved. It's important to identify the barriers up front and then find solutions to break down the barriers. With some thought and creativity, you can turn "I can't" into "I can!"

Step 3 in the planning process involves taking steps to get involved in the recreational activity or activities you've chosen. The first part of this step is to identify those barriers that could prevent you from doing the activity and possible solutions that will help you get involved. Common barriers to physical activity and recreational activities include lack of money, transportation problems, lack of affordable adaptive equipment, and having no one to do it with. Below are some possible solutions to break down these barriers and get you going.

I Don't Have Enough Money . . .

Not having enough extra money to participate in an activity is a factor for many people. Equipment costs and admission fees can really add up! Search for free or low-cost activities in your community. Ideas for finding inexpensive activities include to:

- Check your local newspaper for notices about free or low-cost events, or for discount coupons for events.
- Contact theaters in your area to find out about for special discounts.
- Check with recreational organizations to find out if they will waive membership fees.
- Ask organizations about attending events free if you volunteer.
- Ask about tuition assistance for classes you want to take.
- Become involved with organizations or clubs that will lend you sports gear or other equipment, or ones that will let you use your equipment

while taking classes (see below).
- Join a local wheelchair sports team. Teams usually have sports chairs to lend or contacts on how to get a sports chair

I Can't Get There . . .

Public transportation's accessibility has improved. In major metropolitan areas, subways and buses are accessible for people in wheelchairs. Buses are equipped with ramps and lockdowns for wheelchairs. Subway trains are accessible with elevators available to get to and from the train. Contact your local public transportation office and inquire about travel training in your area. In Washington, D.C., the Washington Metropolitan Area Transit Authority offers travel training. Sure, problems still exist with broken elevators and ramps, but many people successfully use public transportation to get around everyday.

As required by the ADA, cities also offer paratransit services. These low-cost services provide curb-to-curb transportation for individuals with disabilities who qualify. For example, in the Washington, D.C., area, MetroAccess provides this service for a small fee. (At this time, it is $2.50 each way plus $1 per zone). This service can be used for a trip to a friend's house, a shopping mall, or a movie! Check with your county or city government for information about paratransit services in your area. When you use paratransit services, be sure to schedule well in advance and allow ample time to be picked up so you can get to your destination on time. As you become more independent with your wheelchair skills, using a public bus or subway may be a better option because it allows you to set your own schedule, and it is less expensive.

Also check with local taxi services. Many offer accessible service. Additionally, if you're planning to attend a sports clinic or support group meeting, check with the leaders and see if carpooling is a possibility.

I Don't Have the Right Equipment . . .

Getting access to adaptive equipment and finding affordable to buy equipment can sometimes be challenging. Check with people at your local sports and recreational organizations for persons with disabilities to see if they have any ideas about where to borrow or buy equipment. Many have adaptive equipment that they loan to members participating in events. If you attend an introductory clinic or class for a sport or other activity that interests you, you can ask the instructors about where you might buy good used equipment.

I Don't Have Anyone to Do It With . . .

This one is relatively easy! Join an organization or club where you will meet people with similar interests. Take a class and have fun learning a new skill with other novices. You might also join a SCI support group where you can meet and learn from others with SCI. Often support group sponsor get-together social events as well. In addition, you might volunteer with an organization to meet folks who share your enthusiasm for a sport or other activity. The more you get out and participate, the more people you will come in contact with. Opportunities for car pooling will also happen.

PUTTING IT ALL TOGETHER: MAKING YOUR RECREATIONAL PLAN

Now that you've thought through the types of activities that interest you, gathered information about where you can do the activities and what adaptations you will need, and determined how you will confront barriers, it's time to make a plan! Use the recreation planning form (Figure 10.5) to get it all down in writing. Figure 10.6 presents an example of how to fill out the form.

TAKE IT ONE STEP FURTHER—BECOME AN ADVOCATE

As you return to your community, you may find that some places you'd like to go are not accessible. If this happens, don't give up and say, "I guess I just can't go there." Even if you've never done so before, become an advocate and remember that you are your best resource. If you had a previous relationship with a place you want to frequent, talk with the owner or management. Explain what is preventing you from coming to the place of business or services. The staff may be unaware that a problem exists until someone speaks up. Often, they will consider making reasonable changes so that you and others can use their facilities.

John Hudson, a Virginia resident who has a spinal cord injury and uses a wheelchair, relates many stories about making his community more accessible so he and others with disabilities can be more active. For example, John succeeded in getting a local mall to add an automatic door opener. Sending the mall staff copies of all his receipts from other malls with a note saying, "This is what I could have spent in your mall if it was more accessible," accomplished this. He not only helped himself, but also helped others. For example, he now sees parents with strollers or small children, people with packages, and people in wheelchairs using the automatic door opener.

John also succeeded in getting the buses in his area to be more accessible. He uses the bus to get to and from work, but most mornings in the past he found he had to wait for a bus with a working lift. Often, two buses without working lifts would go by, and John waited more than an hour to board a bus. After hearing many complaints from John, the bus company sent the supervisor to his stop at 7 a.m. every day. As the bus arrived, the supervisor would ask the driver if he or she had checked to be sure the lift was working. If it wasn't, the driver was written up. After many days of this routine, the drivers started checking the lift and arriving with working lifts.

Marc Fielder, a wheelchair user and attorney with the Disability Rights Council in Washington, D.C., also recounts many personal experiences advocating for greater accessibility of public places. His recommendation is to ask for the minimum that you need to make the facility accessible. He recalls that when he was in college, he advocated for making the classrooms more accessible. When he realized that the expense involved in making every classroom on campus accessible would be huge, he proposed making only certain classrooms accessible. Since there were six students at the university who used wheelchairs, so he proposed making six classrooms accessible. He also proposed moving classes for wheelchair users into those rooms. The administration quickly agreed.

NOW GO DO IT!

Make relaxation and having fun a priority in your life. Remember how important it is—both mentally and physically—for you to be active. No one really wants to stay home and stare at the four walls! In the beginning, everything may seem to be harder, take longer, and be exhausting, but remember, as with everything else you accomplished in rehab, it will soon become easier. As you acquire needed skills and increase your endurance, you can have a full, rewarding lifestyle. Take small steps: go to a movie, out for dinner, to a game, or to a friend's house. Just take the time and plan your activities to ensure your success.

What Can I Do?

As you make choices about physical and recreation activities, be sure to:

- *Find activities you enjoy doing.* If you're having fun, you'll be more likely to stick with it and will do it more often!

- *Be creative*. Where there is a will, there is a way. If you really like to do something, find a new way to do it! Get ideas from therapists and others with similar interests.
- *Plan ahead*. Check on accessibility and plan your transportation.
- *Be flexible*. Don't give up just because your transportation is late. Always have "Plan B!"
- *Find someone to do it with you*. Many activities are more fun with family and friends.
- *Set your goals*. Set reasonable goals for yourself regarding how much you can accomplish in your day. When you meet those goals, set new ones!
- Get connected. Sign up for mailing lists for support groups, special organizations, and clubs. If their newsletters come to your home, sooner or later something will catch your interest.
- *Know thyself*. Be aware of your needs and know your limits!
- *Strive for balance*. Try to balance rest and recreation. Rest will be important during recovery, but too much will set you back. Ask your therapists for ideas for activities and exercises within your limits. Don't reach for the remote!
- *Let others know what you need*. You are your best spokesperson. Let friends and family know when you need help and when you don't!
- *Challenge yourself!* Use your extra time to try a new activity, learn a new language, or see a new place!

Where Can I Find Out More?

To learn more about getting involved in sports, recreation, and other leisure activities, you may wish to contact:

- The therapeutic recreation service at your rehabilitation hospital
- Your local government's recreation department, community centers, and libraries
- Neighborhood fitness centers and swimming pools
- Local clubs that share your interests
- National and local organizations that offer information about competitive and recreational activities and sports for persons with disabilities
- Magazines focused on sports and leisure activities for persons with disabilities

Appendix C provides information about additional resources.

IMPORTANT POINTS TO REMEMBER

- Physical and recreational activities offer many benefits, including the chance to learn new skills, relax, meet and socialize with others, and improve or maintain your physical and mental health.
- Leisure activities include everything from strength training and outdoor sports to shopping and walking the dog.
- Good planning can help you become more active and enjoy your leisure time more. To make a plan, learn about activities you might enjoy, find places or organizations that can help you get involved, and be creative in overcoming barriers that may prevent you from getting started.

—11—
Sexuality

P. CAROL BULLARD-BATES
LAURO S. HALSTEAD

If this was the first chapter you wanted to read in this book, you are not alone. Virtually everyone is interested in sex, but not always for the same reasons. Some want to know, "Can I still do it (have intercourse) or still have an orgasm?" Others want to know, "Will my boyfriend/girlfriend/ spouse still find me sexually attractive, or will anyone want to date me if I'm in a wheelchair?" A big question for many younger people with spinal cord injury is "Will I be able to have children?"

We won't be able to answer all your questions because, for many, the answer depends on you: who you are, your experience with sex, your attitudes about sex, and how much you are able to make changes. At the same time, we can answer many of these questions because, fortunately, in recent years, there has been much research in this area. Also, we can provide much information to you, your family, and loved ones. This chapter discusses:

- Sexual changes
- Sexuality in the hospital
- Becoming sexual again and getting treatment
- Treatment
- Fertility and pregnancy
- Dating, marriage and divorce
- Aging and sexuality
- Medications and sexuality
- Getting help

SEXUAL CHANGES IN MEN: THE BASIC STUFF

How do men get erections or hardening of the penis?

Two types of nerves help men get an erection (a hard-on). One type of nerve creates an erection by thinking or fantasizing about sex. Fantasizing about sex means imagining some activity that is sexually stimulating. This type of erection is sometimes called "psychological." The other type of nerve helps an erection work when you and your partner touch your penis, testicles, or the skin around these areas. This is called a touch or "reflex" erection.

Because a spinal cord injury damages nerves, both types of nerves that help your penis get hard can be injured. How much your erection is affected depends on how badly your spinal cord was injured and the level of the injury. In general, men with less severe or more incomplete injuries (especially when there is a lot of sensation) are able to get a better erection—both the psychological and reflex types—than men who have more complete injuries. Table 11.1 summarizes what we know about the influence of the level of injury on erections if your injury is complete.

Table 11.1. Percentage of Men with Complete Spinal Cord Injuries Who Report Erections

Level of injury	Erection by Touch	Erection by Fantasy
SCI at or above T12	70%-93% of men	0%
SCI below T12	0%	26 % of men

Source: Sipski, ML, Spinal Cord Injury and Sexual Function: An Educational Model. In: Sipski, ML, Alexander, CJ, eds. Sexual Function in People with Disability and Chronic Illness, Gaithersburg, MD: Aspen Publishers, Inc., 1997, p152-153.

These facts can be discouraging, but the good news is that there are other ways you can achieve an erection. These ways are discussed in the "Treatment" section below.

Can I Still Ejaculate?

Ejaculation is the medical term to describe fluid coming out of the penis. Compared with having an erection, ejaculation is often even more difficult after a spinal cord injury. Table 11.2 presents what we know about the influence of the level of injury on ejaculation after both complete and incomplete injuries. You can improve this situation through vibration of the penis. Electrical stimulation will be discussed in the "Fertility and Pregnancy" Section of this chapter.

Table 11.2. Percentage of Men with Spinal Cord Injury Who Report Ejaculation

Level of injury	Ability to ejaculatee
Complete SCI at or above T12	4%
Complete SCI below T12	18%
Incomplete SCI at or above T12	32%
Incomplete SCI below T12	70%

Source: Sipski, ML, Spinal Cord Injury and Sexual Function: An Educational Model. In: Sipski, ML, Alexander, CJ, eds. Sexual Function in People with Disability and Chronic Illness, Gaithersburg, MD: Aspen Publishers, Inc., 1997, p152-153.

When you do ejaculate after a spinal cord injury, you often ejaculate into the bladder instead of out through the penis. This ejaculation in the wrong direction is called "retrograde ejaculation." This doesn't hurt you or affect the orgasm, but it does affect how likely you are to conceive. Fortunately, we have found ways to compensate for the retrograde ejaculation to still allow men to conceive their own biologic child. More information about this is provided later in this chapter.

Can I Still Have an Orgasm?

Orgasms can occur after spinal cord injury. Men describe them as similar, weaker, or different than they felt before the spinal cord injury. Table 11.3 shows what we know about orgasms and spinal cord injury.

Table 11.3. Percentage of Men with Spinal Cord Injury Who Report Orgasm

Level of injury	Ability to achieve orgasm
Complete SCI	38%
All SCIs	42–47%

Source: Sipski, ML, Spinal Cord Injury and Sexual Function: An Educational Model. In: Sipski, ML, Alexander, CJ, eds. Sexual Function in People with Disability and Chronic Illness, Gaithersburg, MD: Aspen Publishers, Inc., 1997, p153.

An important issue is that you probably don't have any big change in your desire to have sex after an SCI. What is more important is how often your partner/spouse wants to have sex, or finding a partner in the first place. You have a lot of control over these issues by how you communicate with your partner and how comfortably you interact with possible partners in social situations. Although you may have intercourse less often after spinal cord injury because of problems with erections, you may enjoy more oral-genital stimulation in addition to touching, kissing, and hugging.

At first you may feel less satisfied with sex after your injury. The changes in your body can be frustrating. Problems with erections can make intercourse more difficult. Your movement is more challenging, and it may be more difficult to use the positions you used before. Your orgasms will be different. If you don't have a partner, it can be hard to start a sexual relationship for fear of how your partner will respond to all these problems. Talking about these issues ahead of time can be helpful. If you are already married or committed to someone, then good communication and experimentation can make all the difference.

SEXUAL CHANGES IN WOMEN

What About My Sexual Responses as a Woman?

Vaginal lubrication has a similar pattern for women with spinal cord injury as for men's erections. Women with injuries at the T12 level or higher tend to respond to touch but not fantasy with vaginal lubrication.

Some women with complete SCIs also are able to reach orgasm with similar feelings and body reactions as women without an SCI. Approximately half of women reported being able to reach orgasm by self-stimulation or sexual intercourse, while only about a third were able to reach orgasm by touching areas other than the genitals.

Here again, the changes in your body can cause you to be disappointed in your sex life and can cause you to have fewer sexual interactions at first. You may be less interested in masturbating, and, at first, you may prefer kissing, hugging, and touching rather than intercourse. Almost all women with SCI feel sexual feelings when they kiss with their mouth and lips. Fewer report arousability of their clitoris (32%).

Although problems with lubrication and orgasm can be a challenge after an SCI, they do not have to ruin your sex life. We will discuss ways to return to your sex life in spite of these challenges in the section called "Becoming Sexual Again."

Will I Have a Change in My Periods After an SCI?

Yes, you often do miss your menstrual cycle for five months or more after an SCI, but there are usually not many changes in your flow after it returns. You might notice more or less pain, but most women do not notice a big change in the amount of menstrual flow. You can experience hormonal changes that may explain why your menstrual cycle changes.

SEXUALITY ISSUES IN THE HOSPITAL

What Happened to My Privacy?

One challenge you will face in the hospital is the loss of your personal privacy. When you have had a spinal cord injury, the most private areas of your body become public as nursing staff have to catheterize you, give you suppositories, and stimulate your rectum to help you have a bowel movement. Nothing seems sacred or private in these situations, and they can be humiliating at first. Particularly if you have little hand function, you may also be concerned that your partner or a family member might need to do these personal care tasks when you get home.

All of these concerns are important to share with your partner so you can have an honest view of how he or she will handle this aspect of your care in the future. When you consider your intimate relationship and how it can be affected by these aspects of your care, you may be concerned. It is always best to separate these aspects of care as much as possible from times when you are sexually involved with each other.

How Can I Find Out about My Sexual Functioning in the Hospital?

Everyone is different in their level of interest in sexuality as they recover from spinal cord injury. At first, many people feel they are most focused on their ability to move and what areas of their body are getting stronger. They appear not to be worried about their sexual functioning until they are closer to going home. Others have said they started thinking about their sexual functioning from "day one."

You can use different means to discover what level of sexual functioning you have after an injury. If you have hand function, your hospital stay is an important time to experiment with masturbation to see if you can have an erection or an ejaculation if you are a man, or whether you can become lubricated with stimulation and have an orgasm if you are a woman. You can have your loved one help in the stimulation if you do not have hand function. You will also notice if you are being catheterized or bathed if you develop an erection or lubrication.

One of the most important things to realize at this time, however, is that you can learn to appreciate a sexual encounter even if you are not able to function sexually in the same way as before your injury or feel your genital region. While at the rehabilitation hospital, you can request the "family room" for privacy and experiment with each other to discover more about what you appreciate in touching and sharing with each other. Most rehab hospitals also have videotapes that will help you and your partner understand the changes in your sexual relationship, so you can communicate better and work through the changes. Your psychologist, social worker, nurse or doctor will also be important resources for information in this area since they know your specific injury and what will likely be possible for you as you recover.

BECOMING SEXUAL AGAIN

Experimentation and Creativity Are Key!

After a spinal cord injury, many people notice increased arousal from areas of their body above the injury level. Paraplegics may notice more arousal from their nipples and above, and quadriplegics may notice more arousal from their face, neck, and ears. If you have an incomplete injury, you and your partner need to discover what areas still give you pleasure.

In beginning your sexual interaction, it is important to be in a place where you will not be disturbed and where you both feel relaxed and unrushed. If you have a personal care attendant, you may want him or her to help you into comfortable, sexy clothing rather than expect your partner to help. Do not try to make love when you are exhausted. Spend some time just talking and telling each other what you appreciate about each other.

Take time to touch each others' bodies in any way that feels relaxed and comfortable, using words and nonverbal sounds that help to tell each other what feels good. Since most women enjoy foreplay, which gives them time to become lubricated and "turned on," the longer that phase is, the better for the woman. Focusing on touching the clitoral area for the woman and the penis for the man will help you to discover whether touching does stimulate erection or vaginal lubrication, but stimulation of your body above your injury can produce arousal also.

Sexual arousal is often as much mental as physical. You can enhance your pleasure by using all your senses to imagine yourselves in a beautiful place outdoors, such as the beach or beside a lovely lake with the sun's warmth on your bodies. Imagine what you can feel as your partner touches you; what you can hear in that special place, such as waves coming to shore; and what you can see, such as birds drifting on the wind currents above you.

Watching your partner touching you in different places can also arouse you. Having your hand on your partner's hand so you can imagine his or her touch even if you can't feel it can increase your pleasure. Beautiful music in the

background and pleasantly scented creams or lotions can put you further into
an aroused state. (Be sure not to get these creams into the woman's vaginal area
or the head of the man's penis, however, since they can be an irritant.)

Positioning is also important for the best comfort. Here again, experimentation helps. Some quads feel more comfortable in their wheelchair or another
type of chair because they have more mobility against gravity if they are seated.
Paraplegics have more options, although lying on their backs is the least
exhausting. Changing positions and places where you make love can help your
sexual interaction maintain its novelty and help each of you to enjoy it more.

You can have sex with a catheter in place. Just fold the catheter down along
your penis and place a condom over it. For women, your catheter can be taped
to your stomach before having sex.

Don't Give Up!

One researcher said, "It is what you do with what you have rather than what
you have that counts," and "There is always another, day, time or occasion." In
other words, one unsatisfactory sexual interaction does not have to control the
rest of your interactions. You have your whole life to develop the best lovemaking you can with your partner, and you can always try new things and
experiment with what you both enjoy. If intercourse is too difficult, try oral-genital or manual stimulation in different areas, as well as deep kissing and hugging
your loved one. Lie on different textures and make love by candlelight to make
the whole experience more romantic. Looking into each other's eyes as you
touch and hold each other can say so much that other interactions can not.

What Do I Have to Watch Out For with Sex?

After sexual interactions, it is important for you to wash your genital area as
soon as you can to prevent urinary tract infections. It is important to keep your
genitals clean and use extremely careful techniques when catheterizing yourself
to keep everything sterile. Try to hold off on sex if you have a urinary tract
infection. Doing so will help avoid a worse infection and prevent giving any
problems to your partner.

TREATMENT

As a Man, How Can I Improve My Sexual Function?

Many opportunities exist for treatment of erectile problems after spinal cord
injury. Talk with your spinal cord doctor or a urologist about your options.
One of the most widely known medications is Viagra. When taken once

daily as required, Viagra is more likely to improve the quality of your erections and satisfaction with your sex life if your injury is between T6 and L5.
Even if you have a high thoracic or cervical spinal cord injury, Viagra may
be beneficial. Men with incomplete spinal cord injuries may have better
results with this medication. Table 11.4 presents some other possible treatments.

Table 11.4. Medications for Problems with Erections

Medication(s)	Pros	Cons
Viagra,Cialis, Levitra	• Better erections for T6-L5 SCI • May have better effect with incomplete injuries • Viagra lasts 12-24 hours • Cialis and Levitra last 72 hours and are more powerful	• Cannot be used with high or low blood pressure • Some drug interactions • Should not be taken with Nitroglycerin
Penile injections (Papaverine, Prostaglandin E 1)	• Strong erection • for 1-2 hours	• Risks include priapism (blood fails to drain from penis), bruising, scarring, and infection • Seizures • Declining quality of erections • Can not be used more than once a week
MUSE (pellet placed in penis)	• Strong erection	• Risks include infection, burning sensation, decreased blood pressure, and fainting

What about Improving My Sexual Functioning as a Woman?

Unfortunately, there has been little research on treatment of female sexual
dysfunction in both women with and without spinal cord injury. However,
we do know a lot of practical things. For example, if you don't have natural
vaginal lubrication, you can still have sexual intercourse using water-based
lubricants like KY Jelly. You may feel sad, frustrated, or depressed because
you have lost the physical and orgasmic feelings you experienced before your

injury. You may feel more lonely because your spouse or partner may not understand your perspective if the relationship has not changed much from his side. Communication is the key to overcoming these feelings. It may also help you to experience a sense of acceptance of the changes and confidence that your sexual life can be fulfilling again.

If We're Having Problems, Where Can We Get Help?

Finding a good sex therapist who has expertise with disability can be particularly helpful to a couple going through the negative phases of sexual adjustment as described above. Such therapists can be difficult to find, though. Talk to your social worker, psychologist, or nurse at the rehabilitation hospital about whom they would recommend to help you.

Once you find an experienced sex therapist, he or she should be able to suggest techniques that can be helpful in reestablishing your sexual relationship. These techniques can include focusing on changing your negative thinking to positive thinking, relaxation training, use of imagery when you are making love, and improving your communication about your sexual encounters.

FERTILITY AND PREGNANCY

Should I Change Birth Control Methods after an SCI?

The type of birth control you use after an SCI is important because pregnancy is a risk. It is important to choose a method that is comfortable for you, easy to use, and safe. Several types need to be considered carefully because of the risks involved in using them. For example, birth control pills can have a side effect of blood clots, particularly if you have circulation problems, which is the case with SCI, because your loss of muscle movement reduces your ability to circulate your blood. The good news is that levels of estrogen in birth control pills are lower now so the risk of blood clots is lower today than in the past.

Your risk of blood clots is greatest in the first six months, so doctors do not recommend taking birth control pills during that time. If you smoke, you have a greater risk of having heart attacks and strokes if you take birth control pills. Also, if you have undiagnosed breast cancer, birth control pills can make it grow faster. The good news is that birth control pills can protect you from ovarian cancer and cancer of the lining of the uterus.

Many women like to use intrauterine devices (IUDs) because their use doesn't require a lot of preparation or thought. A risk is that IUDs may cause infections, especially in the first few months after insertion. Infections of the uterus, fallopian tubes, or ovaries can lead to pelvic inflammatory disease, which can lead to serious, long-term problems such as infertility and tubal pregnancies. If you have no feeling below your waist, you may not be able to tell that you have this painful disease, so your doctor will not recommend an IUD with your SCI.

You may want to consider an implant (Norplant) placed under your skin. Implants release a synthetic form of progesterone and can provide birth control for five years. A long-acting shot of progesterone every three months is another possibility. Blood clots are not a problem with these progesterone birth control methods.

You can also consider cervical caps, diaphragms, and female condoms for birth control but their pregnancy prevention rates are not as high as other techniques. Their success rates depend in part on how consistent you are in using them and in replacing the spermicidal cream or jelly. Use of these devices also requires good hand strength and coordination. If you don't have enough strength, it is important to see if your partner is willing to be involved with placing these for you. You can even be creative and integrate this step into your lovemaking.

Male condoms are simple to use and help prevent passing on sexually transmitted diseases. [The importance of this protection cannot be stressed enough, if you have sex with a person whom you do not know well, or you have no real knowledge of their sexual interactions in the past.] This problem is especially true if the person is taking drugs or is in recovery from drug and alcohol addiction.

Can I Have Children after an SCI?

You will be happy to hear that usually the ability to have children is not affected, but women with SCI tend to have fewer children than women who are able-bodied. It makes sense that if you have a lot of weakness from your SCI, you are less likely to become pregnant because you realize the difficulty you would have in caring for your child.

If I Get Pregnant, What Problems Will I Have Because of My SCI?

You can have a number of problems with SCI during pregnancy, many of which you are at risk for anyway when you are not pregnant. These problems include urinary tract infections, anemia, worsening **spasticity**, **pressure sores**, **autonomic dysreflexia**, worsening respiratory function, and preterm labor. Finding a doctor who has had some experience with SCI patients and pregnancy is important. You and your doctor need to determine how you can know when you begin labor in spite of your not being able to feel in your stomach area. The length of labor is usually the same as that of able-bodied women, although you might go into the hospital later because it is harder to recognize when you are in labor. Chapter 12 provides more details about pregnancy, labor, and delivery after spinal cord injury.

Can I Still Father a Child?

As a man with an SCI, having your own children is an important issue. You will probably have a lower sperm count than an able-bodied man, and your sperm are less active. Even if you are able to ejaculate into your partner, it will be more difficult for your partner to become pregnant. If you cannot ejaculate normally, a number of techniques are available to make pregnancy a possibility for you and your partner.

Some couples have been successful in using natural, at-home techniques if the man can ejaculate through his penis, even though his erection is not adequate to have intercourse. Masturbation (stimulation of your penis by your partner or with a vibrator) can sometimes produce an ejaculation. (When using a vibrator, it is important to watch out for signs of autonomic dysreflexia and redness that may appear on your penis. If you see signs of skin breakdown, stop using the vibrator until the skin is well healed.) Your partner can catch your semen in a well-washed diaphragm or cervical cap and then insert it into her vagina as usual. If you don't have a diaphragm or cervical cap, you can collect the semen in a clean cup and then use a syringe (which your doctor can give you) to take up the semen and insert it into her vagina, as close to the cervix as possible.

You can determine your partner's probable ovulation time by taking her temperature and examining the type of mucous inside her vaginal area as is done for natural family planning birth control techniques. If no pregnancy results after several months of trying, you have other options.

Vibratory stimulation and electrical stimulation are used by doctors to obtain sperm. These techniques have resulted in many men with spinal cord injury fathering their own biological children since the 1980s. Of the two techniques, vibratory stimulation produces better quality sperm while electrical stimulation is more likely to produce ejaculation. Using electrical stimulation, the man's prostate and seminal vesicles are stimulated through the rectum, and ejaculation usually occurs after 10 to 15 stimulations. Be aware that this method can result in problems, such as autonomic dysreflexia.

A vigorous finger massage of your prostate and the back part of your urethra through your rectum after the electrical stimulation can also produce some semen. If there is no visible ejaculation from the penis, your doctor will check to see if you ejaculated into your bladder. If so, you will then have a "bladder washout" with a solution that helps sperm to function well. Your sperm can then be obtained from the solution and examined to make sure they are healthy enough for use in artificial insemination (see below).

More recently, doctors have obtained sperm without ejaculation from the testicle, or epidymis (a structure that sits on top of the testicle and stores sperm). These techniques result in fewer sperm available for artificial insemination. It also requires injecting your sperm directly into the woman's egg, as described below.

Another possibility for you to consider is the use of donor sperm. This technique involves emotional issues for both you and your partner and requires careful discussion before making a decision.

How Is Artificial Insemination Done?

Artificial insemination involves several techniques. For all of these techniques, the woman is given medication to control the timing of ovulation (release of eggs) so eggs can be collected. For the intrauterine insemination technique, the man's washed, concentrated semen is used. Just before ovulation, the hormone HCG is given to cause ovulation in your partner. Your semen is placed in a small intrauterine insemination catheter (tube) that is injected high into the woman's uterus. It usually takes an average of two to three cycles to obtain a pregnancy. This technique may also used to place the semen into the fallopian tube where the egg is usually fertilized. A catheter guides the semen through the vagina using ultrasound.

What Is *In Vitro* Fertilization?

For in vitro fertilization, the eggs are placed in a dish with the man's sperm so that the sperm will fertilize several eggs. Usually more than four or five fertilized eggs are then placed into the woman at a time. The fertilized eggs are placed as high as possible in the fallopian tube with the hope that they become attached to the uterus to begin a pregnancy. One of the problems with this technique is multiple births (such as twins or triplets), which would present extra challenges for you as a couple.

Another technique for fertilization is called ISCI (IntraCytoplaSmIc, or Ich-See) injection. In a lab, a single sperm is injected directly into the egg to make sure that fertilization occurs. The eggs are placed into the woman as described above. Unfortunately, artificial insemination approximately doubles the risk of low birth weight babies and birth defects. These major birth defects probably occur before birth and involve structural, chromosomal, and genetic defects, including musculoskeletal, cardiovascular, and genitourinary defects that often require surgery. We do not know what part of the process of artificial insemination produces these problems.

It is important for you to make an informed choice about any procedures you choose to attempt to have a baby. You also have to consider the cost of artificial insemination, which is not paid for by insurance, and may run to many thousands of dollars. It is also important that you check with the doctor you plan to use and determine what his or her experience is with the techniques used, what the side effects and risks are that he or she most frequently has observed, and what he/she predicts may be problems for you with your level of injury. Also check on the doctor's success rate in achieving pregnancy.

DATING, MARRIAGE, AND DIVORCE

Will I Ever Find a Partner after an SCI?

Many people with recent spinal cord injuries wonder how they can begin to date again and appear attractive to potential boyfriends or girlfriends. If they have a boyfriend, girlfriend, or spouse, they also fear that they will be abandoned because the injury is too difficult for that person to handle. The emotional changes that can occur after an SCI, such as initial embarrassment about being seen in a wheelchair, anger, frustration, anxiety, and depression can all affect your motivation to get out of the house and into activities you enjoy. The best way to find a partner or to maintain a good relationship with your partner is to continue doing the things you want to do, ones that you most enjoy. This includes getting back to work or school, if possible, and being involved with recreational interests. If previous recreational activities are not possible for you, choose activities you can still do that you will enjoy. The kind of people you will meet while you are active with your own interests will be ones with whom you will more naturally connect.

Being assertive is also important in finding a partner. Being open and honest in how you respond to others helps you to find people who will be open and honest with you. One of the most important things you can find in a partner is someone with whom you can feel totally comfortable to be your true self. If you feel like you have to cover up your real feelings that are negative because the person cannot handle them, then he or she will not be a good match for you.

Because friendship is essential to a good relationship, it is important to try to establish friendships with people in whom you may be interested. This approach can be a lot less threatening than asking someone on a date right away. Since you probably already have friends you did things with before your injury, you can ask someone to go out with you and your friends to a movie or to a friend's house. Some people with SCI find it easier to make friends of the opposite sex because they are no longer seen as a threat and it is an excellent way to really get to know someone. Later, you can see if he or she is the kind of person with whom you want to share a long-term relationship.

How Do I Find the Right Person for Me?

It's helpful to think through the kind of person you would like to meet as a partner. What values are important to you? What characteristics in a person do you admire and respect? What are the essentials that you need to find in a partner? It is important to identify these qualities so that when you are tempted to be with someone who does not fit these essentials, you can remember their importance and keep looking. For example, if your faith in God is important to you and essential to share with a partner, then you might look for potential partners in a church, synagogue, or mosque. If you value an artistic talent, then you might want to take an art class and develop friendships with people in the class.

Will Some People Take Advantage of Me Sexually?

It is also important not to allow anyone to take advantage of you as a disabled person. Some people may see a disabled person as an easy target for sex. Hospitals have shown some concern about abuse of patients occurring when they are not able to defend themselves. Be sure to report anything that happens to you that you are not comfortable with, no matter what it may be, including any unwanted sexual advances by hospital or other medical staff, friends, or family members. No matter what you may be threatened with, if you inform someone about this inappropriate behavior, it is essential you do so to protect yourself and anyone else the person may be hurting. Do not let yourself suffer in this type of situation by remaining silent, no matter what you fear the consequences may be.

Another issue is that some people with SCI may feel so desperate to have any relationship that they are not very careful about whom they choose to be with sexually. This problem can be serious because you may feel used by certain people, which can be an experience more painful than being alone. In these situations, if you don't use protection, you can become infected with sexually transmitted diseases. These diseases, which include hepatitis B and C and HIV (the virus that causes AIDS), can be chronic and can affect your health and life seriously.

If you feel used, ask yourself why you allowed it to happen. By recognizing your own insecurities, you can begin to deal with them more directly and start thinking about how important your self-respect is to the rest of your life.

If you were abused in your past by parents or others, developing your own positive sense of self is important. Developing your own positive self will prevent you from seeking out abusive relationships without realizing it. Getting a mental health professional to help you with this process is usually very important.

What Can I Do if I'm Scared My Partner Will Leave Me?

If you are in a relationship you have had for years at the time of your SCI, you may be questioning whether your loved one can take the stress of dealing with the huge changes that have happened in your life. These issues should not be swept under the rug. Bringing them out in the open and seeing how your partner deals with them is very important. It is a bad sign if your partner does not want to talk about them with you. Communication is essential to any good relationship, yet many couples have never been able to share with each other at a deep level. Their most important problems in the relationship have not been handled and resolved. Getting help from a pastor or mental health professional may be very important to you if you and your loved one are in this situation because your stress levels increase so much on both sides after one of you has had a spinal cord injury. If you cannot decrease these stress levels by talking with each other regularly, your relationship will be difficult.

How Can I Deal with Problems in My Relationship?

Some relationships end in divorce or break up after an SCI. Most of these relationship problems stem from a troubled relationship before the injury, and the SCI put it over the edge. If your partner was not fully committed to you before your injury, then he or she will have a difficult time dealing with this additional problem in your lives together. Even if the commitment was solid and communication was good between you, the stress of the SCI can make it feel that you are at a breaking point in your relationship in the early stage as you recover. We all are more difficult to get along with and communicate with when we are tired or frustrated about something. Think of the frustrations you and your partner go through every day since your SCI and realize that this stress takes a toll on both of you. Be kind to each other when either of you is feeling burned out. Try to evaluate how you can support each other and take time to be together, just the two of you.

How Do I Deal with the End of My Relationship?

Divorce or the death of a spouse are traumatic and overwhelming events in any person's life, but these events can be faced with courage and perseverance. Both involve intense feelings of loss, sadness, and often depression and anxiety. It is difficult to understand at the time you are experiencing these events in your life and wondering how you will survive. You may even wonder if life is worth living. If you become very depressed and feel like killing yourself, you need to find a mental health professional for help, and you may need to take an antidepressant medication.

The most important thing to do for yourself is grieve over the loss of the relationship with friends and family and keep in touch with the people who love you. Finding groups that support those going through divorce or bereavement can be an important resource to prevent you from becoming too isolated and lonely. It helps to know that others have the same intense feelings and to be able to share these feelings with those who understand them firsthand. At times like these, you may stop taking good care of yourself and your body. You may also have to set up more home care and community resources for yourself with your partner gone. A mental health professional at your local rehabilitation hospital can help you to identify your needs for support and find the organizations that can provide that support.

Chapter 3 provides more information about adjusting to relationship changes after spinal cord injury.

AGING AND SEXUALITY

What Changes in My Sexual Functioning Will I Notice as I Get Older?

It is important to realize your sexual function changes with age. Not much research has been done on sexuality in people with SCI as they age. However, we do know that as men age, they experience physical changes such as testicular atrophy, low sperm count, and sperm abnormalities. Your sexual functioning also changes with age. You may have a decrease in your libido. You may develop even more problems with erections. The refractory period, or the time between getting erections, may get longer. If you can ejaculate, it may take longer for you to do so, it and it may be less intense and shorter.

As females age, they experience menopause and changes in hormonal levels. Your menstruation becomes less intense and regular and eventually stops completely. The end of your periods marks the end of being able to have children, although your fertility decreases significantly before menopause occurs. Your vagina becomes dryer, thinner, and more fragile. If you are not sexually active, your vagina can become narrower, and the entrance can become partially blocked. As a result, your sexual functioning can also be affected. You can have a loss of interest in sex and pain with intercourse if you have some sensation in your vaginal area. Your vagina is less lubricated (moist) and takes longer to become lubricated. Your genitals also become less engorged as you age. If you are able to have an orgasm, you can develop more problems with orgasm and your orgasm contractions may be less, especially if you are not as sexually active as previously.

Can I Stay Sexually Active as I Grow Older?

Despite these changes as you age, the good news is that you can remain sexually active. If you are sexually active now or want to be, you will stay sexually active as you age. Most women feel the quality of their relationships depends on how they feel their sex life is going. As a woman, it is important to make your sex life the best it can be. Do not be afraid to talk about what you want and need from your partner. As a man, don't let fatigue, boredom, illness, overweight, or performance anxiety interfere with having a good sexual relationship. Your partner will understand if your sexual functioning changes, and you can always give pleasure to your partner even if you can not have an erection or ejaculation.

Medical issues, such as hypertension, heart problems, and diabetes, can also interfere with sexual functioning as you get older. If these are a problem for you, talk to your doctor and find out if there are treatments that can reduce these effects.

It is important to have this part of your life with your partner remain strong as you age, no matter what sexual problems you suffer. Talk these problems out and tell each other what is important to both of you. Staying physically close and open to what is possible in your relationship is essential to remaining emotionally close to each other. Being patient and discovering what works as time goes on means everything to maintaining the romance in your life, no matter what your age.

MEDICATIONS AND SEXUALITY

Can Medications I Take Make My Sexual Functioning Worse?

Many medications affect sexual functioning. Table 11.5 shows you some medications that can reduce your sexual functioning.

If you are taking any of these drugs or any others and are having sexual problems, it is important for you to talk with your doctor. Find out whether the sexual changes may be caused by the drugs and if medication changes may reduce these effects. This approach is a much better idea than stopping the drugs without your doctor knowing, which can put you at risk for more medical or emotional problems.

YOUR IMAGE AS A MAN OR WOMAN

It takes time after a spinal cord injury to rebuild your self-image and begin to

Table 11.5. Medications and Their Effects on Sexual Function

Medication Type	Effects on Sexual Function
Antihypertensives (high blood pressure medication)	Yes, many affect sex drive, erections and orgasm
Atenolol	No
Clonidine (Catapres)	No for women, patch is better for men
Nadolol (Corgard/Corzide)	No for women
Labetalol (Normadyne/ Trandate)	No for women
Hydralazine (Hydra-Zide)	No for women
Thiazide diuretics	Yes, affect sex drive, erections, and ejaculations
Nicardipine	No
Cholesterol-lowering drugs	Men with high cholesterol can have problems with erection
Pravastatin (Pravachol)	No, can improve erections
Lovastatin (Advicor/Altocor/Mevacor)	No, can improve erections
Digoxin	Yes, after two years can affect sex drive, and erections
Antidepressants	Yes, can affect sex drive, orgasm, and ejaculation. Can take Yohimbine to reduce sex effects for serotonin reuptake antidepressants
Bupropion (Wellbutrin/Zyban)	No
Trazodone	No
Nefazodone (Serzone)	No
Anti-anxiety drugs	Yes
Tranquilizers(Alprazolam, Diazepam)	Yes
Buspirone (Buspar)	No
Anti-psychotic drugs	Yes
Lithium	No
Detrol	May affect erections (anticholinergic)
Neurontin	May be affected due to sedation effects
Baclofen	May affect erections (anticholinergic), sedating

feel confident and strong emotionally again. You can begin or continue a close relationship with a loved one by being honest about your and your loved one's struggles, fears, and joys. Recognize the gifts you bring to the relationship and look for ways to share love, encouragement, and caring with your loved one or with a new partner no matter how limited you may be physically.

Having experienced a major life trauma, you can become a person who has more empathy for others. Realize how precious each moment can be in your own life and in your life with your partner. Many people who have suffered an SCI feel they have learned much about themselves, what is important to them, and what is most meaningful to them from the experience of the injury. This personal and spiritual growth makes you wiser and more in tune with yourself and others. It also makes you a more interesting and mature person to whom people are naturally attracted.

Sex is the natural outcome of a caring relationship that enhances that sense of closeness and commitment to each other. Although commitment may be difficult for you to consider early on in your recovery because of fears of being rejected and abandoned, it is what most of us long for in our lives. Sexuality is a remarkable gift and a true expression of the love and commitment we want to express in deep ways. Whether you are able to have erections or orgasms in the same way as before your injury, each time together can be a time to express that sense of yourself and how important your loved one is to you in your life. The physical closeness, kissing, and looks into each others' eyes help you to say "yes" to what your relationship means to each other. It also helps you to rebuild the sense of trust and love you may forget as you deal with the challenges each day brings. Be kind to each other and to yourself as you continue in this journey.

What Can I Do?

If you feel you need help understanding your sexuality or improving a sexual relationship:

- *Communicate with your partner.* If you are married or in another relationship, talk with your partner about each other's feelings, needs, desires, and physical abilities. Communicating regularly can help you understand each other's perspectives and develop stronger connections as a couple.
- *Talk with a professional.* Ask your rehabilitation doctor, nurse, psychologist, or social worker for advice about how to adjust and address the physical or emotional aspects of your sexuality. If needed, he or she may be able to recommend a qualified sex therapist who has expertise in working with persons with disabilities. A rehabilitation professional should also be able to

advise you about where to find help with fertility and other issues.

- *Focus on your concerns.* If you decide to see a sex therapist, talk with him or her about your most important concerns as an individual or as a couple. If you are married or in a relationship, the therapist will likely want to talk with you and your partner together and separately, since you may not feel comfortable discussing some issues at first. The therapist will also be able to suggest techniques, such as relaxation training, to improve your sexual relationships.
- *Be open and honest.* Issues you may be uncomfortable talking about must be discussed eventually if they are central to your sexual problems. It may take time for you and your partner to become totally honest about the key issues that are preventing you from having the best sexual relationship you can have.

Where Can I Learn More?

To learn more about sexuality, including after spinal cord injury, you may wish to contact:

- Your rehabilitation doctor, nurse, psychologist, or social worker
- Your primary care physician
- The Spinal Cord Injury Information Network (www.spinalcord.uab.edu)
- The National Spinal Cord Injury Association (www.spinalcord.org; click on Resource Center)
- SexualHealth.com
- American Association of Sex Educators, Counselors, and Therapists, to find a sex therapist (www.aasect.org)

Appendix C provides information about additional resources.

IMPORTANT POINTS TO REMEMBER

- Men and women with spinal cord injury experience sexual changes, but they can have satisfying, active sexual relationships.
- Experimentation, creativity, and open communication with one's partner can help improve sexual satisfaction and function. Treatment, including medications and therapy by a qualified professional, can also help.
- Women and men with spinal cord injury can become parents. When needed, fertility treatment and assisted reproduction techniques often can help couples conceive and give birth to their own biological children.

—12—
So You're Having a Baby?

JUDI ROGERS
SUZANNE L. GROAH

"My son is five years old now, and being a parent during those five years has been a remarkable journey—just as it is for all new parents. In fact, the whole process has been easier than I expected it would be." –LaShonne

Having a SCI does not prevent a woman from becoming pregnant or being a parent. Any woman, with or without a SCI, may choose to become a mother. While this chapter addresses many of the issues that a woman with SCI may face during pregnancy, it is written primarily for women who are, or want to become, pregnant and for men who want to gain a better understanding of the impact of pregnancy on a woman, both physically and emotionally.

Because functional abilities vary from individual to individual after SCI, a broad range of abilities and disabilities must be addressed when discussing pregnancy and delivery. This chapter provides information that may help you plan for a pregnancy, whether you and your partner are pregnant now or considering getting pregnant in the future. It discusses:

- Choosing a doctor to manage your pregnancy and delivery
- Common pregnancy side effects
- Pregnancy side effects related to your spinal cord injury
- The role of your **rehabilitation team** in your pregnancy
- Recognizing signs of labor
- Labor and delivery
- Breastfeeding

Whatever your motivations are for being a parent, you can use this chapter as guide for decision-making. We begin with finding a doctor who can care for you before, during, and after pregnancy.

FINDING A HEALTH CARE PROVIDER

It is not uncommon for health care providers to have limited knowledge of pertinent SCI issues and no experience treating individuals with SCI. While a given health care provider may have some limited experience treating women with disabilities, it is likely that he or she has not treated a woman with SCI. Pregnancy and SCI issues are typically not taught during medical school or nursing curriculum. Therefore, it may require some work to find a health care provider who has experience in this area, or you may have to educate your health care provider about some of your unique needs.

You have several options when choosing a health care provider for pregnancy care. An obstetrician/gynecologist (often referred to as "OB/Gyn") is a doctor who specializes in the medical and surgical care of women during pregnancy, childbirth, and after delivery. This type of physician has the most training in pregnancy and childbirth issues. A perinatologist is an OB/Gyn who specializes in the care of the mother and the fetus, who may have a higher chance of complications. Additionally, many times family practitioners and general practice doctors take care of women for routine pregnancy needs.

Other professionals offer services to women, such as certified nurse midwives (CNM) and doulas. A CNM is a specially trained registered nurse, who has experience in providing obstetric and newborn care. Midwives work with obstetricians, who are available to assist if complications occur during pregnancy, labor or delivery. A doula is a person who specializes in helping families through the childbearing year. Because they do not provide any clinical care, you still need to choose an obstetric health care provider since the services of a doula are often not covered by insurance.

While there is no evidence to date that there is any increase in complications in babies born to mothers with SCI, the pregnant woman with SCI is at risk for certain complications. For this reason, in most cases it is probably best that you choose an obstetrician or perinatologist who has experience treating women with SCI. In some cases a general or family practitioner may be amply qualified to take care of your obstetric needs, especially if that person has experience working with others with SCI and if you have a mild injury and are not at risk for many complications (such as autonomic dysreflexia). When choosing a primary obstetric health care provider, you need to weigh the following factors:

• Do you prefer an OB or are you comfortable with a qualified generalist or midwife?

- If you prefer an OB, would you feel more comfortable with a perinatologist?
- What priority do you put on your health care provider having experience treating other women with SCI?
- How far away is you health care provider?

In addition to the health care provider performing your obstetric care, building a pregnancy team can be a good way of optimizing your care. Other members of your team might include your urologist (bladder specialist), your physiatrist (physical rehabilitation doctor), and your physical and occupational therapists. Each of the team members can help manage specific problems associated with pregnancy that you may encounter. If you can't find team members who have experience working with people with SCI, then having doctors and therapists who are interested in learning the issues is critical. To find doctors and therapists in your area, talk with other women with SCI or contact the organizations listed below and in Appendix C of this book.

THE FIRST VISIT

Because it will take some time and energy to find doctors and therapists, ideally you should start identifying these professionals before you get pregnant. The benefit of this approach is that you can have an appointment with you obstetrician for a preconception visit, which is a doctor's visit that occurs before you conceive. Your doctor will have some recommendations for you even at this early stage. These recommendations may relate to your diet, taking prenatal vitamins that have enough folate and other critical vitamins, or the safety of the medications you are currently taking. He or she may also check to see if you are anemic. An initial examination may be included in this initial visit.

During your first visit, you can gain much information by just talking with the doctor and office staff and assessing the accessibility of the office. One topic you might want to discuss is the type of delivery you may have. Having a SCI doesn't necessarily mean that you will need a cesarean section. (See the "Labor and Delivery" section below for more information.) If your doctor hasn't cared for women with SCI before, he or she may not be aware of this fact, and you may need to educate your doctor on this point.

In addition to general questions about pregnancy, other issues to consider related more to SCI and accessibility might include:

- Is the exam table accessible?
- Is it easy to be weighed? (Many offices do not have an accessible scale.

Finding a way to be weighed accurately throughout your pregnancy is critical.)

• Is it easy for you to bring in urine specimens?
• Will there be an easy way to get help if you need it while you are alone on
  the exam table?
• If you are able to stand and/or walk to some degree, are there support bars
  in the bathroom? (You may not need these most of the time, but by the
  sixth month of pregnancy having support bars can be necessary and helpful.)
• If you use a wheelchair, is there enough room to turn your chair in the
  examining room and/or bathroom?
• Is there enough room in the examining room and/or bathroom to allow
  you to close the door and maintain your privacy?

COMMON PREGNANCY DISCOMFORTS—WHAT CAN I EXPECT?

Every woman wonders what pregnancy will be like, regardless of whether she
has a SCI or not. While pregnancy is a truly wonderful, memorable, and special time in your life, there are also aspects of pregnancy that you might prefer to forget. Most women experience some type of pregnancy discomforts.
You will not know which discomforts you will experience because they
depend on many factors, such as how the baby is lying in the uterus and your
hormonal levels. You can't predict if you will experience these discomforts,
how long they may last, or how severe they will be until the pregnancy
occurs. Furthermore, these problems tend to vary with each person and each
pregnancy.

In addition to the "usual" discomforts associated with pregnancy, your
SCI will put you at risk of other discomforts and/or problems. Dealing with
these pregnancy discomforts can be more complicated, though, because of
your SCI. Therefore, it is best to be as knowledgeable as possible and plan
ahead. Also, your doctor may or may not be familiar with problems and discomforts that are specific to SCI. It is your responsibility to educate her
about these, to the best of your ability.

Dr. Amie Jackson of the University of Alabama did a comprehensive
study comparing women who had been pregnant both before and after a SCI
(Jackson, 1996). The study found that complications such as morning sick-
ness, anemia, toxemia, and vaginal bleeding did not change between
"before" and "after" groups. In other words, SCI did not affect many of the
common pregnancy symptoms.

In *A Disabled Women's Guide to Pregnancy and Birth* (Rogers, In Press), one
of the authors reports on a survey about problems encountered during pregnancy of women with SCI. She found that the most common first trimester

complaint was nausea, followed by fatigue and leg spasms. In the second trimester, leg **spasms** were the most common followed by impaired **mobility** and **transfers, urinary tract infection,** and **edema** (swelling of the feet and lower legs). In the third trimester, impaired mobility and transfers, edema, back pain, and spasms were the major problems reported. Other complaints reported consistently, but to a lesser degree, included constipation, heartburn, other urinary problems, and breathing issues. Of 16 pregnancies in women with SCI T6 and higher, 4 reported autonomic dysreflexia in the third trimester.

Most of these complaints are actually common complaints of all women who are pregnant. Some secondary complications of SCI are also typical of pregnancy and are likely to be exacerbated by pregnancy. Therefore, many of the problems are not new, but because of your SCI, you may find additional ways to deal with these old problems. The sections below describe common problems and discuss how to cope with them.

Fatigue

Fatigue is very common in women during pregnancy. The obvious way to handle fatigue is to rest when you feel the need, but this solution is often easier said than done. Other solutions might be to:

- Schedule short rest breaks during the day. By actually scheduling them, you may be more committed to rest even if life keeps you busy.
- If you work outside of your home and don't have a private office, you may want to inquire if there is a room that can be used for rest.
- If you have a wheelchair that tilts or reclines, use that mechanism to rest in addition to using it for pressure relief.
- Carry a small pillow to lean against a piece of furniture.
- Stay in bed for longer periods of time.
- Consider additional attendant care.

Spasticity

While many pregnant women experience muscle cramping, women with SCI are more likely to have some type of **spasticity**. In the survey of women with SCI, 48 percent of the women who were interviewed reported having muscle spasms. This spasticity can be increased because of the pregnancy, it can be a symptom of another problem such as bladder infection, or it can even be the first symptom of labor. Therefore, it's important for you to monitor your spasticity carefully and consider what else might be causing a change in spasticity.

Unfortunately, most muscle relaxants typically used for SCI spasticity are not considered safe for the developing fetus. Some women have found that taking calcium and/or B12 vitamins seems to decrease their spasms. Another option is the Baclofen Pump™, which is considered relatively safe during pregnancy. If you currently take medications for spasticity and you are unsure about their safety in pregnancy, consult with your doctor before you get pregnant to discuss what your other options are to help control spasticity.

Table 12.1 provides further information about medications typically used after SCI and their safety during pregnancy and lactation. Medications listed in Category A and B are considered safe during pregnancy (There are essentially no Category A medications, and Category B medications include prenatal vitamins and Tylenol, among others). Category C medications are those in which some adverse effects have been seen in animals, but they have not been shown to be harmful to fetuses. If the pregnant woman will benefit from the drug and the benefit outweighs the risk to the fetus then it is generally used. Category D drugs have some significant risks and should be used only in serious or life-threatening circumstances.

Table 12.1. Medication Safety During Pregnancy

Medication Purpose	Medication	Safety Category	Safety During Pregnancy	Safety During Breastfeeding
Anti-spasticity	Lioresal (Baclofen)	C	• Some birth defects possible (in animals) • No human information	• 0.1% of dose gets into the milk • Approved by American Academy of Pediatrics for use during breast-feeding
	Diazepam (Valium)	D	• Some birth defects (facial deformity) and behavioral changes in animals • If taken in third trimester, baby may have "floppy infant syndrome"	• Can accumulate in breast milk • Regular dosing not recommended during breast-feeding

(Table 12.1 continued)

	Dantrolene (Dantrium)	C	• Very little information available	• No information available
	Tizanidine (Zanaflex)	C	• Slowed development in animal studies • No human information	• It is possible, yet unknown whether this drug accumulates in breast milk
Bladder relaxant	Oxybutynin (Ditropan)	B	• Some abnormalities in animals when mother is taking very high doses	• No information available
Antibiotics	Ciprofloxacin	C	• Because of musculoskeletal problems in animals, use not recommended in pregnant women	• Recently considered compatible with breastfeeding
	Trimethoprim-sulfamethoxazole (Bactrim, Septra)	C	• Some abnormalities in animals, but none reported in humans • Do not use near delivery due to the risk of serious jaundice	• Can use during breastfeeding except when baby is premature, is jaundiced (yellow), or has G6PD deficiency
	Nitrofurantoin (Macrobid)	B	• No animal or human abnormalities reported	• Approved by American Academy of Pediatrics for use during breastfeeding
	Ampicillin	B	• No abnormalities reported	
	Tetracycline	D	• May cause severe discoloration of teeth	• The American Academy of Pediatrics has classified it as usually compatible with breast feeding
Other medications	Gabapentin (Neurontin)	C	• No information available	• Unknown whether and to what degree it is found in breast milk

(Table 12.1 continued)

	Calcium chan-nel blockers (Nifedipine)	C	• Some abnor-malities in ani-mals • Used in third trimester for preterm labor	• Compatible with breast feed-ing
	Prazosin	C	• No human information available	• Accumulates to a small amount in breast milk

Constipation

All pregnant women are prone to constipation during pregnancy, but con-stipation can be more of a problem for women with SCI. After a SCI it takes longer for your intestinal muscles to push stool through your gastrointestinal tract, putting you at greater risk of constipation. Pregnancy also causes con-stipation because your growing uterus puts pressure on your rectum making it more difficult for stool to pass. Pregnancy hormones often cause some con-stipation, and the usual prenatal multi-vitamin is high in iron, which can be constipating.

Reevaluating your bowel care program often is helpful during pregnancy because of the effects of pregnancy on the gastrointestinal tract. Of routine-ly used medications, Docusate (Colace) and Bisacodyl (Dulcolax) are con-sidered safe during pregnancy. To reduce constipation, eating a diet high in fiber, including fruits and vegetables, can help.

It's helpful to understand that not all fiber is created equal. Fiber is divid-ed into two types: soluble and insoluble. Soluble fiber dissolves in water, forms a gel-like substance in the intestines, and increases the water content in the stool. It has even been shown to lower blood cholesterol. Examples of soluble fiber include oat bran, oatmeal, beans, corn bran, carrots, apples, cit-rus fruit, legumes, and barley. Insoluble fiber, more commonly known as roughage, is fiber that cannot be dissolved in water. It helps to prevent con-stipation by swelling and softening the stool and stimulating the intestines to move. Examples of insoluble fibers are wheat bran, whole cereal grains, and vegetables. Dairy, animal products, and fatty foods contain very little or no fiber. For constipation, the fiber in wheat bran and oat bran seems to be more effective than similar amounts of fiber from fruits and vegetables.

When increasing the fiber in your diet, also increase your intake of water because fiber absorbs water. Also, experts recommend increasing fiber intake gradually, rather than suddenly, to give your intestines a chance to adapt to the change in your diet. It is always wise to increase fiber in moderation because a very high fiber intake may reduce the absorption of some nutrients. If increasing the fiber and water in your diet doesn't solve the problem, you may want to add an over-the-counter fiber supplement (with psyllium) or, with your doctor's approval, a stool softener such as Colace™.

Urination Problems and Bladder Infection

The need to urinate more often and an increased risk of bladder infection are common to all women during pregnancy. Changes in how well your bladder empties and risk of infection also occur in pregnant spinal-cord-injured women. **Self-catheterization** can be much more difficult during pregnancy because your pregnant belly blocks your vision. One solution for this problem is to use a mirror (which can be found in **adaptive equipment** catalogs) to increase your ability to guide the catheter.

Urinary leaking because of increased pressure of the growing uterus on the bladder or even mild bladder spasms can occur as well. To minimize urinary leaking when using intermittent catheterization, one urologist recommends dissolving Ditropan in sterile water and injecting this solution directly through the catheter and into the bladder. This medication can decrease bladder spasms, which cause urinary accidents, without negative effects on the fetus. If you are considering this option, it is a good idea to discuss it with your doctor first.

Because of either of the above difficulties with intermittent catheterization, some women have reported having to switch to an indwelling catheter during pregnancy. The drawback to this solution is that indwelling catheters tend to put you at greater risk of infection. Other concerns with indwelling catheter use is that the bladder may lose its elasticity, or ability to stretch and hold larger amounts of urine, or the catheter may slip out of the urethra, perhaps because of either frequent bladder spasms and/or the baby pushing on the bladder.

Prevention of bladder and kidney infections is crucial during pregnancy because this can lead to preterm labor. Ways to prevent infection from occurring include increasing your water intake, making sure you fully empty your bladder throughout the day, and avoiding use of an indwelling catheter, if possible. If you have any concern that you might have a bladder or kidney infection, see your doctor immediately so that you may have a urine sample tested for the appropriate antibiotic.

The penicillins, including ampicillin, tend to be quite safe during pregnancy. Similarly, the sulfa medications, bactrim, and sulfa are safe during the majority of pregnancy, but should be avoided in the late third trimester. If you develop a kidney infection during pregnancy, it is probably a good idea to get periodic screening urine cultures to check for a developing infection.

Some experts have also suggested all women with spinal cord injury get peri-odic screening urine cultures throughout pregnancy because of the risk of infection.

Check with your doctor or a pharmacist for information about the effects of antibiotics on the developing fetus. If you have repeat infections, be sure to discuss the use a prophylactic (preventative) dose of antibiotics with your doctor. While this approach has been found to be helpful after initial or repeat infections, this issue is controversial if you haven't had infections. It is unclear if the risk of taking preventative antibiotics outweighs the risk to the fetus.

Autonomic Dysreflexia

Autonomic dysreflexia is a spinal cord injury-specific problem that can occur during pregnancy for a variety of reasons. As you know, people who have a spinal cord injury at approximately the T6 level and above are at greater risk of experiencing autonomic dysreflexia. This condition is a reaction of the autonomic (involuntary) nervous system to certain irritating stimulation. Symptoms include high blood pressure, change in heart rate, skin color changes (pallor, redness, blue-gray coloration), and profuse sweating. (For further information, see Chapter 1.)

During pregnancy, you may experience autonomic dysreflexia caused by a bladder infection, bladder distention (from increased extra fluid intake), increased fluid from the baby, excessive pressure on the skin, or other com-mon causes of dysreflexia. To minimize the chances of getting autonomic dysreflexia, be sure to keep your catheterization volumes below 500cc if you use intermittent catheterization. In achieving this level, this you may find that you need to catheterize more frequently. Table 12.1 lists a few drugs used for autonomic dysreflexia. Generally, you want to try to identify what irri-tating stimulus is causing the dysreflexia and remove it. Medications have been successfully used to control autonomic dysreflexia in pregnant women, although extra consideration must be given to preventing hypotension, or the blood pressure falling too low. This is because the developing baby actu-ally tolerates high blood pressure better than low blood pressure.

Blood Clots

Although you had a high risk of blood clots in the first months after your spinal cord injury, this risk does not remain significantly high for the rest of your life. Theoretically, pregnancy should put you at greater risk of blood clots because of the hormones associated with pregnancy and immobility. Despite this fact, very few cases of blood clots have been reported by pregnant women with spinal cord injury. For this reason, treatment with medications to prevent blood clots is not recommended. It is important, though, to remember the symptoms of blood clots and to see your doctor immediately if you suspect that you may have one. (See Chapter 1 for more information about blood clots.)

Breathing Problems

Many women experience pulmonary, or breathing, changes during pregnancy because a pregnant woman's expanding belly takes up some of the room in her abdomen, limiting the amount her lungs can expand. It is also because of the extra energy demands of pregnancy. Additionally, if you have a high thoracic or cervical spinal cord injury, your lung function is limited as well. If you have a cervical level of spinal cord injury and you don't have much spasticity, one of the more favorable positions for breathing is lying flat on your back. Unfortunately, because the weight of the uterus might restrict blood flow while laying flat, your doctor will instruct you that you shouldn't lie on your back beyond approximately the 20th week of pregnancy. Instead, you will have to lie more on your sides. Given this, especially if you have a high thoracic or cervical spinal cord injury that affects your breathing, it is probably best to have your doctor check your lung function periodically. A simple breathing test, called a vital capacity measurement, can be done quickly and easily in the doctor's office.

Anemia

Anemia is a common problem encountered by pregnant women. Research has found that in non-spinal-cord-injured persons, anemia results from dilution of the blood, which is actually beneficial to pregnant women. While mild anemia is generally not considered to be a serious problem, the major consideration for women with spinal cord injury is that severe anemia may increase the risk of skin breakdown. Treatment for anemia usually involves increasing iron intake in the diet and/or through the use of an iron supplement. In severe cases, a blood transfusion may be needed. Careful treatment is recommended, though, because of the risk of constipation associated with iron supplementation.

Pressure Sores

While some people believe that women with spinal cord injury have an increased risk of developing **pressure sores** because of the extra weight of pregnancy, we have not seen any evidence of this risk. One study found that only 6 percent of pregnant women with spinal cord injury experienced a pressure sore (Jackson, 1996). Interestingly, many women with spinal cord injury who were interviewed found that their skin condition improved during pregnancy.

It seems that, no matter which type of spinal dysfunction a person has, there is anecdotal evidence that pressure sores are more likely to heal during pregnancy. This phenomenon of certain conditions or diseases improving during pregnancy has been observed in other diseases, and in this situation, the improvements may be caused by the changing hormone levels that occur during pregnancy, increased blood volume that occurs as a result of pregnancy, and/or perhaps partly because of the improved diet that most women adopt during pregnancy. Regardless, it is safer to maintain a healthy fear of pressure sores since the consequences can be catastrophic or even deadly.

In nearly all cases, a pressure sore is a preventable complication of spinal cord injury. Whether you are pregnant or not, it is important to continue to perform your twice daily skin checks, eat a healthy diet, drink a healthy amount of water, and do your weight shifts every 15 minutes to 20 minutes. Additional considerations during pregnancy include using a larger wheelchair to accommodate your growing body (described in greater detail below) and suggesting that your doctor incorporate skin checks into your regular doctor appointments.

FINDING A WHEELCHAIR THAT FITS ALL OF YOU

Most insurance companies restrict payment for a new wheelchair to no more than once every five years. Therefore, since your body size will obviously change as a result of pregnancy, you need to plan ahead with regard to the fit of your wheelchair. No one can predict how big you will become during pregnancy, so it is wise to order a chair that gives you more flexibility.

Ideally, you should have both a power chair and a manual chair. A manual chair is more convenient because you can travel in any car rather than relying on a van. "Wheeling" your manual chair also helps you to maintain good physical conditioning. Later in pregnancy your center of gravity changes and your lungs don't have as much room to expand, so you may find it more difficult to push the chair up an incline. In the latest stages of pregnancy, any mobility may become more difficult because of your growing belly and fatigue. Therefore, a properly fitting chair for your changing body, or even a power wheelchair, can prevent putting further undo strain on your body.

When ordering a power wheelchair, you should consider the features that you might use while pregnant even if you don't need them now. For example, the tilt-and-recline features can help you change position in order to relieve pressure on your skin. You may also be comfortable enough to rest in the chair rather than getting into bed. However, when a wheelchair is in the tilt-and-recline position, much more space is needed to move around. If you want to stay in the reclined position, it can be a problem in a small space. An **occupational therapist** or a **physical therapist** can help you decide the features you may need.

THE BENEFITS OF OCCUPATIONAL AND PHYSICAL THERAPY

Physical therapy and occupational therapy can be beneficial both at the beginning of pregnancy and at or about the end of the second trimester. Early on, before your body has undergone many of the changes associated with pregnancy, it is helpful to practice baby care tasks and organize your baby care equipment with help from family, friends, or even an occupational therapist (OT). For example, in the early months of pregnancy, you can learn and practice transferring a baby to a diapering surface, and find a carrier such as a front pack or a sling that would work best for you. (See Chapter 13 for more information.)

Toward the end of the second trimester, you may find that your sense of balance has changed, and you may need to experiment with different techniques to transfer. If you were able to walk before your pregnancy, you may need a wheelchair toward the end of pregnancy. Working with a physical therapist (PT) can help maintain safety throughout pregnancy and can help you regain the ability to walk after delivery.

A PT can also help you deal with muscle spasms (especially the calf muscles), which are another common pregnancy discomfort. A PT may be able to reduce the muscle spasms by stretching and ranging the leg and/or teaching an attendant to range (move and stretch) the leg, especially the calf, every day. A PT may also recommend other methods such heat or ice. In addition, the PT can help with techniques to reduce muscle spasm during labor and can help you find different positions for labor and delivery.

LABOR AND DELIVERY—WHAT SHOULD I KNOW?

Because of certain risks of secondary conditions associated with spinal cord injury, it's a good idea to talk with your doctor about special considerations during labor and delivery—and to do it well before labor begins. For example, your doctor needs to be aware that frequent position changes are needed to avoid skin breakdown. In addition, bladder overfilling should be avoided with frequent bladder emptying or placement of an indwelling catheter.

Knowing When Labor Begins

The uterus receives nerve input from the T10-T12 nerves. Theoretically, if your injury is complete at the level of T10 and above, you likely will not feel labor pains. In reality, many women with higher levels of spinal cord injury do perceive labor—but in different ways than able-bodied women do. You might feel intermittent gas pains, abdominal tightening, backache, pelvic pressure, and/or an increase in spasticity. If your injury is at the T6 level or higher, you should pay special attention to and possibly be periodically monitored for autonomic dysreflexia. Possible labor signs may include:

• A bloody show—You may see a bloody, mucous discharge that often occurs hours to weeks before labor starts.
• Breaking of the bag of water—Only about 15 percent of women break their "bag of water" at the start of labor. If you have leaking around the catheter, it may be difficult to distinguish between urine and amniotic fluid. By having litmus paper on hand you can be prepared to distinguish between them. Urine is acidic and will turn the litmus paper red. Amniotic fluid is basic and will turn the litmus paper blue. In situations in which the liquid is a combination of the two (urine and amniotic fluid), smell can help distinguish the two.
• Labor pain—This is different for everyone but may feel like period cramps.
• Autonomic dysreflexia—If your injury is at T6 or higher.
• Back labor pain—One-third of all women experience this classically severe pain, which is caused by the back of the baby's head facing the spine so that the hard part of the head compresses some of the lower back spinal nerves. You may experience this as severe back pain, feeling "unwell" or you may feel generally uncomfortable.

Another way to know that you are in labor is to feel your abdominal muscles with your hands (uterine palpation) to check for tightening. A home monitor also may be used to help detect the beginning of labor, although monitors have not been found to be helpful for some women with other pregnancy difficulties.

Preterm Labor

The information available is somewhat limited, but preterm labor occurs either with approximately the same or slightly greater frequency in women with spinal cord injury. Therefore, it is important to stay in close contact with your doctor, especially as you enter the third trimester. Some experts recommend more frequent doctor visits, or even weekly cervical examinations, from the 28th week through the time labor has started. In any case, it is important for you to self-monitor using the techniques listed above.

Dealing with Dysreflexia

If you are at risk for, or frequently get, autonomic dysreflexia, you may want to consider epidural anesthesia, a method of labor-pain relief. An epidural can prevent or avert autonomic dysreflexia and should be started when labor begins. Ask your obstetrician to schedule an appointment with a member of the anesthesiology team a month or two before your expected delivery date. It is important to keep a copy of your records in case you go into labor before your due date or if a different anesthesiologist works with you. Be sure to notify your doctor if you have any sensation around your birth canal. You want to make sure to get appropriate pain control (if you want it).

Also, the likelihood of autonomic dysreflexia increases if labor is induced (begun) with medications, rather than waiting for labor to start naturally. For this reason, you and your doctor can plan to have an anesthesiologist nearby. Contractions brought about by induction medication are stronger than usual. Talk with your doctor about this well before your expected delivery date.

Vaginal Versus Cesarean Delivery

Many women with spinal cord injury can give birth vaginally (through the birth canal) because the uterus works as automatically as your heart. Generally you don't need to use abdominal (stomach) muscles to push out the baby. Special considerations for those having a vaginal delivery include:

- Frequent position changes to prevent skin breakdown
- Bed delivery is preferred to on the delivery table due to risk of skin breakdown
- Considering the side-lying position with the upper leg flexed or support from two people due to inability to use stirrups because of spasticity or contractures
- Frequent bladder emptying or use of an indwelling catheter

The alternative to vaginal delivery is cesarean section or C-section. This surgery involves delivery of the baby through an incision near the mother's pubic line, rather than through the birth canal. As long as there are no medical reasons that would favor a C-section, vaginal birth is often a healthier choice for you and your child. Although SCI itself is not a reason to have a C-section, a number of medical reasons are associated with spinal cord injury

that may increase the need for a C-section. In addition to the usual obstet-
rical reasons, if you have had your spinal cord injury for a long time, you
may have a contracted or tight pelvis, which makes vaginal delivery much
more difficult because the shape of the pelvis makes it difficult for the fetus
to travel down the birth canal. C-section can be a life-saving surgery if you
have autonomic dysreflexia that is not improving with medications or
anesthesia. C-sections are so commonplace today that we tend to forget
that they are major abdominal surgery. As a result, recovery often takes
longer than vaginal delivery. During recovery, you may experience more
difficulty with transfers, self-care, and some baby care tasks. Be sure to discuss the pros and cons of the different types of delivery with your doctor.

WILL I BE ABLE TO BREASTFEED?

There are advantages and disadvantages to both breastfeeding and bottle-
feeding. Babies can be healthy and happy with either method. (See Table
12.2 for decision-making guidelines.) Women who are limited in the physical care they can provide their babies, are very motivated to breastfeed. In
this situation, nursing can be a special way to connect with your baby.

There are several challenges to take into account, some of which are
unique to spinal cord injury. These challenges include low milk production, autonomic dysreflexia, spasticity, breast infection, and positioning
the baby.

Low Milk Production

If your injury is at T4 and above, you may have difficulty with milk production. In spite of limited milk production, some women continue to
nurse and supplement their milk with formula. You may also find that one
breast produces more milk than the other and/or your baby may have a
preference for one side more than the other. One suggestion in this situation is to have the baby nurse on the side he doesn't prefer first when he is
hungriest and his suck is the strongest. Milk production issues are not an
uncommon nursing problem. Suggestions to increase milk supply include
to:

• Drink plenty of water (the rule of thumb is to drink an 8 ounce glass of
  water each time you nurse).
• Rest.
• Drink fenugreek tea. (Be aware of unwanted side effects, which may
  include gas, maple syrup smell of urine and sweat, loose stools, low blood
  sugar, uterine contractions, and lowering of blood glucose levels).

- Consume brewer's yeast
- Eat oatmeal together with fenugreek.
- Take the prescription medication Metoclopramide (Reglan). Be aware that this medication is also prescribed for constipation, so it may cause unwanted bowel movements.

Autonomic Dysreflexia and Spasticity

Autonomic dysreflexia and/or spasticity can be triggered by overly full breasts (engorgement) or the baby latching onto the nipple. It is important, therefore, to be prepared to nurse or pump when these problems arise. Autonomic dysreflexia and increased spasticity can also be early warning signs of breast infection. Other signs of a breast infection may include breast pain, redness of the breast, tenderness to touch, fever, malaise, and other body aches. It is important to get medical attention if you think you may have a breast infection since this condition is treated with antibiotics. It is important to continue nursing if you do have a breast infection. This often helps to clear the infection, and your baby will not get the infection from you.

Positioning

One of the keys for successful nursing is finding both a comfortable position and using a nursing pillow, challenging tasks for women regardless of disability. Options might include a pillow placed on top of a lap tray, an adapted sling to help hold the baby while nursing, or side-lying in bed.

If you decide to bottle-feed, bring bottles to the hospital that are easy for you to hold because hospitals often stock only small glass bottles. To hold an 8-ounce bottle easily, you can use a universal cuff made for a telephone receiver. It may be a good idea to try out some bottles that friends or family may have before your baby is born. You don't want to have to worry about how to hold the bottle when you're just getting used to holding a baby!

Whichever method you choose, burping the baby can be problematic. You can try the following techniques to burp your baby:

- Sit the baby on your lap facing out and stroke upward on the baby's tummy.
- Sit the baby on your lap facing out, lean the baby over your crossed arms, and rock the baby slightly forward on your arms.
- Lay the baby on his right side and roll the baby slightly onto his or her tummy.

ADOPTION MAY BE AN OPTION

If you and your partner can't get pregnant or you choose not to carry a baby, adoption is a good alternative. Many adoption agencies are sensitive to the issue of disability.

Table 12.2. Breastfeed or Bottle-feed? Advantages and Disadvantages for Parents with Spinal Cord Injury

Type of Feeding	Advantages	Disadvantages
Breastfeeding	• Colostrum (first milk released) contains antibodies • Breast milk is more digestible • Baby may be less likely to develop allergies • Nursing releases hormone to shrink uterus • No cost for formula with breastfeeding only	• Baby may need to be fed more often • Mother may need to postpone certain medications • May cause vaginal dryness affecting sexual relations • Can increase autonomic dysreflexia • Mother may feel more confined • May be too difficult or uncomfortable to nurse in public • Baby may be more likely to develop jaundice • Other people cannot help with feedings
Bottle-feeding	• Other people can feed the baby, allowing mother to sleep through the night, go to appointments, etc. • Easier to feed baby (easier to position baby, inverted nipples are not a problem) • Mother's milk production is not a factor	• Baby does not get health benefits of breastfeeding if bottle-fed only • Preparation and cleaning of bottles • Adapted equipment may be needed in order to hold the bottle can be • Cost of formula

Table 12.3. Pregnancy Planner

Whom should my OB and I consult with?	Possible specialists:
• Do I have a disability specialist doctor? • Do I need my medications evaluated and/or changed?	• Physiatrist (if specializing in spinal cord injury care, may be able to address all of the issues below)
• Do I have problems with bladder infections? Do I have problems with breathing? • Do I have internal special medical devices, i.e., Baclofen™ pump?	• Urologist • Nephrologist (kidney specialist) • Pulmonologist (breathing specialist) • Anesthesiologist
Do I need a new or additional mobility aid?	**Possible devices:**
• If I gain a lot of weight during my pregnancy, will my wheelchair continue to fit and not cause skin breakdown? • Can I independently transfer out of the wheelchair to lie down when I am experiencing fatigue or dizziness? • Will the wheelchair provide clearance under tables, desks, or other potential baby-care surfaces? • What mobility devices may assist with my physical fitness during pregnancy so I don't lose function? • During late pregnancy can I push myself up an incline?	• Larger wheelchair • Power chair with tilt-and-recline

What Can I Do?

To help ensure a successful pregnancy and birth, be sure to:

• Educate yourself and your partner. Talk with other women with spinal cord injury who have given birth and read as much as you can about pregnancy

and birth, including for women with spinal cord injury.
- Find the right doctor. Look for an obstetrician or perinatologist with whom you think you can work and who is amenable to caring for you.
- Build a team. Ask your doctor to work as a team with urologist, physiatrist, and occupational and physical therapist.
- Be a self-advocate. Be sure to talk with your doctor and other health care providers about your specific needs and issues that might arise during pregnancy and childbirth. Voice any concerns, ask questions, and contact your doctor if problems or potential problems arise.

Where Can I Learn More?

To learn more about pregnancy and birth for women with spinal cord injury, you may wish to use the following resources:

- Through the Looking Glass (www.lookingglass.org)
- Your obstetrician
- Your physiatrist (physical medicine and rehabilitation doctor)
- An occupational therapist or physical therapist

Appendix C provides information about additional resources.

IMPORTANT POINTS TO REMEMBER

- Women with spinal cord injury can become pregnant and give birth, including by vaginal delivery. Breastfeeding is also an option for mothers with spinal cord injury.
- While pregnant, women with SCI may have fatigue, constipation, and other discomforts experienced by women without spinal cord injury. They may experience urinary and bladder problems, autonomic dysreflexia, pressure sores, and other challenges that require special medical care.
- A team approach to prenatal care can help prevent problems and ensure a healthy pregnancy and successful birth experience.

Acknowledgment

Most of the information presented here is derived from Judi Rogers's research for the second edition of A *Disabled Women's Guide To Pregnancy and Birth*. Judi Rogers is an occupational therapist at Through the Looking Glass (TLG). Her work at TLG has provided her with vital experiences and information on parenting. In addition, her work has given her an opportunity to make contacts that led her to some of the 90 women interviewed for her book. The book covers 22 different types of disabilities. Of these, there were 22 women with some form of spinal dysfunction.

REFERENCES

Jackson, A. B. Pregnancy and Delivery. In: D. Krotoski, M. Nosek, and M. Turk, eds. *Women With Physical Disabilities Achieving and Maintaining Health and Well-Being*, Baltimore, MD: Paul Brooks Publishing Company, 1996: 92.

Rogers J. *A Disabled Women's Guide To Pregnancy and Birth Pregnancy and Birth*, New York: Demos Publications (In Press), 2005.

—13—

Parenting After Spinal Cord Injury: From Rehabilitation to Home

CHRISTI TULEJA
JUDI ROGERS

"What children most need from their parents are unconditional love, unlimited time, and the knowledge that we will be there for them unfailingly." –Robert

After a spinal cord injury you will face many new challenges throughout your life. In this book, you have also learned that although fertility is altered, especially for men with spinal cord injury, the ability to conceive a biologic child is still possible. This chapter discusses the next step: raising children. The primary focus of this chapter is parenting during the early years with an emphasis on baby and toddler care. Discipline, school years, and family recreation are also briefly discussed. In this chapter you will learn about:

- Baby care, including useful baby care equipment, accessories, and home readiness
- Child cooperation and discipline
- Parenting school-age children
- Family recreation possibilities

PARENTING—A REWARDING PROCESS

Regardless of whether you have a spinal cord injury or not, raising children is one of the most rewarding and challenging experiences of your life. It may surprise some people, but individuals with disabilities around the world have been parenting and grandparenting successfully for generations. Like other aspects of living with spinal cord injury, parenting is a process of discovering what works and what doesn't. Some of the greatest challenges can occur during the first year of a child's life when the physical demands of parenting are greatest. After the first year the child can participate more, and parenting becomes less physical and more psychological in nature. Out of necessity, parents have come up with nontraditional ways to care for babies since baby accessories and home environments can create barriers rather than reduce them.[1, 2]

Resources are increasingly available for parents. The Internet has provided ways to get immediate information and to connect you with other parents. Recent research has looked at how helpful specially designed or altered baby equipment and accessories can be for parents.[3, 4] For example, modified equipment can bring a parent and child close for caressing, nuzzling, and eye contact. It can make tasks easier and help prevent secondary disabilities such as neck and back problems.[5] The research also shows that having support from individuals or professionals, who believe you can be involved in your baby's care, can boost confidence and tremendously affect the willingness to take on more baby care responsibilities.

BABY CARE

Caring for a baby is the first of many parenting experiences. During baby care, moments of intimacy and interaction occur that you will cherish for the rest of your life. It is important to discover your own personal care style and move beyond conventional ways of caring for babies and toddlers. New ideas of how to perform baby care activities can come from your own ingenuity, as well as from other parents within the disability community, the Internet, videotapes of parents completing baby care tasks, or a trained occupational therapist. (See Appendix C for resources.) If you are someone who has lived with spinal cord injury for a considerable amount of time, you have likely already developed strategies for everyday living that can be useful in baby care. By planning ahead, being creative in handling challenges as they come up, and getting a little support from family and friends, you can be involved in care or be the primary caregiver for your baby.

The Rehabilitation Unit—Getting Reacquainted with Your Baby or Toddler

You may have had a period of separation from your baby or toddler for a variety of reasons related to your spinal cord injury. If you already had a baby or toddler at the time of your spinal cord injury, then your initial hospitalization and rehabilitation may have caused a separation. Likewise, if you've been injured for a while, a medical complication resulting in hospitalization could have caused a separation. You can expect your baby or toddler to go through a period of adjustment as he or she transitions back into your care.

As early as possible, have your baby or toddler visit daily or as regularly as possible. Encourage the occupational therapist to include baby care in your therapy. Communicate your wishes with your doctor, therapist, and other key rehabilitation team members, and tell them how important and extremely motivating it to be with your baby or toddler. During the initial visits with your baby, focus on activities that foster your relationship. The following are some examples of activities to do with your baby either during rehabilitation or at home:

- If you have a high (cervical) spinal cord injury, you can feel and nuzzle your baby by having someone place your baby near your neck where you have sensation. Use supportive pillows under and around the baby to maintain the position.
- Find positions that are comfortable for the two of you to talk and play in. For example, you can face each other lying down together on a plinth (a flat raised cushioned surface) in the therapy room.
- While sitting up in the hospital bed, use pillows, foam wedges, or a baby car seat to allow your baby to be supported upright and facing you and near enough to exchange gazes. Have your family bring your baby's favorite toys, such as rattles, to the hospital for your visit. Use your mouth if you are unable to use your hands to secure the toy and attract your baby's attention.
- Tie a couple of toys to a hat and wear it. Shake the toys with your head to engage your baby.
- Use facial expressions to draw your baby toward you. Stick your tongue out and wait to see if your baby imitates you and stick his or her tongue out, or stick your tongue out and when your baby reaches for it, slip it back into your mouth. Close and open your eyes or slowly alternate blinking your eyes.
- Connect and find intimacy with your baby through bottle-feeding. (See Appendix D for adaptation suggestions.)
- Sing, talk, and imitate your baby's sounds to enjoy each other and get reacquainted.

The following are examples of activities that you can do together with your toddler:

- Play computer games designed for young children. You can participate by playing together, cheering your child on, or helping them think out what to do.
- Hold a paintbrush with your mouth and paint with your child.
- Use switch-operated toys (for example, battery-operated toys that have been altered to be used by a simple touch-see resource) designed for children with disabilities. These toys may be available from a hospital pediatric department.
- Read or make up stories together.
- Audiotape yourself reading an age-appropriate book so that your toddler can go through the book at home with your voice.

Once you feel that you and your child are more comfortable, include more baby care in your visits. You should find that practicing baby care goes more smoothly as your child becomes reacquainted with you.

Baby Care Problem Solving

You may find the Baby Care Planner (Appendix D) to be helpful in figuring out which baby care activities you can do and which might be challenging. The planner lists all the baby care activities and steps within each activity. You and your family or occupational therapist together can find ways to complete each step. The first activities—holding, positional changes, and carrying—and moving along with lifting and placing (which is listed under each baby care task) are important since they are part of all baby care activities. Many parents will tell you that these activities may be more difficult than the task itself. For example, lifting and placing a child into a highchair can be more difficult than the actual spoon-feeding. Through The Looking Glass research[6] also finds that most parents find "transitional tasks" (holding, positional changes, etc.) to be the most challenging and deserving of the parent's attention first.

Don't feel you have to have solutions to everything right away. Choose one or two baby care activities that are most important to you. Later you can build on your experiences by adding more baby care responsibilities. Initially, think about how to be involved in your baby's care rather than how to be independent. For example, at first you could have someone bring the baby to you, then you feed your baby a bottle. Your confidence will develop as you do more baby care. As stated earlier, ask your occupational therapist to incorporate baby care activities into your intervention plan since you are really working on two goals at the same time: learning to do baby care and increasing your strength and endurance. If you are separated from your child because of hospitalization, you may want to practice with a weighted doll to build your strength, techniques, and confidence between visits with your child.

Some general guidelines about goal-setting in relation to your level of injury and parenting the baby or toddler are as follows. Generally speaking, if you are a wheelchair user and have good use of your hands (T8 or below), focus on developing solutions to inaccessible baby care surfaces, such as the diapering surface or crib. If you have use of your hands but some trouble with your trunk (C7/8 to T8), you will still need accessible surfaces and strategies on how to pick up and place your baby without falling over. If you have little or no use of your hands (C5 to C7/8), you will need accessible wheelchair surfaces, lifting tricks, and solutions for doing small motor tasks such as using diapering tabs and zippers. Table 13.1 offers adaptation suggestions.

For the most part, if you are independent in self-care activities, you have the skills to care for your child independently. This statement does not mean that you can't care for your child if you are not independent, but you will need a few more helpful gadgets, such as modified baby care equipment and some unique baby-handling skills.

Baby Care Equipment and Accessories

When searching for equipment that helps with baby care, first look at commercially available products. More and more companies are designing products for ease of use that may be helpful for a parent with a physical disability resulting from spinal cord injury. One such product is the *Arms Reach Co-Sleeper* from Arms Reach Concepts®. This bassinet opens on one side and attaches to the parents' bed, removing the need for the parent to get out of bed in order to nurse or comfort the baby. Some commercially available baby equipment can be beneficial if used differently than intended. For example, the Boppy™ nursing pillow can give a wheelchair user the means to support a newborn on their lap.

You may find that baby care products on the market will not match your modifications of equipment or a newly designed piece of equipment is necessary. For ideas on useful baby care products, modifications, and newly created baby care equipment, refer to *Adaptive Baby Care Equipment: Guidelines, Prototypes & Resources.*[7] This resource provides pictures and descriptions of more than 50 baby care ideas and examples developed at Through the Looking Glass. Although these products are not for sale, Through the Looking Glass can offer local face-to-face assistance or assistance over the phone.

If you need to make or modify a piece of baby care equipment, look to occupational therapists, woodworkers, sewers, welders, plastics workers, engineering students, wheelchair repair shops, and anyone skilled in using heavy-duty sewing machines (shoe-repair, sail or parachute makers). Safety should be the priority in developing the equipment. Once you have begun using the equipment, family and professionals need to routinely monitor the modifications for broken or worn-out parts, loose bolts, ineffective Velcro™, etc. The child's growth and development, or a change in your functioning, may make a previously safe adaptation unsafe. Figure 13.1 suggests strategies and equipment, based on your abilities, that can help you care for your baby. You can keep track of your own ideas by putting them in your Baby Care Planner (Appendix D).

Getting Your Home Ready

It cannot be overstated that being organized and prepared helps baby care activities go smoothly. Having all diapering items together on your diapering surface or in one container can save energy and time, which is especially important with a toddler who may not want his diaper changed in the first place. Placing items at reachable levels minimizes bending or reaching. If organization is not your strength, find a friend, family member, or occupational therapist to assist you in streamlining your baby care process.

Consider placing the diapering table, highchair, and other baby care accessories near each other, decreasing the need for you to go from room to room to do various activities. Create a gated or corralled play space for the child in the same area. Your mobility aids (such as your wheelchair or walker) and your child care equipment can take up a lot of room. Therefore, look for baby care products that are compact and serve many purposes.

As your child becomes able to crawl and move around, childproofing becomes necessary. Childproofing can be one of the more challenging areas to problem-solve since restricting the child can also mean restricting you. However, the more you childproof your house, the less you will need to say "no" to your child and the more freedom he or she will have to play. The best solution for childproofing is obviously removing unsafe or breakable items from the area. When that's not possible, childproofing gadgets on the market can be helpful for parents with some hand function. One example is the First Alert" "Swing and Lock" one-handed release safety gate that has no bottom bar and is more accessible for a wheelchair user. If that doesn't work for you, look to creating your own safety system such as a dowel gate.[8] Another suggestion would be to purchase from your local hardware store a "Draw-Catch" lock and insert a carabiner (an oblong metal ring with a spring clip) in the place of the key lock. This device creates a two-step lock, which most children take time to figure out or give up all together.

Managing In-Home Help

Whether it's family, friends, or paid assistance, you need to decide how you will make use of the help in your home. Would you prefer them to do household chores so you can save energy for caring for your baby? Or would like them to assist you directly in caring for your baby—or a mixture of both household chores and baby care? Remember that being responsible for a baby care activity can take many forms. It does not necessarily mean you must physically perform the task. Some parents do none of the physical aspects of an activity, yet they oversee the task. They direct the helper and continue to interact and play with their baby throughout the activity. Other parents do parts of the physical tasks and direct the rest. Such teamwork allows the parent to be involved and free to focus on the interaction with his or her baby. Remaining involved while someone else is physically doing the task says to the child that you are central to their care. Being central and the person who says "how things go" becomes important for later discipline. Keep in mind that it's your love, responsiveness, and the time you spend with your child talking or playing that develop your connection with your baby.

The following are example of ways you can be central in the baby care while others physically help you:

- You decide what clothes to put on, what food to offer, and what the nap schedule will be.
- When the baby cries, you can figure out why: for example, whether the baby needs to be fed, to have a diaper changed, or to be offered a different toy.
- When your child is hurt or upset, you can be the one who comforts him or her. Your helper can assist by bringing the child to you and/or supporting the child on your lap while you either verbally or physically do the consoling.
- You talk about your child's needs during doctors' visits and school meetings.
- You decide on when and how to discipline a child.

On the other hand, every parent, with or without a disability, needs a break at some time. It is important to remember that time dedicated to you is very important and will help your relationship with others, including the relationship with your child. During those times that you

Table 13.1. Modified Baby Care Gear and Adaptive Strategies

Parent Abilities	Baby Care Task	Baby Gear/Tricks
Walking with mobility aid (e.g., walker, cane)	Hold while moving	-Use a four-wheel walker with a baby car seat secured to it
	Transferring (lift and place) child	-Sit for transfers. Use lifting harness for extra support of child, or for leverage. -When the child is able, supervise them in climbing up to your lap or surfaces instead of lifting.
	Diapering	-Sit while diapering at a table or half card table with commercial concave diapering pad on top.
	Bedtime	-Arm Reach Co Sleeper®, Side Away Crib -Wooden port-a-cribs can also be adapted and are smaller than standard cribs.
	Bathing	-Sit down while bathing at the sink or baby tub on a counter. -If you have a roll-in shower, a plastic bin on the floor, only big enough for your child to squat. Secure bin to the floor with nonstick stripping.
Manual wheelchair user with good upper extremity and trunk control.	Hold while moving	-Snugli Early Care Sling™ (infants only) -Covered foam wedge attached to the parent's waist. Good for

(Table 13.1. continued)

Parent Abilities	Baby Care Task	Baby Gear/Tricks
		doing many different activities. -Standard front pack. -Parent-child seat belt for children who can sit up.
	Transferring child	Use lifting harness for extra support of child. -When the child is able, supervise them in climbing up to your lap or surfaces instead of lifting. Lifting harness can also be secured to your wheelchair seat belt with climbing carabineers.
	Diapering	Same as above Have a bin full of novel toys available.
	Bedtime	Surface same as above.
	Bathing	Same as above
Wheelchair user with limited hand function /decreased trunk control.	Hold while moving	Snugli Early Care Sling™ (infants only), covered foam wedge attached to the parent's waist. Parent child seat belt when child can sit up. -With professionals' assistance attach an infant car seat onto motorized wheelchair.
	Transfer (lift and place)	-Use lifting harness (infant) to lift with one arm and stabilize self with the other. -When the child is able,

(Table 13.1. continued)

Parent Abilities	Baby Care Task	Baby Gear/Tricks
		supervise them in climbing up to your lap or surfaces instead of lifting.
	Feeding	Use pillow under bottle or the Bottle Bundle® by Little Wonders to secure bottle. -Create a Universal cuff for bottle or child's spoon.
	Burping	-Sit the baby on your lap facing out and stroke upward on the baby's tummy. Sit the baby on your lap, facing out, lean the baby forward over your crossed arms. -Roll the baby on his/her tummy and pat. -Lay the baby on its right side and roll slightly onto tummy.
	Diapering	-Use same surface as above, adapt child's seat belt with a Velcro closure. -Attach toy mobile to diapering surface. -When using disposable diapers, use packing tape or bag twist ties (be sure baby can't remove) to make finger loops on diapering

(Table 13.1. continued)

Parent Abilities	Baby Care Task	Baby Gear/Tricks
		tabs, or use teeth to manipulate tabs. With cloth or disposable diapers use diaper wraps adapted with key rings on tabs. -Use diapering wraps, made by such companies as Kushies, which are easy to attach key rings to.
	Bed time	Same as above
	Bathing	Participate while someone else performs.
General Information for all levels	Taking temperature	Use pacifier with thermometers built in (Pacifer Plus®).
	Giving medicine	-During infancy have someone prepour dropper amount into a cup to store. -Use chewable Tylenol tablets with toddlers. Have someone remove from packaging ahead of times.
	Dressing	-Buy one size larger, it's easier to put on. -Buy clothes with zippers (attach key ring) or clothes with elastic such as sweats. **Baby Gear/Tricks-** Dressing on your lap with the child facing outward. -Encourage your child to assist you.

(Table 13.1. continued)

Parent Abilities	Baby Care Task	Baby Gear/Tricks-
	Dressing	Place the least amount of clothes as possible on your child. -Only snap the most essential snaps and leave the rest undone. -Onesie with Velcro closure- Baby Headquarters™ Begin training your child to lift his butt as early as 3 months of age. Say "butt up" when doing.
	Transfer (lift and place)	Before lifting them up say "one, two three-up". Then lift your child. This allows them to prepare their bodies for the transfer.
	Community	Walking fanny pack or harness with tether. Gerber® Harness and Handstrap.

*See Adaptive Baby Care Equipment: Guidelines, Prototypes & resources for additional details on equipment.

need a break or need some time for yourself, don't be afraid to let your family or friends know that you want or need them to take over.

CHILD COOPERATION

Another challenge to baby care can be the lack of cooperation from your child during activities. If your child does not want to work with you, any task can turn into a drawn-out struggle. One idea is to give the child a favorite treat or toy during critical times. For example, during diapering, which can take longer with a physical disability, keep a small bin of toys, soft books, or a small cloth picture album that your child can play with or look through while you change his/her diaper. The trick is to keep the toys interesting by saving them for use only when a distraction is needed.

As parents, we easily become accustomed to doing things for our children, such as lifting them up or getting objects for them. Instead, try to think about what your child can do physically by his or herself. The following are some examples for children who can crawl:

- Your toddler can crawl onto an accessible diapering table from your lap.
- Your toddler can climb up onto your lap from the floor or the couch so that you do not have to pick her up.
- By 9 months of age, when cued, a baby may be able to arch his back and push his legs against the surface, bringing his bottom up so that you can slip a diaper under him.
- Your toddler may be able to walk instead of being carried.

Encourage these behaviors early so your child becomes accustomed to your care style. This strategy takes nothing away from you as a parent. Instead, it contributes to the child's sense of independence and teaches him that he can do things in the world successfully.

Discipline with Toddlers

A common mistake that some parents make is to blame their disability during difficult times when discipline of a child is required. Most of what you will face, or are facing, is common to all parents. However, there are some unique aspects to disciplining with a physical disability. Able-bodied parents often use physical means to discipline toddlers, such as picking them up and removing them from the situation. There are alternatives, but they take more thought because we don't see these techniques used as often. Here are some examples:

- Save your stern voice for safety issues. Use a firm voice when it really counts or your child will begin to ignore the serious tone of your voice.
- Toddlers naturally love to play chase, but they can get themselves into places where wheelchair users cannot follow. Therefore, it is a good idea to change the game from "chase the baby" to "chase the parent." Start by playing this game in your home. When the baby starts heading in a different direction, say, "Catch mommy (or daddy)." Once your child is familiar with the game, you can try it outside of the safety of the home.
- To keep your child near you when you are outside the home, use a walking harness. Several companies make these, including The Kid

Keeper™ from One Step Ahead or Gerber's Safety Harness and Hand Strap. The walking harness allows the child to explore without totally getting away from you.

- When you leave home, bring a few toys along so that when a youngster picks up something they cannot have, you have something else to offer. If they are bored while you shop or use the ATM, you can have a treat to give if they behave.
- When a child has a tantrum, simply move away and wait it out. This removes the "fuel" from the tantrum and the child usually calms down. If this occurs within your home, go to another room. Of course, your home needs to be fully child-proof so that you feel safe leaving the room.

If you understand your child's temperament, it will be easier to figure out ways to manage your child in and outside the home. The book *Temperament Tools* [9] offers ideas about how to manage your child when he or she acts out or has behavior that is to handle. Talking to other disabled parents about discipline may also provide you with more ideas, and you will find out that nearly everyone finds this challenging. If you don't know other parents in your community, become part of the Parent to Parent Network sponsored by Through the Looking Glass. The network can match you up with another parent with a disability in a similar situation.

SCHOOL-AGE CHILDREN

Parents with school-age children may face several issues: inaccessibility of the school building, difficulty assisting with homework, and challenges in participating in extracurricular activities. Many school buildings are supposed to be accessible but are not, making it difficult to enter the school to talk with your child's teacher and be part of school life. You can talk with the school district to make your child's school more physically accessible, for example, by building a ramp or having your child's classroom be located downstairs. School accessibility gives you the opportunity to become a classroom volunteer, to meet other parents, and get to know what happens in the classroom.

Volunteering in the classroom also allows you to get a sense of what occurs among the students. For example, teasing is common among children. It is important to remember that children will tease about anything, so do not be surprised if your child is teased about your disability. One good comeback to teach your child is, "So what?" This seems to stop children in their tracks. Another way to reduce teasing is to ask to talk with students in the classroom about your disability and allow them to ask questions, a great introduction for the students on disability issues.

Another potentially challenging area is homework. One obstacle in helping your child may be your inability to write letters or numbers. Explain your situation to your child's teacher so that he or she might accept a different format for homework assignments. Use a computer to go over homework concepts in math, reading, or writing. **Assistive technology** centers, especially those that work with disabled children, may be helpful. They can provide alternative formats for homework programs, such as "Math Pad" and "Math Pad Plus" by Intellitools^{TM}, which provides a way of doing math problems without paper and pencil. The special education department at your child's school may also have these programs.

As your child gets older and more independent, you will want to meet their friends and their friend's families. Since most homes are inaccessible, you might suggest that your first play date with their parents be at your house or at a restaurant. Then, the next time the classmate wants a play date, you can feel more at ease in letting your child go. Since you can't enter their home, check in frequently with your child about how comfortable he or she is there and what kind of supervision is given. Some parents restrict their child's play to school classmates because they are able to talk with other parents about the family and their experiences in the home.

FAMILY RECREATION TIME

Many places and organizations offer adaptive sports for winter and summer. Adaptive winter ski schools provide lessons and adaptive ski equipment for all levels of abilities. Summer sports include kayaking, sailing, and sit-down water-skiing. Adaptive sports can provide a family camp-like experience for the whole family. You can choose vacation spots where adaptive sport programs are available, allowing everyone in your family to participate.

In addition to organized sports there are now several types of adaptive outdoor equipment that make parks and beaches accessible. For example, the Beachcomber, made by Roleez$^{®}$ is a set of wheels that can be switched with the wheels on a manual wheelchair so that you can be pushed on the sand. The Beach Cruzr^{TM} is a motorized beach wheelchair. The Mobi-Mat^{TM} is a rollout mat that allows a wheelchair user to travel over rough terrain. Inquire whether your city or town might be able to buy the mats to make local parks accessible to all community members.

Accessible toys and games can be found in stores. For example, a toy called "Velcro Catch," appropriate for age six and up, is an eight-inch mitt that serves as a paddle and comes with a Velcro ball that sticks to the mitt. The ball can be removed from the paddle with a swipe of your palm or forearm. If you like card games, there are commercially available shufflers and card holders, or you can make your own cardholder by turning a shoe or game box upside down and securing the cards between the lid and the box. Children love computers and they can be easily adapted to match your functional abilities. Check with assistive technology centers for adaptation ideas. Regardless of the type of play you choose, remember that what children really want is your love, time and undivided attention. It is you they want!

CONCLUSION

Many parents with grown children believe that their disability has shaped their child's character in a positive manner. They report that their adult children are compassionate and empathic toward others, independent and self-reliant, determined and resourceful individuals who persevere through great odds.[10] Adult children will tell you that their childhood experiences were enriching and invaluable. [11, 12] They learned the importance of persevering by watching a parent overcome obstacles in his/her life. No matter if you are doing all of childcare or involved in aspects of care, what's most important is not how much of the physical task you are doing but the quality of the relationship with your child.

What Can I Do?

As you make plans to return to caring for your baby or young child, be sure to:

- *Find ways to get reacquainted with one another.* Have your baby or toddler visit you while you're still in the rehabilitation unit and find ways to include baby or child care activities in your therapy.
- *Engage your child.* Find creative ways to connect with your baby or toddler, for example, by singing, reading, or playing with toys together.
- *Be a problem solver.* Use the Baby Care Planner (Figure 13.1) to find strategies and equipment to solve problems and determine how you can be involved in caring for your baby.
- *Learn from others.* Talk with other parents with disabilities and with professionals experienced in working with parents with disabilities to gather ideas for tips and tools.
- *Ask for help when needed.* All parents need help at some point. Make a plan for getting the child care and household help you will need and

don't hesitate to ask your family and friends if you need extra help sometimes.

• *Stay involved*. Regardless of your physical abilities, stay involved in your child's care and upbringing as much as possible. Take part in child care activities, and be sure to spend time having fun with your family.

Where Can I Learn More?

To learn more about child care and parenting after a spinal cord injury, you may wish to contact:

• An occupational therapist or the occupational therapy service at your rehabilitation hospital
• Organizations such as Through The Looking Glass (www.looking-glass.org)
• Other parents with disabilities
• Your local Center for Independent Living (visit www.ilru.org for a directory of these centers)

Appendix C provides information about additional resources.

IMPORTANT POINTS TO REMEMBER

• Raising children can be one of life's most rewarding and challenging experiences. Women and men with disabilities can be effective parents, regardless of physical limitations.
• Planning ahead to find solutions to problems, get appropriate baby care equipment and accessories, get your home ready, and arrange for needed in-home help can enhance your ability to adapt to your role as a parent with a disability.
• What children want most is their parents' love, time, and undivided attention. A positive, caring relationship with your child is more important than your ability to perform the physical tasks involved in child rearing.

REFERENCES

[1]Garee B, ed. *Parenting Tips for Parents (Who Happen To Have a Disability) On Raising Children*, Bloomington, IL: Accent Special Publications, Cheever Publishing, Inc., 1989.
[2]Kirshbaum M. Parents with physical disabilities and their babies. Zero Three 1988; 8(5): 8-15.

[3]Tuleja C, Rogers J, Vensand K, DeMoss A. *Continuation of Adaptive Parenting Equipment Development*, Berkeley, CA: Through the Looking Glass, 1998.

[4]Kirshbaum M., Olkin R. Parent with Physical, Systemic, or Visual Disabilities. Sexuality and Disability 2002; 20(1):7-28.

[5]Tuleja C, Rogers J, Vensand K, DeMoss A. *Continuation of Adaptive Parenting Equipment Development*, Berkeley, CA: Through the Looking Glass, 1998.

[6]Tuleja C, DeMoss A. Babycare assistive technology. Technology and Disability 1999; 11: 71-78

[7]Vensand, K., Rogers, J., Tuleja, C., & De Moss, A. *Adaptive baby care equipment: Guidelines, Prototypes & Resources*. Berkeley: Through the Looking Glass, 2000.

[8]Vensand, K., Rogers, J., Tuleja, C., & De Moss, A. *Adaptive baby care equipment: Guidelines, Prototypes & Resources*. Berkeley: Through the Looking Glass, 2000: 56.

[9]Neville H, Johnson DC. *Temperament Tools: Working With Your Child's Inborn Traits*. Seattle, WA: Parenting Press, Inc., 1998.

[10]Garee B, ed. *Parenting Tips for Parents (Who Happen To Have a Disability) On Raising Children*, Bloomington, IL: Accent Special Publications, Cheever Publishing, Inc., 1989.

[11]Stanford P. You poor old soul. Disability, Pregnancy and Parenthood International 2001; 33: 17-19.

[12]Unpublished findings from adult children with parent with disabilities forum- 2002 Berkeley Ca.

14

Secondary Conditions and Other Little Surprises as You Age with Your Spinal Cord Injury

SUZANNE L. GROAH

"I started off this new beginning with apprehension, anticipation, questions, and fear—all of which are normal parts of being human. In 11 years, I have responded by going after one victory at a time." –Tim

So, you have survived your SCI, worked through rehabilitation, and are finally at a point where you feel you are accustomed to life again. Now, what lies ahead—not in the next few days or weeks, but in the coming months and years?

Recently, what exactly happens as people "age" with SCI has been a growing area of interest for researchers, doctors, nurses, and other health care professionals. Whether you have a SCI or not, as you age you will experience new and possibly unanticipated changes. Also, as you well know, there has been an explosion of research investigating new possibilities toward a "cure" for SCI. If we are lucky enough to see that "cure," whether in the next few years or decades down the road, your body needs to be as healthy as possible to support yet another phase of recovery. The better you are able to anticipate changes associated with aging, the better you will be able to adapt to your "new and improved" self.

Changes that arise with age may involve, but are not limited to, medical, functional, social, emotional, and financial changes. Each individual experiences these changes differently, depending on personality, overall health, genetics, and lifestyle. In addition, we are now realizing that the changes a person experiences over time depend on the characteristics of the spinal cord injury, such as the level and completeness of injury and any other conditions that have occurred because of the SCI. This chapter discusses:

- Some typical changes that occur with aging
- How the aging process might be different because of your spinal cord injury
- Considerations as you age with a spinal cord injury

LIFE EXPECTANCY—THE GOOD AND THE BAD NEWS

Let's start with the good news. Decades ago, before the development of specialized centers to treat people with SCI, the life expectancy of someone with an SCI was only a few years. In the past, if you were to have an SCI, you would have been much more likely to die within the first year after injury. If you did survive, you were more likely to die within the first several years because of infections such as pneumonia or bladder/kidney infection. Today, with improved medical care, people with SCI are living much longer lives.

Now the bad news: Life expectancy for someone with an SCI is still not as long as that for people who do not have an SCI (Table 14.1). For example, if you were 20 years old at the time of your SCI, we would expect you to live approximately 37 years if you have C1-C4 tetraplegia, 41 years if you have C5-C8 tetraplegia, and 46 years if you have paraplegia. In contrast, you would be expected to live to 57 years if you didn't have an SCI. You can see the impact that SCI has on your survival.

You may ask, "If we have gotten better at preventing and treating pneumonia, bladder and kidney disease, why won't I live as long than if I didn't have an SCI?" The answer is that we really don't know, and several factors may be involved. For example, people with SCI continue to be at greater risk

Table 14.1. Life Expectancy for Spinal Cord Injury Survivors

Life expectancy for those who survive the first year				
Age at Injury	No SCI	Paraplegic	C5-C8 Tetraplegic	C1-C4 Tetraplegic	Ventilator Dependent
20 years	57.2	46.2	41.2	37.1	26.8
40 years	38.4	28.7	24.5	21.2	13.7
60 years	21.2	13.7	10.6	8.4	4

Source: National Spinal Cord Injury Statistical Center
(http://www.spinalcord.uab.edu/show.asp?durki=21446)

than others of getting overwhelming infection and kidney disease, but we now prevent and recognize these conditions earlier. Although these diseases are still dangerous for individuals with SCI, they result in fewer deaths than they did years ago.

Another factor contributing to the lower life expectancy of people with SCI is "accelerated aging." Several decades ago, people who had SCI generally wouldn't live long enough to develop heart disease, stroke, cancer, and other diseases and conditions associated with aging. People with SCI are now living long enough to develop these conditions. The difference is that we are finding that people with SCI develop certain conditions earlier than people without SCI. This is called "accelerated aging." The sections below discuss a few examples of diseases that are associated with "accelerated aging."

> Accelerated aging is the development of certain diseases or conditions at a younger age or more rapidly than expected.

BLADDER CANCER

Bladder cancer is a good example of a disease that is part of the "accelerated aging" phenomenon. In the non-SCI population, bladder cancer is the fifth most common type of cancer in the United States, with almost 53,000 people diagnosed each year. This means that approximately 17 of 100,000 people will be newly diagnosed with bladder cancer each year. The average age of a person at the time of bladder cancer diagnosis is approximately 68 years. Also, men (who are three to four times more likely than women to develop bladder cancer) and smokers are more likely to develop bladder cancer. In roughly three-fourths of cases, bladder cancer is "superficial." At the time of diagnosis, it often hasn't progressed much, so it tends to respond better to treatment. Many people live for years after a bladder cancer diagnosis.

However, during the past several years, researchers have become aware of a higher risk of bladder cancer among people with SCI. We now know that if you have an SCI, you are more likely to develop bladder cancer over the course of your life. It has been shown that chronic bladder inflammation (or irritation) contributes to bladder cancer, and the most likely source of this inflammation is repeated urinary tract (bladder or kidney) infections and bladder stones. So, it is not as simple as your SCI "causing" bladder cancer, but instead other factors related to the SCI contribute to the higher risk of disease. This statement is good news because it means there may be things you can do to prevent bladder cancer.

Several studies have tried to determine what factors contribute to bladder cancer after SCI. In one study of many people with SCI who were followed for many years, researchers found that those who used indwelling catheters (foley or suprapubic) for most of their lives tended to develop bladder cancer more often than those who never, or only intermittently, used indwelling catheters. In fact, if you have an SCI and use an indwelling catheter, you are 4.5 times more likely to get bladder cancer than if you used intermittent **catheterization**.

Researchers are not sure if there is a direct link between indwelling catheter use and cancer, or if the catheter causes other problems, such as bladder infections or stones, that in turn lead to cancer. This makes sense because we know that indwelling catheters lead to more frequent bladder stones and chronic inflammation of the bladder.

How Much Catheter Use Is too Much?

Research suggests that as little as 10 years of catheter use is associated with a higher risk of bladder cancer. Most people with SCI are injured while in their 20s or 30s, so that means bladder cancer could develop in someone in their 30s or 40s, which is very young compared to the average of 68 years for the general population!

Also, the course of bladder cancer after SCI is often different than the bladder cancer that develops in people without SCI. Generally, bladder cancer after SCI is a much more aggressive and deadly cancer. It is often a different type of cancer. Transitional cell cancer predominates in people without SCI, while other (more aggressive) types such as squamous cell cancer are more common in people with SCI.

We don't know all the causes of bladder cancer, but there is evidence that certain factors might put you at greater risk. Some of these factors are listed in Table 14.2.

Obviously, you can't do anything about your race, age, or gender, but you can possibly decrease your chances of getting bladder cancer by taking the best care you can of yourself and your bladder. A good approach might include drinking plenty of water (while balancing this with your bladder management method), avoiding bladder infections and stones, and possibly most important, stop smoking. You can actually decrease your chances of getting bladder and other cancers by stopping smoking. Also, this might mean rethinking whether a foley or suprapubic catheter is the best option for you. For many people with SCI, this type of catheter is really the best choice. However, some people might benefit by changing to another type of system. For example, some people choose an indwelling catheter early after their SCI because it is the "easiest" option at the time. Consider how much assistance (if any) you need during the day and whether changing to an alternative bladder management method would increase the assistance you need, how

Table 14.2. Risk Factors for Bladder Cancer

Risk Factors You Can't Do Anything About	Risk Factors You CAN Do Something About
• White race • Older age • Male gender • Family history or personal history of bladder cancer	• Long-term use of a foley or suprapubic catheter • Smoking • Frequent bladder infections • Bladder stones • Exposure to certain chemicals, such as some hair dyes, rubber, textiles, paints • Diet high in saturated fat • Infection with *Schistosoma haematobium* (a parasite found in many developing countries, but uncommon in the United States) • Consumption of *Aristolochia fangchi* (an herb used in some weight-loss formulas)

readily you transfer and get dressed and undressed, and your hand function. Your rehabilitation physician or urologist can review other options with you.

Other steps you can take include trying to avoid bladder and kidney infections and periodic check-ups for bladder or kidney stones. (This procedure requires an X-ray or ultrasound and should be done under the supervision of a urologist, your rehabilitation specialist, or your primary care doctor.)

How Do I Know If I Have Bladder Cancer?

Usually, the only indication that early bladder cancer is present is the presence of blood in the urine. In fact, one study found that most people who were diagnosed with bladder cancer reported having blood in their urine at some earlier time. The difficulty is that any type of bladder catheter, especially an indwelling catheter, is more likely to cause bladder irritation, infection or stones, which all may cause blood to appear in the urine.

We are recommending, then, that you advocate for yourself. Ask your health care provider to arrange for bladder cancer screening as early as 5 years to 10 years after your injury if you use an indwelling catheter or if you have other reasons to suspect that your risk of developing bladder cancer is high. Periodic screening is typically done by a urologist and may include a test called cystoscopy, in which a urologist inserts a very thin and flexible scope into your bladder to visually check for any abnormal areas. New tests are being developed that may be better able to screen for bladder cancer in the future.

HEART DISEASE AND STROKE

We know that as people age, the risk of developing heart disease and stroke increases. Recently, researchers have discovered that if you have an SCI, your risk of heart disease and stroke may be even higher than if you didn't have an SCI. Researchers have also found that heart disease and stroke cause more deaths of people with SCI than noted previously partly because of changes in cholesterol levels and blood sugar after SCI.

Good Fats, Bad Fats

Increases in cholesterol levels and blood glucose (sugar) levels are related to a greater likelihood of developing heart disease, stroke, and diabetes. Cholesterol actually has a purpose, which is to move fat to where it is needed in the body. So, your body needs a certain amount of cholesterol, but too much is bad and increases your risk of heart disease and stroke by clogging up blood vessels. You have probably heard that there is a good cholesterol (high-density lipoproteins, or HDL) and a bad cholesterol (low-density lipoproteins, or LDL). Generally, LDL is the clogging, or bad, cholesterol and HDL is the unclogging, or healthy, cholesterol.

An easy way to remember the difference is that HDL is the healthy cholesterol and you want that number to be high, whereas LDL is the lousy cholesterol and you want that number to be low. On average, people with SCI are four times more likely to have low HDL levels. A low HDL can actually put you at greater risk of heart disease. Fortunately, you can increase your HDL cholesterol by not smoking, losing weight or maintaining a healthy weight, and being physically active.

Another type of cholesterol that we have learned more about recently is Lp(a). This is a type of LDL cholesterol, and, like LDL cholesterol in general, it is lousy because it also causes arteries to clog. The last type of fat in the blood is triglycerides, which are a form of fat that is made in your body and comes from food. People with heart disease or diabetes and those who are obese tend to have high triglyceride levels.

DIABETES

Sugars, starches, and other foods are the basic fuel for cells in the body. Insulin is a hormone produced by the body that is needed to change these sugars, starches, and other food into energy. Insulin actually takes the sugar (glucose) from the blood and transports it into the cells where it is used as fuel. If the body does not produce insulin, or if insulin is not used properly, then diabetes, or high blood sugar results.

There are several different types of diabetes. In Type 1 diabetes, the body does not produce insulin. This type of diabetes is usually diagnosed in children and young adults, and was previously known as juvenile diabetes. Type 2 diabetes is the most common form of diabetes and occurs in adults. In type 2 diabetes, either the body does not produce enough insulin or the cells ignore the insulin (called insulin resistance).

With both types of diabetes, glucose can build up in the blood instead of being used by cells. This, in turn, causes the cells to be starved for energy. Down the road, excess glucose in the blood may damage body organs, such as your eyes, kidneys, nerves, or heart. You may not have realized this, but diabetes is the most common cause of blindness in people ages 20 to 74, the most common cause of serious kidney disease (end-stage renal disease), and the most common cause of non-traumatic amputation.

How Do I Know If I Have Diabetes?

Unfortunately, it is often difficult to tell if you have diabetes unless you get tested. The most frequent symptoms of diabetes are frequent urination, excessive thirst, extreme hunger, unusual weight loss, increased fatigue, irritability, and blurry vision. It is a good idea to ask your health care provider to test you if you think you might have diabetes or pre-diabetes. Pre-diabetes is a relatively new term used to describe a state in which blood glucose levels are higher than normal but not as high as those seen in diabetes. To determine if you have diabetes or pre-diabetes, you need to have a fasting plasma (blood) glucose (FPG) test or an oral glucose tolerance test (OGTT). Also, it is a good idea to have the glucose levels in your blood checked periodically to screen for early disease. If your blood glucose levels are high, then your health care provider will do an FPG test or an OGTT to determine if you have the disease. Table 14.3 lists the glucose levels doctors use to diagnose pre-diabetes or diabetes for each of these tests.

What Causes Diabetes and What's the Connection with SCI?

We're not really sure what exactly causes diabetes, but heredity, lack of

Table 14.3. Glucose Levels Indicating Pre-Diabetes or Diabetes

Level	Pre-Diabetes	Diabetes
Fasting Plasma Glucose (FPG) Test	100 – 125 mg/dl	126 mg/dl or higher
Oral Glucose Tolerance Test (OGTT)	140 – 199 mg/dl	200 mg/dl or higher

Source: American Diabetes Association (http://www.diabetes.org/about-diabetes.jsp)

exercise, and obesity seem to play roles. We do know, however, that after SCI you are more likely to develop pre-diabetes or diabetes. We think that changes in body composition and exercise level as a result of the SCI are responsible. Body composition is the distribution of body components that can be broadly organized into fat mass or lean body mass. Lean body mass includes:

• Muscles
• Tendons
• Ligaments
• Bones
• Skin
• Organs

We also know that after SCI your body changes fairly rapidly, and not necessarily for the better. Because of the paralysis associated with the SCI, the body becomes less active, and most types of exercise become more difficult. With this "imposed" physical inactivity, we see a change in body composition characterized by a higher proportion of fat and a corresponding lower proportion of muscle than was present before the injury. Although unproven, this change in body composition can mean that, although you do not look overweight, your body thinks and acts like you are. This change in body composition could be responsible for changes in your body's metabolism of glucose and insulin resistance. Therefore, it is important to have your health care provider check periodically for any indication of pre-diabetes or diabetes.

What's the Connection Between SCI and Cardiovascular Disease?

What does the following equation equal?

high LDL cholesterol + low HDL cholesterol + high triglycerides + diabetes = ?

These are basically all risk factors for cardiovascular disease, which includes heart disease and stroke. We know that often after SCI HDL cholesterol decreases because of lack of exercise, LDL cholesterol increases, and diabetes is more likely. Combining these risk factors with less exercise and perhaps other risks, such as smoking, and you could have a very high risk of heart disease and stroke.

A change that occurs after SCI that might actually be protective against cardiovascular disease is the change in blood pressure observed in some. High blood pressure (hypertension) is a common condition that is a significant risk factor for cardiovascular disease. The good news is that often after SCI, especially if you have a tetraplegia or high paraplegia, blood pressure is actually lower, which might protect you to some extent from cardiovascular disease. Nevertheless, all factors considered, SCI most likely puts you at a greater risk for cardiovascular disease. Therefore, it's important to eat a balanced diet, exercise to maintain a healthy weight, stop smoking if you smoke, and make sure your cholesterol and glucose levels are periodically checked.

WHAT DOES ALL OF THIS MEAN FOR ME AND WHAT CAN I DO ABOUT IT?

By now, you are getting the hint that you are at risk for diabetes, heart disease, and high cholesterol—not only because of aging, but also because you have a SCI. In addition to practicing healthy behaviors such as eating a nutritionally balanced diet, drinking a lot of water (and balancing this with bladder management), maintaining a proper weight and not smoking, it is important to be physically active and exercise to help prevent disease and to keep you feeling energized and good about yourself.

How Much Should I Exercise?

Everyone is asking this question. Researchers are searching for the answer, but we have much more to learn. The American College of Sports Medicine currently recommends that people exercise at least 30 minutes on most days. Of course, we actually don't know if this is the correct amount of exercise if you have an SCI.

We always have to keep in our minds that things might be different because of the SCI. As you know, your arms and shoulders are now doing a lot more work than they were not meant to do. They are really doing the work of your legs and look how much bigger and stronger peoples' legs are! You might not think about it, but you need to be able to move your shoulders freely to brush your hair and teeth, wash your hair and face, put some food in the microwave, take milk out of the refrigerator, and drive, among many other activities. Over time, just pushing the wheelchair every day can put a tremendous amount of stress and strain on your arms and shoulders. It is very important to maintain strong and pain-free shoulders because you need them for so many activities, including wheelchair pushing, transferring, and pushing and pulling objects. As you can imagine, shoulder pain is very common in people with SCI. It is such an important issue that an entire chapter is dedicated to it. (See Chapter 15).

Now I'm Really Confused

The message we're trying to convey is that more exercise is not necessarily a good thing when you have an SCI. You do want to exercise as much as you can so you can get the health benefits, such as decreasing your risk of diabetes, heart disease, and high cholesterol. Above all, you may want to exercise because you enjoy it and have a good time. However, you don't want to exercise to the point that you have overused your arms and shoulders, and you can't even push your wheelchair or transfer by yourself. When you decide to exercise, keep in mind that it's important to try to combine different types of exercise so you don't overuse the same muscles and joints. Also, it is very important to remember to keep your shoulders balanced, a topic that is discussed in detail in Chapter 15.

OSTEOPOROSIS

Osteoporosis is another piece of the "accelerated aging" puzzle. Nearly all people with SCI develop osteoporosis, or bone mineral density loss. You may be familiar with osteoporosis if friends or family have had it. In people who have not had an SCI, osteoporosis typically occurs in older women, usually worsening after menopause. Severe osteoporosis is fairly uncommon in men. This bone mineral density loss occurs throughout the body, and the result is that bones break more easily. In people without SCI the broken bones usually occur in the spine, hip, or wrist. (Do you know an older woman who got shorter with age or started to walk hunched over?) The osteoporosis that occurs in conjunction with SCI is similar to that seen in people without SCI, with a few key differences:

• Men *and* women are equally affected.
• You get osteoporosis much younger.
• The broken bones tend to occur in the legs, usually around the knee.

Why do these differences exist? To answer this question, let's look at what exactly happens to your bones after you have an SCI.

Boys and girls are born with approximately the same bone mass, which increases steadily during childhood. During puberty, your bone mass increased dramatically, with up to a four to six-fold increase in the rate of bone development in the spine and a doubling of the rate of bone development in the arms and legs. You had the greatest amount of bone mass when you were an adolescent. This bone mass typically remains stable until you are/were in your 40s. Slow bone loss—at a rate of about 1 percent loss per year—begins to occur when you are in your 40s or 50s. Genetics are responsible for much of the variation in bone mass among people. Other factors that influence how much bone you have are listed in Table 14.4.

Table 14.4. Non-Genetic Factors Affecting Bone Mass

Factors That Increase Bone Mass	Factors That Decrease Bone Mass
• Physical exercise	• Sedentary lifestyle
• Heavy body weight	• Smoking
• Good nutrition	• Poor nutrition

The SCI Connection

We know that immediately after SCI, bone resorption, or breakdown, begins to occur within days. Although we cannot see this breakdown on X-rays for months after the injury, chemicals resulting from bone being broken down are found in the blood and urine immediately after SCI. This bone loss is greatest in the first month after the injury, but the loss persists for several years after the injury.

We don't know exactly what causes the osteoporosis; probably there are several causes. We do know that when you exercise, muscle pulls on bone, actually helping the bone become stronger. After SCI, muscles that are no longer able to function properly because of paralysis, cannot pull on the bone to keep it strong.

So, when we look at the bone mass of people with SCI we actually see that loss of bone mass correlates with the severity of the SCI. For example, if you are a paraplegic using a wheelchair, you likely have had bone loss in your legs but not your arms. The muscles in your arms are still functioning and pull on the bones to keep them strong when you do many activities, such as pushing your wheelchair and transferring. Even the bones in your spine remain strong because in maintaining your posture, some or all of the muscles in your back are pulling on those bones keeping them strong even when you sit. If you are active and have paraplegia, the bones in your arms and spine may be even stronger than before your SCI —or they may be stronger than those of people without SCI because of these activities. If you have tetraplegia, you likely have lost bone mass in your legs and possibly in your arms and spine as well.

What Can I Do?

Researchers are trying to find ways to prevent bone loss or even restore bone mass that has already been lost after SCI. Although we have seen some limited success, it seems that preventing bone loss is more likely than building new bone from bone that has already been lost. Thus far, we also haven't found good treatments to restore bone mass that has already been lost after SCI. The best advice is to do everything you can to prevent further bone loss. This includes to:

• Stop smoking.
• Get moving with exercise.
• Eat a healthy and balanced diet, including getting the recommended amount of calcium and vitamin D. Vitamin D is made in the skin when you are in the sun and can also be found in fortified milk, fatty fish, and fish oils.
• Consider estrogen supplementation if you are a postmenopausal woman.

In addition, some treatments that may help prevent bone loss include:

• Medicines called "bisphosphonates" have been shown to prevent or slow bone loss in people with SCI and postmenopausal women without SCI.
• New drugs that may be used in the future to prevent bone loss include the "statins" (currently used to reduce high cholesterol) and PTH (parathyroid hormone).
• Novel types of exercise, such as functional electrical stimulation (FES), in which electrodes are applied to the skin and an electrical stimulation causes the muscles to contract, pulling on bone.
• New rehabilitative techniques such as assisted standing or walking.

ROUTINE MEDICAL MONITORING CAN HELP AS YOU AGE

You might be asking yourself what you should be doing and what preventive measures you should be considering as you age with your SCI. Most importantly, you want to stay in touch with a health care provider who specializes in treating people with SCI. This person, whether a doctor, nurse, or other health care professional, should be knowledgeable of the latest advances in the care and treatment of people with SCI. It is also important for you to stay knowledgeable about your condition, so you can assist your health care provider in developing the best health promotion and disease prevention plan for you. Table 14.5 describes how often you should have specific check-ups and tests. These recommendations are flexible depending on your individual characteristics and risks.

Table 14.5. Recommendations for Preventive Care

Age-related Recommendations	Frequency	For Men	For Women
All ages	Daily	Skin checks	Skin checks
	Monthly	Testicular self-examination	Breast self-examination
	Yearly	Check up with health care provider	Check up with health care provider
	Yearly	Weight check	Weight check
	Yearly	Blood pressure check	Blood pressure check
	Yearly	Flu shot if SCI T8 or higher	Flu shot if SCI T8 or higher
	Yearly		Gyn exam with Pap smear
	Yearly	Urologic evaluation	Urologic evaluation
	Yearly	Cystoscopy if indwelling catheter use 5-10 years or more	Cystoscopy if indwelling catheter use 5-10 years or more
	Every 2-5 years	Vital capacity if SCI is T12 or higher	Vital capacity if SCI is T12 or higher
	Every 2-5 years	Vision evaluation	Vision evaluation
	Every 2-5 years	Equipment and seating evaluation	Equipment and seating evaluation
	Every 10 years	Pneumovax vaccine if SCI T8 or higher	Pneumovax vaccine if SCI T8 or higher
	Every 10 years	Tetanus booster	Tetanus booster

(Table 14.5. continued)

35 to 40 years and older	Yearly		Breast exam by health care provider
	Yearly	Rectal exam	Rectal exam
	Yearly	Heart disease risk assessment	Heart disease risk assessment
	Every 2-5 years	Cholesterol and lipid check	Cholesterol and lipid check
40 years and older	Yearly		Mammogram
50 and older	Yearly	Prostate exam by health care provider	
	Yearly	Prostate specific antigen test	
	Every 2-5 years	Colonoscopy	Colonoscopy

DON'T FORGET ABOUT FUNCTION

Although most of this chapter has focused on health and medical changes that may occur with age, another important consideration that should not be overlooked are "functional changes." By that we mean the ability to take care of yourself, your caregiver's ability to assist you when needed, your ability to push your wheelchair, transfer, bathe, etc. An important impact of the "normal" changes associated with aging and those associated with aging after SCI is your ability or inability to maintain your current level of function. It is important to remember that just as medical problems can curtail your activities at any point during your life, the medical, emotional, or psychological changes that occur with aging can likewise hinder your activity level or even function. Further, if a family member provides some of your care, you also need to consider the impact of that individual aging. The cases below are not uncommon for someone with SCI.

Case #1

Tom is a 55-year-old man who has had a T4 SCI for 20 years. He lives with his wife, and his two children are in high school. He drives to work every day and exercises several times a week. Recently, transfers and other activities have become more difficult because of shoulder pain. Since the pain started 4 months ago, he has not exercised, has gained several pounds and has missed several days of work.

This is a very common scenario in a highly functioning person with SCI, in which shoulder pain can lead to a cascade of problems. Beyond the obvious solutions, such as seeking medical care to get the shoulder problem treated, someone in this or a similar situation might want to consider reevaluating the type of exercise that was done and that still can be done to maintain health, transfer techniques, and the use of different of even new equipment. Perhaps eliminating some stressful transfers, adding a slide board or a lift, and even considering beginning to use a power wheelchair might help Tom maintain his activities, health, and happiness.

Case #2

Jane is a 50-year-old woman with a T10 SCI since 1975. She is a very successful lawyer but has missed work and other social activities for the past several months because of occasional bowel accidents. She very much loves her job and her activities but now is very limited because of the embarrassment of having a bowel accident.

Bowel problems are problems that are most likely to limit someone's participation in work or other activities outside of the home. The result is social isolation and can eventual depression. Bowel changes are very common with aging. It is important to realize the impact of bowel problems and to make adjustments in your bowel routine so that bowel accidents don't have a major impact on your quality of life and overall health.

Case #3

Jerry is a 60- year-old man with a C6 SCI. He and his wife do not have children, volunteer often, and are socially very active in their community. His wife provides all of the assistance that he needs, such as helping with transfers, bathing, dressing, bowel care and driving. His wife recently was diagnosed with cancer and has been having difficulty taking care of herself, much less Jerry.

Whenever a family member provides care and assistance, the health and wellness of the caregiver has a very strong impact on the health and wellness of the person receiving care. Ideally, as you and your partner/caregiver age, it is probably best to anticipate that aging of the caregiver will affect that person's ability to provide care. Developing alternative plans for care giving early, before problems arise, is in everyone's best interest.

These cases represent commonly seen situations after SCI. The best advice to give is to be aware and knowledgeable of the changes associated with aging and actually prepare for them ahead of time. Again, this might include:

• Reevaluating how you currently do your functional activities

• Assessing your caregiver situation and making sure you have back-up plan(s)
• Considering changing from a manual to a power wheelchair (this is best initiated several years before you really "need" it and the transition can be very gradual)
• Reassess all of your equipment

WHERE IS THE "NEW AND IMPROVED" ME?

We all need to remember that as we age, regardless of whether we have an SCI or not, our bodies change. The better we anticipate and plan for certain changes and the more we take care of ourselves, the happier, healthier, and more fulfilled our lives will be. As promised, there is a happy ending to this story. Despite the changes that occur "normally" with aging and those that occur at least in part because of your SCI, most people with SCI report that their quality of life is the same or only slightly lower than that of their non-disabled counterparts.

Keep in mind, too, your quality of life does not depend on the severity of your injury. Rather, it is related to coping skills and staying involved in your community. This involvement might include participating in leisure activities (see Chapter 10), work, family life, and other enjoyable activities. Being able to participate in these community activities over the course of your life means taking the best care you can of your mind, body, and soul.

What Can I Do?

As you make choices about physical and recreation activities, be sure to:

• *Be aware.* Learn to recognize signs of aging and accelerated aging and talk with your doctor if you have questions.
• *Get regular checkups.* Talk to your doctor about how often to get preventive care checkups and medical tests that can detect signs of problems as you age.
• *Eat well.* To help prevent cancer, heart disease, stroke, and diabetes, be sure to consume a low-fat, high-fiber, high-cholesterol diet that includes needed vitamins, minerals, and calcium.
• *Drink fluids.* To help prevent bladder cancer and other problems, be sure to drink plenty of water and other fluids.
• *Quit the habit.* If you smoke, try to quit or talk with your doctor about how to quit.
• *Exercise.* Be sure to include physical activity into your daily schedule.

Where Can I Learn More?

To learn more about aging with an SCI, you may wish to contact:
• Your primary care physician or physiatrist
• Other members of your rehabilitation team
• The Natinoal Spinal Cord Injury Associatioin (www.spinalcord.org)
• The National Institute on Aging (www.nia.nih.gov)

Appendix C provides information about additional resources.

IMPORTANT POINTS TO REMEMBER

• People with SCI are living longer than ever before. As a result, they are now developing diseases and conditions such as heart disease, cancer, osteoporosis, and diabetes that are often associated with aging. Doctors have found that people with SCI experience "accelerated aging"—development of certain diseases or conditions earlier than people without SCI.
• Regular medical checkups by a health care provider who specializes in treating people with SCI can help detect signs of health problems so they can be addressed or prevented early.
• Frequent exercise, eating a healthy diet, not smoking, and getting medical help when needed can promote health and well-being.

This chapter was supported in part through a grant from the U.S. Department of Education, National Institute on Disability and Rehabilitation Research, Grant #H133B031114.

15

The Impact of Spinal Cord Injury on the Shoulder

MATT ELROD, P.T., M.Ed., N.C.S.
ALISON LICHY, P.T., M.P.T.

"As a spinal cord injured individual, you will rely strongly on your arms and especially your shoulders, i.e. for transfers, pressure relief, and general mobility. To avoid injuries to your shoulders, exercise that strengthens and maintains flexibility is crucial." --Brenda

Let's start with some basic facts about you and your body. It is human nature to want to move. Most movement to get from one place to another occurs with the use of legs. If you move from the bed to a chair or want to get something from the refrigerator, we typically use our legs. Your legs were made to support the weight of your body and for more continuous use. Your arms were made to move in many different directions, but not to support as much weight as your legs.

If something happens to cause you to be unable to use your legs, things change. You are forced to use your arms in ways different than they where intended to be used. Your arms are forced to become the major moving force to get out of bed, get a snack, and do lots of other activities, but there can be a cost to your arms picking up the slack. Unfortunately, the cost can have a profound impact on your functioning, health, and quality of life.

Because of the importance of your shoulders on many aspects of life, we have dedicated a full chapter to this part of your body. It is important to remember that shoulder function and problems are complex and often require working with your health care provider and rehabilitation team.

This chapter provides general information about the impact of spinal cord injury on the shoulder and recommendations to prevent problems and maintain your shoulder health. It discusses:

• Shoulder anatomy
• Common shoulder problems
• Exercises and functional mobility related to the level of spinal cord injury

SHOULDER ANATOMY

Before we dive into the specifics of shoulder problems and how to prevent them, let's make sure that you understand how the shoulder is built and how it works. Think of the shoulder as a ball and socket made of bones, with a lot of extra parts (muscles and ligaments) that keep it moving in a controlled fashion. The bony structures of the shoulder include the shoulder blade (scapula), the upper arm (humerus), and the collarbone (clavicle). These structures must stay in proper alignment for the shoulder to function and move normally. The muscles and ligaments hold the bones together and in proper position. Movements of the shoulder occur when muscles that are attached to the bones of the shoulder shorten or lengthen. This is a complex balance that, when disrupted at any step, can cause limitations in movement, decreased strength, and/or pain. Let's take a closer look at the bones of the shoulder. We will start from the top and work our way down the arm.

Your Shoulder Bones

The clavicle (collar bone) is a small bone that attaches the sternum (chest bone) to the scapula (shoulder blade). It's the bone you can feel sticking out toward the top of your chest. The humerus (upper arm bone) is the long bone of the arm that connects the elbow and shoulder. Toward your shoulder, the humerus ends in a ball, which is the ball of the ball and socket shoulder joint.

The scapula is a large, flat, triangle-shaped bone that lies in your upper back between your spine and shoulder. You can see the triangular outline of the scapula if you look in the mirror and bring your arms forward and back. The portion of the scapula that lies near the shoulder joint is shaped like a baseball glove. It is the socket part of the shoulder's ball and socket joint. Another way to think of it is the glove that holds the ball part of the humerus in place.

Your Shoulder Joints

A joint is where two or more bones meet and where movement between these bones occurs. Some other joints in the body include the elbow, wrist, hip, and knee. Muscles, ligaments, and tendons help hold joints together.

Ligaments, which are not flexible, hold bones to bones and tendons attach muscles to bones.

Your Shoulder Muscles

Now for the fun part—muscles. Muscles contract to pull, rotate, and move body parts to move in different directions. Table 15.1 lists and describes the muscles involved in shoulder health. There are probably many more than you expected. You don't need to memorize the names of all of these muscles, but it's important to understand that many muscles must function properly and together to keep your shoulder in the best shape possible. You can refer to the table when you think about doing exercises to strengthen or stretch a given muscle.

Table 15.1 Muscles Involved in Shoulder Health

Muscle	Bones to Which the Muscle Attaches	What the Muscle Does	Location of the Muscle
Trapezius (This muscle is close to the skin and can be felt with little difficulty)	Attaches the vertebral bones to the shoulder blade, running from the head to the mid-spine	Moves the shoulder blade up, down and inward	
Levator scapulae (This muscle is under the trapezius and is difficult to feel.)	Attaches the shoulder blade to the upper neck	Lifts the shoulder blade upward	
Serratus anterior (This muscle is located under the scapula and is difficult to feel.)	Attaches the underside of the shoulder blade to the ribs	Helps position the shoulder blade properly during arm movement	

(Table 15.1 continued)

Muscle	Bones to Which the Muscle Attaches	What the Muscle Does	Location of the Muscle
Rhomboid (2 parts) 1. Minor 2. Major (They are located under the trapezius and is difficult to feel)	Attaches the shoulder blade to the spine	Keeps the shoulder blade stable during arm movement	
Deltoid (3 Parts) 1. Anterior 2. Middle 3. Posterior (This muscle is close to the skin and can be felt with little difficulty)	Attaches the shoulder blade to the collar bone and arm	Lifts the arm forward, backward and up, and rotates the arm inward and out	
Coracobrachialis (This muscle is deep and difficult to feel)	Attaches the shoulder blade to the upper arm	Moves the arm forward and inward	

(Table 15.1 continued)

Muscle	Bones to Which the Muscle Attaches	What the Muscle Does	Location of the Muscle
Rotator cuff 1. Supras-pina-tus 2. Infraspinatus 3. Teres minor 4. Subscapu-laris (These muscles are deep and difficult to feel)	Attaches the shoulder blade to the upper arm	Keeps the shoulder joint in proper posi-tion during arm movement	
Pectoralis major (This muscle is close to the skin and can be felt with lit-tle difficulty)	Attaches the chest to the upper arm	Brings the arm in toward the body and twists the arm inward	
Pectoralis minor (This muscle is difficult to feel because it is under the pec-toralis major.)	Attaches the ribs to the scapula	Helps stabilize the scapula and helps with deep breathing	
Latissimus dorsi (This muscle is close to the skin and can be felt with lit-tle difficulty)	Attaches the lower part of the back to the upper arm	Moves the arm backward and twists the arm inward	

(Table 15.1 continued)

Muscle	Bones to Which the Muscle Attaches	What the Muscle Does	Location of the Muscle
Biceps brachii (This muscle is close to the skin and can be felt with little difficulty)	Attaches the top of the shoulder blade to the upper arm and lower arm (past the elbow)	Lifts the arm out to the side of the body and up	
Triceps brachii (This muscle is close to the skin and can be felt with little difficulty)	Attaches the back of the shoulder blade to the upper arm and lower arm (past the elbow)	Moves the arm backward	

You have likely heard about the rotator cuff group of muscles. The rotator cuff is actually a group of four small but very important muscles. These muscles are the supraspinatus, infraspinatus, teres minor, and subscapularis. Looking at the photo of the rotator cuff muscles in Table 15.1, you can see how they stretch across the upper shoulder to support the joint. Together, these muscles are very important in holding the shoulder joint together. If cared for properly, the rotator cuff can keep your shoulder healthy and functioning well. If injured or not cared for properly, the rotator cuff can be a source of shoulder pain and instability.

MUSCLES AND FUNCTIONING

You've seen how muscles move and/or support the shoulder joint. Now let's look at how they actually work together to help you get around. As stated above, when you rely on your arms to propel your body, the muscles around your shoulder are being used more than you ever used them before and more than they were designed to be used. For this reason, it is important to be aware of which muscles control and stabilize your shoulder and move your arm. If you can't control your shoulder when moving your arm, you could have pain when using your arms (for example, when you're pushing your wheelchair or moving from the chair to the bed).

Different muscles are active depending on which part of wheelchair-pushing you are doing. The serratus anterior, trapezius, and rhomboid muscles stabilize and position the scapula when you are propelling your wheelchair backward and forward and when turning. To reach backward and get a strong grip on the wheel, you must move your arm backward using the middle and posterior portion of your deltoids, and your supraspinatus, teres minor, and infraspinatus (three muscles in the rotator cuff group). You also must extend your elbow with your triceps as you grab the rim of the wheel. As you propel the wheel forward, you rotate your arm inward with the increase use of your pectoralis major and pectoralis minor, anterior deltoids, and subscapularis (a muscle in the rotator cuff group). To get a forceful push, you increase your use of the coroacobrachialis, biceps, and anterior deltoids. Did you imagine that so many muscles were involved in this relatively simple task?

Another daily task involving your shoulders is doing transfers. Depending on your level of injury, strength, and the surface you are transferring to, you will do various types of transfers. Transfers from one surface height to a higher surface height require more strength and balance than transfers between surfaces at the same height. If done incorrectly, such transfers can increase the stress on your shoulders, leading to pain or problems with your shoulder and limiting your ability to do transfers safely and independently. Your therapists will teach you which types of transfers are best for you based on your functional level.

COMMON SHOULDER PROBLEMS

There are many types of shoulder problems. Basically, a problem arises when there is a problem in any of the bones, muscles, tendons or ligaments mentioned above. Less commonly, problems arise because of nerve or blood-flow issues. Here we focus on muscle, ligament, and tendon problems because they are more commonly encountered after spinal cord injury.

Shoulder Pain

If you have to depend on your arms to get out of bed, dress, do self-care, and get you where you want to go everyday, you are at risk of having shoulder pain. The good news is that most shoulder pain can be prevented. Pain in the shoulder typically occurs because of problems in the nerves, bones, muscles, ligaments and/or tendons.

You might experience two types of pain: neuropathic pain, or nerve pain, and musculoskeletal pain (pain from muscles, ligaments, tendons or bones). Both neuropathic and musculoskeletal pain can be controlled. Neuropathic pain is typically treated by medications or other techniques, such as relaxation techniques, stretching, or biofeedback. Your rehabilitation team will discuss the specifics of the treatment with you and they will work with you to determine the best treatment.

Musculoskeletal pain happens because of muscle; bone; or ligament damage, imbalance, and/or overuse. There are three common types of musculoskeletal pain: impingement pain, muscle pain, and degenerative joint pain.

Impingement pain is caused by pinching of the tendons or muscles of the shoulder. This type of pain typically occurs at the top of the shoulder blade where the muscle connects to the top of the arm. The tendon can become irritated, swollen, and painful. This can limit the use of your shoulder, most commonly for activities in which you reach above your head.

To prevent impingement, it is important to be aware of three important things: proper posture and equipment, scapular stabilization, and proper use of your muscles. Proper posture and equipment is different for each activity that you perform. For example, the proper posture for pushing a wheelchair starts with how you sit in the wheelchair. The ideal position has the middle joint of your middle finger located in the middle of the wheel when you are sitting in your chair with your arms straight and hanging down by your side. Not every person can achieve this position. It is dependent on your level of injury and your comfort with balance in the wheelchair. Scapular stabilization, or your ability to maintain a stable base for your shoulder muscles to work from, is the second key part to preventing impingement. Finally, proper use of your muscles must be considered. This is probably the most complicated. It is important to have your physical therapist help determine if you have the proper timing and strength of muscles for activities that you are performing.

Muscle pain is typically associated with generalized muscle soreness or muscle strain. Generalized muscle soreness usually occurs from overdoing an activity. The pain starts about 24 hours after the activity and goes away after about three days of normal activity. Muscle strain or tear usually comes from a sudden burst of movement. The pain starts immediately, does not go away, and is constantly there when you do tasks that use that muscle. Muscle strain can also result from overuse of certain muscles or incorrect positioning. Contact your health care provider if the pain doesn't diminish after a few days or if you're unable to use your arm. To prevent muscle pain, be sure to start activities slowly and don't overdo activities.

Degenerative joint pain comes from a gradual breaking down of the bones, muscles, tendons, or ligaments in the shoulder. Over time, if you have pain or misuse your shoulder and don't address the problem, you could experience painful degenerative changes. You should contact your health care provider if you are concerned about degenerative joint pain.

Weight gain can contribute to any of the above-mentioned problems by increasing the stress placed on your shoulders. It takes more strength and control to move your body if you are carrying extra weight. If you don't have the strength to handle the increase in weight you may fatigue more easily or incorrectly use your shoulder muscles, leading to problems or pain with daily activities.

Muscle Balance and Imbalance

Muscle balance means that the muscles surrounding, supporting, and moving a particular joint are relatively equally strong. Muscle balance is needed to correctly position the bones and joints of the shoulder. This balance allows for optimal use of your shoulder. Muscular imbalance occurs when one or more muscles are stronger (or weaker) than the other muscles controlling the joint. The result is that correct movement does not occur. When the joint cannot move correctly, you are more likely to injure the joint or have pain in the joint because certain muscles, ligaments, or tendons may become injured (such as in a rotator cuff strain or tear). You also may be at risk of early arthritis (from the bones rubbing together during movement).

All of these problems can cause pain and limit the use of your shoulder. If you are doing activities over and over again with incorrect use of the shoulder, you are more likely to injure the joint or have pain when moving your arm. Because you rely on your arms for bed mobility, transfers, wheelchair mobility, and other daily tasks, once you injure your shoulder or movement becomes painful, this could significantly limit your ability to perform daily activities and limit your independence.

Muscle imbalance may happen because you work some muscles harder than others. In addition, after a spinal cord injury, muscle imbalance may happen because some muscles aren't able to contract since they don't receive needed information from the brain. If you can't contract a muscle, it will become soft and smaller. You may have heard this called muscle wasting or atrophy. After a spinal cord injury, muscle imbalances can be anticipated based on the level and completeness of the injury (discussed in greater detail later in the chapter).

Your rehabilitation team will teach you about appropriate transfers, bed mobility, and wheelchair set up to help prevent shoulder injuries. This information is very important when performing your daily routine and activities.

Subluxation

Subluxation of the shoulder happens when the arm slides out of place from the shoulder. This is basically a "partial dislocation" of the shoulder. Subluxation typically results from the muscles of the shoulder being too

weak to support the weight and position of the arm. The instability can lead
to pain caused by improper positioning of the shoulder. This problem is very
common after spinal cord injury, especially in people whose injury is high in
the cervical area. You can work to prevent shoulder subluxation by strengthening of your shoulder muscles and using proper positioning.

Contractures (a shortening of muscles and/or tendons producint deformity)

Contractures may occur when the shoulder joint becomes too tight and is
unable to move through the normal range of motion. This can make it hard
to do activities such as bathing and dressing that require full range of shoulder motion. This problem is common after spinal cord injury, especially in
the early days or during other times when you might be lying in bed more
than usual. Contractures can be prevented by actively moving your shoulder
through the full range of motion, or by having someone assist you with
stretching of the shoulder complex.

THERE'S MORE—SHOULDER ISSUES AND YOUR SPINAL CORD INJURY LEVEL

Now that you know the basic anatomy of the shoulder and common shoulder problems after spinal cord injury, it is useful to know how the shoulder is
affected by different levels of injury. As you learned in Chapter 1, 31 pairs of
spinal nerves exit from the spinal cord to connect with the muscles of your
body. The signals sent through these nerves tell the muscles to move, inform
the brain when you are moving, or when you feel something (sensation).
Eight cervical nerves go to the muscles in your neck, shoulders, chest, and
arms. Table 15.2 shows the spinal cord levels from which the muscles get
information.

So, what does this mean? Because muscles get information from more
than one level in the spinal cord, and we know what these levels are, we can
expect the following according to the level and completeness of your injury:

- Most muscles *above* your injury level should have normal strength or full
  movement.
- Muscles *at* your level of injury may be partially functioning or weak.
- Most muscle *below* your level of injury will be weak (if your injury is
  incomplete) or have no strength or movement (if your injury is complete).

For example, the trapezius receives information from the cervical nerve
C2, C3, and C4 levels, and the biceps receives information from C5 and C6.

Table 15.2. Nerve/Spinal Cord Levels From Which Muscles Get Information
(Note: The smaller type size indicates fewer signals being sent to the muscle by the
individual nerve. C = Cervical and T = Thoracic)

Muscle	Nerve/Spinal Cord Level
Trapezius	C2, C3, C4
Levator scapulae	C3, C4, C5
Serratus anterior	C5, C6, C7, c8
Rhomboid	c4, C5
Deltoid	C5, C6
Coracobrachialis	C6, C7
Rotator cuff muscles	c4, C5, C6, c7
Pectoralis major	C6, C7, C8, T1
Pectoralis minor	C7, C8
Teres major	C5, C6
Latissimus dorsi	C6, C7, C8
Biceps brachii	C5, C6
Triceps brachii	C6, C7, C8, T1

Therefore, if your spinal cord injury is at C4, you should have full function
of you trapezius but no function of your biceps.

The section below is intended to provide information based on a specific
level of complete injury and explain what muscles work at each level. In
addition, ideas for strengthening and/or stretching various muscles depending on your level of injury are listed. Your physical and/or occupational therapist will assist you with exercises that are appropriate for you, depending on
you strengths, weaknesses, and level of injury. They will also assist you in
proper technique or modifications of the exercise as needed. If you have an
incomplete injury, you may experience these same problems, but to a lesser
degree.

If You Have a C4 Complete Injury

If your injury is at the C4 spinal cord level, you have minimal movement of
the muscles that position your shoulder blade and very little movement of
the muscles that move your arms. This lack of movement puts you at risk for
shoulder and/or neck problems. Because of the inability to position the
shoulder and arm, proper use of adaptive equipment is key for proper shoulder positioning and independent power-wheelchair control. Overuse and
pain of the upper portion of the trapezius are common because the trapezius

is one of the fully functioning muscles. If your neck muscles, including the trapezius are weak, this could result in your head being positioned too far forward. In addition to causing shoulder pain, this can affect your breathing by decreasing airflow to your lungs.

It is also important to support your arms when in the wheelchair to maintain proper positioning of the shoulder. This support helps to prevent shoulder subluxation (see above). Subluxation could result in painful shoulders or injury and limit your range of motion during daily tasks such as bathing and dressing.

Maintaining the best neck and shoulder position possible involves using your upper, middle, and lower trapezius, and your partially innervated (receiving information from a given level of the spinal cord) rhomboids. It is very important to strengthen the muscles that are able to move to keep the shoulder blade in a downward position and not over-strengthen muscles that bring the shoulder blades up. Specifically, the lower and middle portions of the trapezius and the rhomboids should be strengthened and trained to keep the shoulder blades down and in. At the same time, the upper trapezius and levator scapulae should be trained to relax. See the exercises at the end of the chapter for details on strengthening the trapezius and levator muscles.

Table 15.3. Common Shoulder Problems and Typical Cause for Individuals with C4 Complete Spinal Cord Injury

Common Shoulder Problem	Typical Cause of Shoulder Problem
Painful shoulders and neck	• Upper trapezius overuse • Head being positioned too far forward
Shoulder subluxation (shoulder coming out of the socket)	• Improper (rounded shoulder) sitting position • Weak posterior shoulder and scapula muscles • Tight chest, upper trapezius and anterior shoulder muscles
Shoulder impingement (Pinching)	• Improper (rounded shoulder) sitting position • Weak posterior shoulder and scapula muscles • Tight chest, upper trapezius and anterior shoulder muscles
Limited range of motion	• Shoulder pain • Tight muscles (contactures)

Table 15.4. General Recommendations to Prevent Common Shoulder
Problems for Individuals with C4 Complete Spinal Cord Injury

Action	Activity	Comments
Strengthen muscles	• Middle and lower trapezius • Rhomboids • Rotator cuff muscles	These are the muscles that are typically weak.
Stretch muscles	• Upper trapezius • Levator scapulae • Pectoralis muscles	These are the muscles that are typically tight.
Instruct caregiver how to correctly assist with:	• Rolling in bed	• Do not roll on top of your shoulder. Direct your caregiver to position your shoulder on the side that you are rolling toward by positioning the scapula out or forward from under the weight of your body. • Ensure that your top arm is positioned in front of your body toward the direction that you are turning. • Instruct your caregiver not to pull your arm.
	• Transfers	• Maintain neutral neck (neck position straight in line with the back) • Support trunk • Support elbow
	• Sitting position	• Maintain neutral neck • Support trunk • Support elbow
	• Bed position	• Maintain neutral neck • Support arm when in bed

If You Have a C5 Complete Injury

If your injury is at the C5 level, you have some movement of the muscles that position the scapula and minimal movement of the muscles that move your arms at the shoulders and elbows. Therefore, you want to strengthen the muscles to keep the scapula in a downward position and not over-strengthen the muscles that bring the shoulder blades up. Specifically, the lower and middle portions of the trapezius and the rhomboids should be strengthened and trained to keep the shoulder blades down and in. At the same time, the upper trapezius and levator scapulae should be stretched and trained to relax.

At this level of spinal cord injury, you have movement and stabilization control of your shoulder, but limited arm movement. Wheelchair propulsion is difficult at this level and can be tiring and/or painful if done incorrectly. If pushing is done incorrectly, this may lead you to overuse other muscles, such as the levator scapulae, upper trapezius, biceps brachii

Table 15.5. Common Shoulder Problems and Typical Cause for Individuals with C5 Complete Spinal Cord Injury

Common Shoulder Problem	Typical Cause of Shoulder Problem
Painful shoulders and neck	• Upper trapezius overuse • Head being positioned too far forward • Pushing a wheelchair incorrectly due to weak muscles, poor position and/or improper technique • Inability to stabilize scapula
Shoulder subluxation (shoulder coming out of the socket)	• Improper (rounded shoulder) sitting position • Weak posterior shoulder and scapula muscles • Tight chest, upper trapezius and anterior shoulder muscles • Inability to stabilize scapula
Shoulder impingement (Pinching)	• Improper (rounded shoulder) sitting position • Weak posterior shoulder and scapula muscles • Tight chest, upper trapezius and anterior shoulder muscles • Inability to stabilize scapula
Limited range of motion	• Shoulder pain • Tight muscles (contactures)

Table 15.6. General Recommendations to Prevent Common Shoulder Problems for Individuals with C5 Complete Spinal Cord Injury

Action	Activity	Comments
Strengthen muscles	• Middle and lower trapezius • Rhomboids • Rotator cuff muscles • Serratus anterior • Deltoid • Teres major	These are the muscles that are typically weak.
Stretch muscles	• Upper trapezius • Levator scapulae • Pectoralis muscles • Teres major	These are the muscles that are typically tight.
Use proper positioning during:	• Rolling in bed	• Do not roll on top of your shoulder. Direct your caregiver to position your shoulder on the side that you are rolling toward by positioning the scapula out or forward from under the weight of your body. • Ensure that your top arm is positioned in front of your body toward the direction that you are turning. • Instruct your caregiver not to pull your arm.
	• Transfers	• Maintain scapula in a down and back position
	• Sitting position	• Maintain appropriate support of elbow when in wheelchair • Maintain scapula in a down and back position
	• Bed position	• Maintain neutral neck • Support arm when in bed

Table 15.7. Common Shoulder Problems and Typical Cause for Individuals with C6 Complete Spinal Cord Injury.

Common Shoulder Problem	Typical Cause of Shoulder Problem
Painful shoulders and neck	• Upper trapezius overuse • Head being positioned too far forward • Performing activities that involve the shoulder incorrectly due to weak or tight muscles, poor position and/or improper technique. • Inability to stabilize scapula
Shoulder subluxation (shoulder coming out of the socket)	• Improper (rounded shoulder) sitting position • Weak posterior shoulder and scapula muscles • Tight chest, upper trapezius and anterior shoulder muscles • Performing activities that involve the shoulder incorrectly due to weak or tight muscles, poor position and/or improper technique. • Inability to stabilize scapula
Shoulder impingement (Pinching)	• Improper (rounded shoulder) sitting position • Weak posterior shoulder and scapula muscles • Tight chest, upper trapezius and anterior shoulder muscles • Performing activities that involve the shoulder incorrectly due to weak or tight muscles, poor position and/or improper technique • Inability to stabilize scapula
Degenerative changes to bones and joints	• Overuse of shoulder during movement activities • Performing activities that involve the shoulder incorrectly due to weak or tight muscles, poor position and/or improper technique
Limited range of motion	• Shoulder pain • Tight muscles (contactures)

Table 15.8. General Recommendations to Prevent Common Shoulder
Problems for Individuals with C6 Complete Spinal Cord Injury

Action	Activity	Comments
Strengthen muscles	• Middle and lower trapezius • Rhomboids • Rotator cuff muscles • Serratus anterior • Deltoid • Teres major	These are the muscles that are typically weak.
Stretch muscles	• Upper trapezius • Levator scapulae • Pectoralis muscles • Teres major	These are the muscles that are typically tight.
Use proper positioning during:	• Rolling in bed	• Do not roll on top of your shoulder. Direct your caregiver to position your shoulder on the side that you are rolling toward by positioning the scapula out or forward from under the weight of your body. • Ensure that your top arm is positioned in front of your body toward the direction that you are turning. • Instruct your caregiver not to pull your arm.
	• Transfers	• Maintain scapula in a down and back position
	• Sitting position	• Maintain scapula in a down and back position

or deltoid, which can also cause neck and/or shoulder pain.

Transfers in and out of a wheelchair are also difficult at this level and can increase the stress on the shoulders leading to shoulder problems if done incorrectly. It is important to have strong deltoids to perform a level transfer at this level and to prevent future shoulder problems. A sliding board may assist you with your transfers.

If You Have a C6 Injury

If your injury is at the C6 level, you have some movement of the muscles that position the scapula and some movement of the muscles that move the elbow and wrist. It is important for you to strengthen the muscles to keep the scapula in a downward position and not over-strengthen muscles that bring the shoulder blades up. This action of the scapula is what will keep the muscles and tendons from being pinched and irritated during arm movement. In addition, you should be able to move and use the rotator cuff muscles. These muscles should be trained so that they don't tire easily during activities.

You should also be able to rotate your arm and shoulders inward. This lets you roll the wheel of your wheelchair forward in an efficient movement pattern. You will use the teres major, deltoids, latissimus dorsi, biceps brachii, rotator-cuff muscles, and occasionally the pectoralis major to move the wheelchair.

At the C6 level of injury, you should have enough control and strength of your serratus anterior to help with transfers, although you don't have the nerve innervation to your triceps needed to straighten your elbows. Therefore, you'll need to rotate your arms outward to maintain straight elbows to support your weight during transfers. You will need to maintain strong anterior deltoids to maintain this rotated position to lock your elbows straight and a strong serratus anterior to allow you to push your body up for your transfer. If you are incorrectly using your shoulder and not stabilizing the joint, you could cause injury by putting too much stress on the shoulder joint.

If You Have a C7 Injury

If your injury is at the C7 level, most of the muscles that position and move your shoulder blades, arms, and wrists (but not hands) are functioning. Your weak muscles include the pectoralis minor, which stabilizes the shoulder blade, and the pectoralis major and latissimus dorsi, which bring the arm in toward you and assist with arm rotation. The latissimus also is an important muscle in extending your arm behind you. Therefore, you

Table 15.9. Common Shoulder Problems and Typical Cause for
Individuals with C7 Complete Spinal Cord Injury

Common Shoulder Problem	Typical Cause of Shoulder Problem
Painful shoulders and neck	• Upper trapezius overuse • Head being positioned too far forward • Performing activities that involve the shoulder incorrectly due to weak or tight muscles, poor position and/or improper technique. • Inability to stabilize scapula
Shoulder subluxation (shoulder coming out of the socket)	• Improper (rounded shoulder) sitting position • Weak posterior shoulder and scapula muscles • Tight chest, upper trapezius and anterior shoulder muscles • Performing activities that involve the shoulder incorrectly due to weak or tight muscles, poor position and/or improper technique • Inability to stabilize scapula
Shoulder impingement (Pinching)	• Improper (rounded shoulder) sitting position • Weak posterior shoulder and scapula muscles • Tight chest, upper trapezius and anterior shoulder muscles • Performing activities that involve the shoulder incorrectly due to weak or tight muscles, poor position and/or improper technique • Inability to stabilize scapula
Degenerative changes to bones and joints	• Overuse of shoulder during movement activities • Performing activities that involve the shoulder incorrectly due to weak or tight muscles, poor position and/or improper technique
Limited range of motion	• Shoulder pain • Tight muscles (contactures)

Table 15.10. General Recommendations to Prevent Common Shoulder Problems for Individuals with C7 Complete Spinal Cord Injury

Action	Activity	Comments
Strengthen muscles	• Middle and lower trapezius • Rhomboids • Rotator cuff muscles • Serratus anterior • Deltoid • Teres major	These are the muscles that are typically weak.
Stretch muscles	• Upper trapezius • Levator scapulae • Pectoralis muscles • Teres major	These are the muscles that are typically tight.
Use proper positioning during:	• Transfers • Sitting position	Maintain scapula in a down and back position

want to strengthen the muscles that can help you keep your shoulder blades stable, bringing your arms in and rotating them.

If your triceps are strong enough to support your body, you may be able to lift your bottom during transfers and to do uneven transfers (from one surface height to another) without a sliding board. Remember that transfers to a higher surface put more stress on the shoulders and require more strength and balance. To prevent injury from overuse, weakness, or improper positioning, your shoulder muscles must be strong enough to support your body moving from one surface to another.

If You Have a C8 Injury

If your injury is at the C8 level, you have all of your shoulder stabilizing muscles intact and have partial function of your pectoralis major. Therefore, you want to ensure that you strengthen the muscles that can help you keep your shoulder blades stable, bringing your arms in and rotating them. In addition, you need to focus on strengthening the pectoralis major. It helps bring your arm in and in front of you, which increases your force when propelling the wheelchair forward. When strengthening your pectoralis major, it's important to keep a down and back position of your scapula to ensure proper strengthening.

Table 15.11. Common Shoulder Problems and Typical Cause for Individuals with C8 Complete Spinal Cord Injury

Common Shoulder Problem	Typical Cause of Shoulder Problem
Painful shoulders and neck	• Upper trapezius overuse • Head being positioned too far forward • Performing activities that involve the shoulder incorrectly due to weak or tight muscles, poor position and/or improper technique. • Inability to stabilize scapula
Shoulder subluxation (shoulder coming out of the socket)	• Improper (rounded shoulder) sitting position • Weak posterior shoulder and scapula • Tight chest, upper trapezius and anterior shoulder muscles • Performing activities that involve the shoulder incorrectly due to weak or tight muscles, poor position and/or improper technique. • Inability to stabilize scapula
Shoulder impingement (Pinching)	• Improper (rounded shoulder) sitting position • Weak posterior shoulder and scapula • Tight chest, upper trapezius and anterior shoulder muscles • Performing activities that involve the shoulder incorrectly due to weak or tight muscles, poor position and/or improper technique. • Inability to stabilize scapula
Degenerative changes to bones and joints	• Overuse of shoulder during movement activities • Performing activities that involve the shoulder incorrectly due to weak or tight muscles, poor position and/or improper technique.
Limited range of motion	• Shoulder pain • Tight muscles (contactures)

Table 15.12. General Recommendations to Prevent Common Shoulder Problems for Individuals with C8 Complete Spinal Cord Injury

Action	Activity	Comments
Strengthen Muscles	• Middle and lower trapezius • Rhomboids • Rotator cuff muscles • Serratus anterior • Deltoid • Teres major	These are the muscles that are typically weak.
Stretch Muscles	• Upper trapezius • Levator scapulae • Pectoralis muscles • Teres major	These are the muscles that are typically tight.
Use proper positioning during:	• Transfers • Sitting position	Maintain scapula in a down and back position

If You Have a T1 Injury

If your injury is at the T1 level or below, you have full function of your shoulder muscles. Be sure to maintain good posture and to keep your muscles strong because they are important in maintaining a healthy shoulder and decreasing the possibility of injury. Also, keep in mind that you're using your shoulders for mobility more than you ever have before. Preventing problems will help you to continue with your daily routine and recreational activities.

SHOULDER EXERCISES

The following muscle-specific exercises will help you maintain healthy shoulders and prevent injury. Your physical and/or occupational therapist can tell you which exercises are appropriate for you, depending on you strengths, weaknesses, and level of injury. They can also assist you with developing proper technique or modifications of the exercise as needed. If you have difficulty with your exercise program or if you feel it is too easy, talk with your therapist about changing your program. Also, be sure to let someone on your rehabilitation team know if you are experience shoulder pain.

Table 15.13. Common Shoulder Problems and Typical Cause for
Individuals with C8 Complete Spinal Cord Injury.

Common Shoulder Problem	Typical Cause of Shoulder Problem
Painful shoulders and neck	• Upper trapezius overuse • Head being positioned too far forward • Performing activities that involve the shoulder incorrectly due to weak or tight muscles, poor position and/or improper technique. • Inability to stabilize scapula
Shoulder subluxation (shoulder coming out of the socket)	• Improper (rounded shoulder) sitting position • Weak posterior shoulder and scapula muscles • Tight chest, upper trapezius and anterior shoulder muscles • Performing activities that involve the shoulder incorrectly due to weak or tight muscles, poor position and/or improper technique. • Inability to stabilize scapula
Shoulder impingement (Pinching)	• Improper (rounded shoulder) sitting position • Weak posterior shoulder and scapula muscles • Tight chest, upper trapezius and anterior shoulder muscles • Performing activities that involve the shoulder incorrectly due to weak or tight muscles, poor position and/or improper technique. • Inability to stabilize scapula
Degenerative changes to bones and joints	• Overuse of shoulder during movement activities • Performing activities that involve the shoulder incorrectly due to weak or tight muscles, poor position and/or improper technique.
Limited range of motion	• Shoulder pain • Tight muscles (contactures)

Table 15.14. General Recommendations to Prevent Common Shoulder Problems for Individuals with C8 Complete Spinal Cord Injury

Action	Activity	Comments
Strengthen muscles	• Middle and lower trapezius • Rhomboids • Rotator cuff muscles • Serratus anterior • Deltoid • Teres major	These are the muscles that are typically weak.
Stretch muscles	• Upper trapezius • Levator scapulae • Pectoralis muscles • Teres major	These are the muscles that are typically tight.
Use proper positioning during:	• Transfers • Sitting position	Maintain scapula in a down and back position

Middle Trapezius

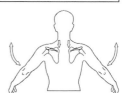

• Lie on your stomach
• Put your arms out to your side
• Squeeze your shoulder blades together
• Lift your arms toward the ceiling

You may need help supporting your arms

Repeat _____ times
Perform _____ sets

Lower Trapezius

• Lie on your stomach
• Put your arms out over your head like a "Y"
• Squeeze your shoulder blade together and down as you lift your arms upwards toward the ceiling
• Keep your neck muscles relaxed and keep your head on the table

You may need help supporting your arms

Repeat _____ times
Perform _____ sets

Rhomboids

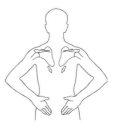

- Lie on your stomach
- Put your hands over back pocket with palm upwards toward the ceiling
- Squeeze your shoulder blade together and down as you lift your arms upwards toward the ceiling
- Do not lift your shoulders toward your head, keep your head on the table

You may need help supporting your arms

Repeat _____ times
Perform _____ sets

Serratus Anterior

Position 1

- Sit in a chair
- Position your arms on a table so that they are supported
- Push your arms forward in a reaching motion
- Do not lift your shoulders, keep your head and neck in a neutral position
You may need help supporting your arms

Repeat _____ times
Perform _____ sets

Position 2

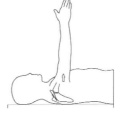

- Lie on your back
- Position your arms toward the ceiling
- Maintain your shoulder and arm position, and relax your neck muscles
- Push your arms forward in a reaching motion

You may need help supporting your arms
You can use an air cast to make this exercise easier

Repeat _____ times
Perform _____ sets

Position 3

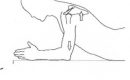

- Lie on your stomach and elbows
- Align elbows under your shoulders
- Push your elbows into the table
- Keep your neck muscles relaxed and head in a neutral position

You may need help supporting your body weight
You can use pillows under your chest and waist to make this exercise easier

Repeat _____times
Perform _____ sets

Rotator Cuff Muscles

Internal external rotation

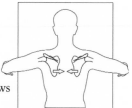

- Sit in a chair
- Position your arms by your side with your elbows bent and thumbs turned away from your body
- Maintain this position as you slowly squeeze your shoulder blades together to rotate your arms outwards
- Slowly return your arms to the starting position
- Make sure you keep your neck muscles relaxed

Do not lift your shoulders
You may need help supporting your arms

Repeat _____times
Perform _____ sets

Empty Can Exercise:

- Sit in chair
- Position your arms by your side with your thumbs turned downwards toward your knees
- Lift your arms upwrds to shoulder height
- Make sure your neck muscles are relaxed.

You may need help supporting your arms

Repeat _____times
Perform _____ sets

What Can I Do?

As you work to maintain your shoulder health and prevent problem, be sure to:

- *Understand your body so you can recognize potential problems.* Develop a good understanding of how your shoulders work and what shoulder problems might arise, depending on your level of spinal cord injury.
- *Be proactive.* Take steps to prevent shoulder problems before they develop. Maintain good muscle balance, position your shoulders properly, and use appropriate assistive equipment. Doing so will prevent pain and allow you to continue doing activities you need to do or want to do.
- *Strengthen and stretch.* Make shoulder exercises a routine part of your life. Review the exercises provided in this chapter and talk with your physical therapist or occupational therapist about which exercises are appropriate for you. Make sure you understand which muscles you are strengthening and why.
- *Avoid overuse.* Don't overdo exercises and other activities that could strain or injure your shoulder muscles.
- *Deal with pain.* If you experience shoulder pain, talk with your doctor or therapist right away so you can resolve the problem and prevent injury.

Where Can I Find Out More?

To learn more about improving or maintaining your shoulder health, you may wish to contact:

- Your doctor
- Your physical or occupational therapist
- Spinal Cord Injury Information Network (visit www.spinalcord.uab.edu and go to "Shoulders" in the A-Z SCI topics index)

Appendix C provides information about additional resources.

IMPORTANT POINTS TO REMEMBER

• The shoulder is a very complex joint with many muscles that help with movement of the arm and shoulder. Different spinal cord injury levels can affect the muscle innervation and amount of possible strength in different shoulder muscles.
• Common shoulder problems among persons with spinal cord injury include shoulder pain, muscle imbalance, subluxation, and contractures.
• Exercises to maintain muscle strength and range of motion can help prevent shoulder problems and pain that might reduce one's ability to do activities of daily living. Maintaining a healthy weight and striving for good muscle balance, positioning, and posture can also avert shoulder-related problems.

This chapter was supported in part through a grant from the U.S. Department of Education, National Institute on Disability and Rehabilitation Research, Grant #H133B031114.

—16—

Reflections of a Senior Physician: How Do You Make Spinal Cord Injury Work for You?

JOHN E. TOERGE

"In wanting to become independent, remember, no one is totally independent. Being independent doesn't mean being able to do everything by yourself. It means knowing what help you need to recruit in order to participate in life." –Price

If you've read much or all of this book, you've learned a great deal about living well with spinal cord injury. You've heard from experts representing different disciplines and perspectives and, we hope, gained useful information that will help you throughout your life. This final chapter offers insightful observations of a physician with many years of experience working with persons with spinal cord injury. This chapter discusses:

- The need to establish consistent, daily care routines
- The importance of communication with your health care professionals
- The impact of changes in your daily routines
- Ways to reduce your risk of complications and other problems
- Ways to build relationships with others

HOW DO YOU DO—THINGS?

Developing Care Routines

Many people will give you and your family advice. Health care providers will provide medical advice and factual information, and people who have been injured for a while will offer practical information based on their first-hand experience. Whom do you believe? In the initial stages, health care providers should be your most important source of information. They can help you develop specific, repeatable, standard routines, which are necessary for survival and self-preservation. The first step in getting past the initial injury is to learn and practice these routines. These routines are health care activities to rebuild, maintain, and preserve your health. They include skin care and monitoring, bladder management, bowel regimens, nutrition, fluids, health care monitoring by physicians, equipment use and maintenance, management of supplies and personnel issues. When these routines have become second nature, you might cautiously try variations to streamline or improve your daily life. With experience, you and your family can decide how best to adjust how you do specific activities and tasks. This lets you develop an acceptable lifestyle for yourself and your family.

Regardless of the modifications you may make, routine activities must occur to preserve your health, safety, and well-being. Variations in care routines can be developed through discussion with your health care providers or other patients who have found reliable methods to deal with specific problems.

Becoming Independent

Spinal cord injury is the ultimate condition of inconvenience. It requires careful planning, knowledge, and most importantly, consistency to avoid complications and unintended outcomes. You and your caregivers share responsibility to understand what needs to be done when. Failure to act appropriately and within specified time frames can result in problems and harm. Having established routines and using lists, timers, and reminders can help you to manage the complexities of spinal cord injury. As consistent routines develop, you may find that your need for these artificial reminders decreases greatly. Understanding your new, post-injury patterns of behavior and physical needs helps you and your caregivers recognize what is now "routine." Alterations in those patterns require a specific response to avoid significant complications.

Open lines of communication with appropriate experts are critical in the early phases of spinal cord injury care. Reassurance may be the only thing you need in some situations. Learning to gauge the degree and urgency of response also is part of the early learning process. You must also learn to recognize when and how to involve health care professionals. A goal of rehabilitation is to help you make the transition from relying on professional health care providers for all aspects of care to ensuring that you and your caregivers can do things on your own. In time, your rehabilitation team members must shift their roles from direct caregivers to advisers who encourage you and build your self-confidence. This process makes you more independent and is remarkably liberating for everyone involved in your care.

Who Teaches Whom?

In the early stages of rehabilitation, your relationship with your health care team is one way, with the team giving you needed information and advice. At this point, your health care providers have information and experience that far outdistance yours. As time goes by, you'll use the information they provide to learn new routines to maintain your health. Based on that knowledge and experience, you'll find that creative ways of managing your care emerge and you begin to customize and refine your routines.

At some point, you and your team members possess roughly equivalent information and background for personal care delivery. Soon, your routines and your understanding about what you need may actually be greater than your team's knowledge of what you need. At that point, you may find yourself helping others to devise creative solutions and actually teaching your health care providers.

Learning to Deal with the Unexpected

One of the most difficult tasks associated with spinal cord injury is the need to amass lots of information, filter that information, test its practicality, and develop appropriate routines. The task is daunting at first. There is too much information to understand or manage in a practical way. Slowly, information about the injury and how it affects each body system becomes clearer, more understandable, and more manageable. Care routines and practical solutions emerge.

The most significant amount of learning occurs within the first six months after injury. Then, over the first six months to several years, you'll develop care and management tactics. You'll be confronted by almost all situations within the first five years after injury. Each of these situations provides the opportunity to learn and develop creative solutions. From these experiences, you and your caregiver will adapt your care to meet the unexpected. Learning to meet and overcome challenges means taking direct responsibility for your own care.

Helping Health Care Providers Know What You Know

There is no greater teacher than the day-to-day activities you and your caregiver encounter. These experiences enhance your confidence and competence. They also provide the context within which professional health care providers can make practical suggestions to help you continue to take responsibility for yourself. It is critical, however, for you and your caregiver to assert your knowledge and competence in exchanges with professional health care providers. Be sure to speak up, and don't let anyone push you into making health care decisions that aren't appropriate for you in a given situation. After all, you are the person with the most information and experience. You need to weigh the information and options to make the best health care decision for yourself. For most individuals, this is a new and awesome responsibility.

Taking an active role in decision-making is an essential role. Failure to do so can lead to negative consequences. Firm insistence, particularly in familiar situations, is the most appropriate way to help health care providers recognize your personal competence. It balances the advice that the professional suggests with your experience and knowledge. Your assertiveness and open communication with your health care providers should enhance your own and their understanding of care options, and your respect for one another. If this mutual understanding and respect don't develop, other health care providers should be sought.

MAKING CHOICES

Established Practice Vs. New Ideas

Change for the sake of change is not appropriate or safe for persons with spinal cord injury. Innovations in care, equipment, medications, and other interventions may prove useful, and information and advice are critical in order to decide when it is judicious to try "new" things. However, you should not be first to try "new" things. Any innovation that addresses a specific need must be evaluated for efficacy. If the benefits are shown to outweigh the potential risks, then you may decide to try a new approach. Again, take care to introduce innovations one by one to monitor their effects. Be sure to keep alternatives or "old" technology available in case you need to revert to them. Your health care providers should be aware of the any experimentation with new technology so they can help monitor the positive or negative effects. This should be done in a collaborative manner.

Conventional Vs. Unconventional Treatment Routines

Routines and approaches to daily care can be conventional or unconventional. For instance, some individuals manage bladder care by alternating use of an indwelling catheter and use of an intermittent catheter. Conventional wisdom suggests that the best management is intermittent catheterization. Mixing this approach with use of an indwelling catheter does not fit the medical model precisely. However, there are times when an unconventional approach to care fits the lifestyle and needs of the specific individual.

In time, you may find some of these unconventional approaches to be effective. However, your health care providers need to be aware of changes in your care routines so they can monitor for any negative effects. You may need to negotiate with your providers to convince them of your rationale for using an unconventional approach. There are times, however, when altering care routines is ill-advised. When someone tells you about the newest and greatest development in spinal cord injury, it is a good idea to have that evaluated with your health care advisors. Many of the "newest" advances have been tried in the past. Generally, this has been met with limited success or may have adverse consequences. Sometimes, the newest and greatest development may be too expensive or not readily available to you. A good rule to follow is not being the first to try things but not be the last to try things, either. When these newest and greatest developments present themselves, that is when traditional advice from your trusted health care providers may prove most useful.

Self-Reliance Vs. Self-Destruction

Self-reliance is a natural outcome of the successful rehabilitation process. Be aware, though, that each element of care is established to meet a physiologic need. A certain amount of latitude in customizing your care is desirable and reasonable. However, unfounded approaches and shortcuts to care routines may actually cause. Although certain efficiencies and shortcuts may be helpful, failure to do the basic routines may be self-destructive. The most common area for individuals to short change is the bowel program. Adjusting the timing or methods you use in your bowel program ultimately may lead to an inability to empty your bowel. What at first appears to be a convenient shortcut may result in surgeries to relieve obstruction, rerouting the bowel or otherwise altering the way the bowel should work. The more surgical procedures you have, the more likely you are to face complications. Therefore, routines must be established to avoid self-destructive behaviors.

Pop Culture Vs. Fact Versus Opinion

Things change. What you learn as the only way to do a certain task today may be different from what is recommended tomorrow. Someone will always come up with a better way to do a task. How do you decide what is right for you? This is difficult. Just as new methods to lose weight are constantly touted, so too are popular suggestions for the newest ways to do routine spinal cord injury care. Much of this pop wisdom is unproven and possibly even dangerous. In other words, the pop culture of spinal cord injury has the potential to do harm. Generally, these approaches have not been around long enough to be tested for safety. Some pieces of equipment like wheelchairs and their modifications have fallen into this category. Certainly, valuable advances have grown out of pop culture ideas and become acceptable practice. This is the ideal outcome, but is not always the reality.

As you sift through information about new approaches, be sure to seek advice from a qualified health care professional about what is known and not known. Also keep in mind that many health care providers and virtually all spinal cord injured persons have opinions as to how best to manage a wide variety of daily care issues. Opinion must be recognized as just that—opinion, not necessarily fact. Opinions are generated from observations, experience, and the intention to do the right thing. Many times, however, there is no way to prove that they are correct, despite the work done to evaluate the results of these approaches. Sorting through the pop culture, facts, and opinions is frequently the most difficult task for the spinal cord injured person. In this instance, your health care professionals' and your own experience is probably the best teacher.

Who Has the Experience?

Yes, experience is the best teacher. Experience is frequently gained by correcting a mistake that you've made. This is the harsh reality for many spinal cord injured persons. As discussed above, you are probably the most qualified person to determine what is best for you. Confidence in yourself is essential, but be careful of becoming overly confident too soon. Learning to live with spinal cord injury in some ways is similar to learning to drive a car. The biggest issue confronting the new driver is overconfidence or lack of understanding of the consequences of certain actions. Like a new driver, your skill and judgment will grow over time. During this process, you must assess your health care providers' experience and weigh the information they share. The best arrangement is a collaborative effort between you and the professional to reach a common goal—your continued health and well-being.

Risk-taking behaviors by both parties must also be assessed. If you are a risk taker, then the practitioner should probably be more conservative. If you shy away from risk, then the practitioner might need to be more eager to encourage change. This delicate balance comes from both individuals listening, talking, and supporting each other.

MAKING CHANGES

Know the Basics—and Explore Your Options

At first, the long list of "must do" tasks given to you by health care professionals is overwhelming and nearly impossible to comprehend. As time goes by and you begin to understand the rationale for each action, you begin to develop practical routines for life. The endless details are still overwhelming, but they start to take shape in the form of specific themes of care related to each body system. During this stage of care, your health care providers seem rigid and unbending in the specifics of routines necessary to maintain the spinal cord injured person. Precision is the goal for making most of these routines work.

Unfortunately, despite their expertise, health care providers may give you the impression that all elements of care are equally important. They also are not particularly good at showing newly injured persons how to "cheat on" or alter care routines. However, once you master the basics of care, variations on those themes may be considered. This is when a dialog between you and your health care professionals is most critical and when you must be a well-informed consumer. Questions about why things are done the way they are and how they can be modified must be met with answers from health care professionals. This initial chance provides variations on the basic themes of health care for each system in the body.

When you go home and reenter the community, new obstacles are presented. This is when additional modifications or variations must be considered. During this period, be sure to keep track of your questions and to explore them your health care team. Frank and honest discussion between you and your health care professional is critical for good decision making, now and in the future.

Is It Dangerous?

When making a change or doing something new, the first assessment should be to ask if the activity is dangerous to your overall well-being. You may be inclined to adopt suggestions from well-intended persons about medications, equipment, or health care routines. Following this advice may cause injury, even though no harm was intended. Sometimes, too, you may decide to change something on your own because you are tired of the continuous demands of routine care.

For example, one of the most common issues is pressure relief for the skin. Few individuals can sit for prolonged time periods without injury to their skin. The short-term consequence of sitting too long in the wheelchair is a skin pressure ulcer. The long-term consequence of sitting in the wheelchair too long is a skin pressure ulcer that does not heal or does not heal correctly. A brief conversation with someone who has endured the healing process of pressure ulcer would scare the most ardent risk taker into watching the pressure relief schedule carefully. Following advice from only reliable sources is the best way to avoid potentially hazardous activities or making dangerous decisions.

What Are the Long-term Consequences?

One of the most important questions to ask at any time is, "What are the long-term consequences of what I'm doing right now?" This is one of the most difficult questions to answer. Based on statistics, we know that sitting too long on skin produces a pressure ulcer. Who will develop a pressure ulcer? We don't know. We also don't know exactly who will develop kidney stones or bladder stones—which can lead to progressive, irreversible loss of kidney function—after changing their catheterization program. The risks cannot be assessed precisely for each individual. Statistics, however, are gathered to get the best idea of what is most likely to happen. It is best to follow the numbers!

Making random changes in your daily care routines can rob you of the vitality you need to enjoy life and meet the demands of daily living. Therefore, we emphasize the importance of establishing and following specific routines to monitor for and avoid complications. These are the health care routines that statistically make the most sense for the largest number of people with spinal cord injury. Every effort should be made to keep statistics on your side.

One Step at a Time

When your routines are firmly established, you can consider attempting changes. You might want to make a change in a routine because you want to find a better way of doing a specific task, you're changing caregivers, you want to travel, or a suggestion has been made by of a reliable source. The cardinal rule is to change only one thing at a time. Because everything else stays the same, any adverse effects can be attributed to the change. When you've been successful with established routines, change must be considered very carefully in order not to adversely affect your health. Once the risks and benefits of change have been analyzed, that change may be instituted and then monitored for its outcome. If the change does not work for any reason, you can immediately return to the original method.

Analyze What Happened When Something Goes Wrong

If anything appears to go wrong, try to analyze why there is a problem. Some things are obvious. Perhaps there is a break in the typical routine that has led to a negative outcome. Perhaps the typical approach to problem-solving has failed. Perhaps your body has changed, dictating the need for change in the standard routines of care.

If experience is the best teacher, then the analysis of why routines do not work is the best way to understand what will work in the future. Despite what may appear to be a negative situation, all efforts should be directed toward discovering why that negative situation developed. Obviously, the same circumstances should not be repeated in the future. If you don't follow your basic health care routines daily, analysis of where the system failed is nearly impossible.

REDUCING YOUR RISKS

High-Risk Times

Times of change in routine are the most high-risk times for persons with spinal cord injury. These changes may include alterations in your diet or fluid intake associated with your bladder or bowel management routines; increased bed rest; increased sitting in a wheelchair; and changes in equipment such as your wheelchair, wheelchair cushion, or vehicle seating also increase your risk of complications.

Changing your caregiver is one of the highest-risk situations you may face. You and a long-time caregiver likely have a comfortable relationship and understanding about your care-delivery needs and expectations. A new caregiver may not be familiar with your routines or have the same skill as the original caregiver. This could place you at risk for injury or complications due to miscommunication or no communication. Therefore, special attention to detail is critical during transitions from one caregiver to another. If a caregiver change is anticipated, many spinal cord injured persons find that videotaping the care activities is helpful to the next caregiver. New, experienced caregivers may have bias regarding how they have performed tasks for other spinal cord injured persons. Videotaping specific to your needs will direct care delivery without controversy. Videotaping details the specifics of care for the new person trying to make the transition to care provider.

In addition, if your living situation changes, new challenges may arise. For example, decreased accessibility of work, community and home, longer distances for commuting or shopping, less personal support from neighbors and decreased access to resources can make this a high-risk time. If a change such as this is anticipated, every effort should be made to make routines similar to those followed in the original living situation.

Furthermore, your relationships with your spouse and friends may change. Some of these changes may be positive. On the other hand, they can present attitudinal or emotional changes that can be psychologically or physically devastating. This can be one of the highest risk times for the spinal cord injured person. This often is a time when a person needs additional support to maintain health and self-esteem.

Finally, changes in vocational or avocational activities may present a positive or negative situation for you. Working or suddenly not working either by choice or change in circumstance may be equally important to the spinal cord injured person. How this is viewed can have major effects on the spinal cord injured patient. Many relationships change because of changes in work and avocational activities. Regardless of the nature of the change, it represents high-risk times because of the change in routines for the spinal cord injured person.

Routine—The Way to Get Grounded Again

What if high-risk events like those described above bring about negative outcomes for you? Again, analysis of how and why the outcomes occurred, and return to standard routines of care, will help. Going back to the basics can help to reestablish your health and well-being. Returning to the basic routines of care that you learned in the early stages of rehabilitation can reduce your risk of further problems. If one body system is under stress, all the other body systems are likely to be under stress as well. Therefore, improving the health and well-being of each individual system by following the basic routines will re-establish your health.

Periodically, a problem with one body system problem results in hospitalization. If this occurs, be sure that all other body system routines are performed consistently and correctly. This can be a significant challenge in the health care system of today. During these times, you might find it helpful to have another person who understands your needs advocate for you and insist that the basic care routines be followed exactly. Otherwise, your overall health care will deteriorate. This is a critical time for collaboration with your health care providers and effective coordination of your care.

BUILDING RELATIONSHIPS

Your Relationships with Health Care Providers

After your spinal cord injury, you should work, with and stay in touch, with a team of physicians and other health care providers throughout the course of your life. Your physicians may include a neurosurgeon, orthopedist, urologist, gastroenterologist, physiatrist, and family physician. Your other health care providers may include a physical therapist, occupational therapist, rehabilitation nurse, psychologist/psychiatrist, social worker, vocational counselor, therapeutic recreation specialist, and case manager. Each of these individuals has a specific role to help you achieve your personal goals. All of them play a role in your acute care, and each may have a specific role at various times throughout your rehabilitation. Each may also have a selected role in dealing with complications or other situations for the spinal cord injured person. Depending on the situation, any one of these health care providers may be the pivotal expert at that time.

It is important to identify a single health care provider as the coordinator of your care. Most likely this will be a physician who can order laboratory tests, radiology, equipment, and other services. Typically, long-term relationships are helpful due to the complexity of the issues most spinal cord injured persons present.

Family, Friends, and Relatives

Relationships with family members, friends, and relatives have special meaning. These relationships range from direct caregivers to supporters and advocates. Spinal cord injury can change your relationships with these individuals, however. While you face significant life changes, family, friends and relatives also face significant changes in their relationships with you. Sometimes these relationships grow stronger. Other times, unfortunately, the injury may damage a relationship with any of the individuals.

Open communication and honesty will help everyone to adjust. Family members, friends, and relatives must recognize that you have not changed inside, despite the change in your physical capacity. This is a major hurdle in many instances. For those who recommit to the relationship, a much stronger bond is often formed. A sense of humor, a sense of the serious, and a healthy dose of genuine mutual respect can help your relationships. The significance of these relationships can never be underestimated. It takes work, but it is worth it.

Personal Care Attendants

Personal care attendants introduce a whole new dynamic into your life. These individuals frequently provide the most intimate care. Recruiting, training, and retaining personal care attendants can be a nearly full time job. While these individuals are clearly employees, you rely on them for your essential daily care. Personal care attendants must be trustworthy, compassionate, honest, and perhaps most importantly, reliable. The long-term relationships with your personal care attendants can be a lifeline to your health and well-being

Because of daily needs, it is important to have backup or duplicate/parallel care assistance in case of emergencies. This is not always easy to accomplish. Often, for better or worse, this backup care falls to family members, friends, and relatives. Coordination of this type of care requires significant attention to detail and planning. You may find that training in management of personal care attendants is helpful.

Payers

Along with many other changes in a spinal cord injured person's life comes management of finances related to health care and other living expenses. In most instances, a claims examiner is involved for the insurance company. These individuals look at the cost of care and elements of care to which you are entitled. This care varies widely with the payer and the policy. The claims examiners interpret the policies and entitlement to care. Because of the catastrophic nature of spinal cord injury, insurance companies often assign a case manager to monitor progression of care. This person may serve as your advocate or in an advocate role for the insurance carrier to limit the liability and costs. He or she may be pivotal in decisions about your care. You and your health care providers must negotiate with the case manager to ensure the appropriate distribution of resources. This frequently requires multiple conversations and significant documentation to be successful.

Case managers may or may not be familiar with the issues associated with spinal cord injury. Frequently, they must be educated as to the needs and expectation for care. Once the case manager understands your needs and the ramifications of not meeting those needs, he or she may become more responsive. If this doesn't happen, direct contact with the medical director of the insurance carrier may be necessary. You may need to educate this person about spinal cord injury and its ramifications. The medical director may be the person to make the final decision about resources provided for care. It is important that you and your health care providers present the most relevant information so good decisions are made at this level. Unfortunately, not all health care insurance policies deal with catastrophic illness in the same manner. Benefits for rehabilitation and other necessities may be excluded.

Your Employer

Spinal cord injured persons who are working often have excellent relationships with their employers. Employment frequently provides structure and meaning in the spinal-cord-injured person's life. Aside from earning a living, work frequently provides a social environment appreciated by all involved. Many spinal-cord-injured persons are good employees because of their organizational skills developed as a result their injury. Certain jobs, obviously, are more conducive than others for return to work after spinal cord injury. Your experience, skills, and education before your injury to some extent determine your ability to return to work, but vocational retraining can open new doors. The desire to work and be employed is the strongest determinant for the ability to return to work.

CLOSING WORDS

It's not easy to endure the effects of spinal cord injury. Maintaining and improving your health, safety, and well-being are keys to enjoying the rest of your life to its fullest. Knowledgeable, reliable advisers can keep you moving in the right direction and help you sift through all of the medical information, personal opinion, and the advice of others so that you can choose the most appropriate course of action at any given time. The experience of others who have been injured previously also can help you make good decisions.

Finally, remember that love, work, and play are the elements of a satisfying life. Seek out each of these to the fullest extent possible to maintain a balanced life. Health is the foundation upon which the remaining balanced life can be built. Stay healthy!

**The Bottom Line: Ten Recommendations for a
Satisfying, Healthy Life**

1. Learn everything you can about spinal cord injury.
2. Learn health care routines and know/practice them effectively.
3. Gather information from a variety of sources, but use this information with caution.
4. Find a support group or another group of reliable health care professionals and others who can advise you.
5. Recognize that "if it sounds too good to be true," it probably is too good to be true—and it may actually be dangerous.
6. Seek professional help early if you suspect a health problem.
7. Make sure someone else knows your health care as well as you do, he or she can act as your advocate or reliable sounding board for changes in your care.
8. Think about changes in your health care from all perspectives before changing anything, then make changes one at a time to determine if they are workable and appropriate.
9. Keep all equipment in excellent working condition and be very cautious to avoid personal injury at times when equipment changes occur.
10. If there is a change in your health care status changes, resume basic, well-proven routines until the crisis passes.

Appendix C provides information about additional resources.

This chapter was supported in part by funding from the U.S. Department of Education, National Institute on Disability and Rehabilitation Research, Grant #H133B031114.

Appendix A: Personal Stories

On Rehab, Work, Independence, Relationships, Awareness, the Good, the Bad, and the Joys of Living
Jennifer Sheehy Keller

From the very beginning, when I was completely paralyzed and being fed intravenously, I had dreams about flying and sliding . . . and dessert. In some dreams, I was flying above people dining in a restaurant and diving down to have a bite of apple crisp or chocolate mousse cake. In one, I was sliding fast down a chocolate mountain onto a graham cracker beach. I had lots of flying dreams. I was never in a wheelchair and I was never paralyzed. Some of my dreams expressed fears I couldn't acknowledge while awake. In my most vivid dream, I was at Kmart in the cashier line. In front of me was a head. He was rolling and smiling, and a cheery salesperson helped him put items on the counter. The cashier rang his items as if there was nothing unusual about a bodyless head being at Kmart. In my dream I remember thinking, is this what I'm like now? A head with a positive attitude and no body? At least I could shop at Kmart.

In the beginning, every morning when I woke up, I would realize I hadn't been cured the night before and I couldn't fly or slide through life. I believed that my dreams were a sign that I would recover completely and walk again. Now, 10 years later, I am still a C5-C6 quadriplegic, paralyzed from the chest down with no use of my hands. To this day, if my wheelchair is in my dream, it is in the room with me or I am dragging it behind me. My dreams no longer mean that I am going to walk again. I no longer have to walk to be recovered, successful, or happy. Now I know my dreams were telling me that I would still have a great life, just with a different way of getting around.

I must preface my story by gratefully acknowledging the ideal foundation I had from family and friends who provided needed assistance—physical, emotional, and financial. My family and friends participated in therapy, helping me work on techniques after hours and on weekends. When I left the hospital, my family juggled their own lives to spend time helping me.

They bolstered my attitude and conversely, were bolstered by mine. Attitude is a fragile suspended sculpture that depends on all creators holding up their parts. Many people don't have the support from others that I had. A strong emotional support system, whether it is from friends, family or both, is critical to successful rehabilitation.

I was injured in 1994 at a time when my life was at a high point. I had completed my first year of business school, drove a cute convertible, and played golf every free minute I had. The only handicap I knew was my rotten putting stroke. I was a marketing intern at Anheuser-Busch, a job my business school colleagues envied. Life was relatively carefree and we all took much for granted. Then, on the Fourth of July, at a neighborhood pool party, I was pushed into the shallow end of the pool and broke my neck. I did not know my life was changed forever; I was completely paralyzed, but still responded like nothing had changed. As the ambulance raced to the hospital, I asked my boyfriend to call work and tell them I'd be late, then reminded him to bring my mascara to the hospital. I had my priorities. I went through 12 terrifying hours of surgery during which my family rushed in from across the country. We all prayed that this paralysis was temporary. The doctors told us that, if it was, I would probably start moving again in three days. My family kept an anxious vigil for the three longest days of my life, asking every couple hours if I could move anything yet. Three days later, nothing. Life as I knew it was over. What was next? Would I ever work or have fun again?

On to Rehab

Before I began rehabilitation at National Rehabilitation Hospital (NRH), the doctors and nurses in St. Louis warned me that I was about to begin the hardest work I would ever do. They were right, but then again, the stakes were the highest I had ever faced. In the process of rehab, I called upon internal resources and developed skills and traits that made me and others who experience spinal cord injuries, better, stronger people. These skills and traits, which remain inherent in me today, include goal setting, perseverance, problem solving, self-confidence, and determination.

Goal setting: I had a list of short-term and long-term goals that I still tick off one by one. My most important short-term goal was to be able to scratch my nose. My long-term goals were to walk and break 80 on the golf course.

Perseverance: It took me a year and a half of practicing every single day to learn how to transfer myself, with a sliding board, from my chair to my bed. In the beginning, my therapist made me practice incremental steps that she promised would eventually lead to one smooth transferring movement. There were many days when I believed that my therapists were the most deluded people in the world. Couldn't they see I was paralyzed? I truly could not imagine how I would eventually string the small steps together into one movement across what seemed an overwhelming distance between my chair and bed. I had to trust that she knew what she was doing, which, of course, she did. Increased function is a maximization of strength, knowledge and practice. I was an inpatient for three months and an outpatient for a year and a half. When I "graduated," I continued to work out two or three times a week with wrist weights, for a few months with a personal trainer then on my own.

Problem solving: When you acquire a spinal cord injury, you are forced to learn new ways of doing even the simplest activity. To do that, you must be open-minded, creative, patient, and directed. I have no hand function, but I was bound and determined to tweeze my own eyebrows and apply mascara. Writing, feeding myself, dressing, and walking the dog all required adaptation that was achieved by trial and error, research, and out-of-the-box thinking.

Self-confidence: You cannot go through rehabilitation without developing valuable skills. Soon you recognize that you are becoming a more capable person, able to conquer obstacles that would defeat many.

Determination: I was adamant about returning to business school and getting back on track with my life. I was also determined to walk again. Never underestimate the power of denial. It is a very effective coping mechanism that, when used the right way, can be an energizing, productive force. Today, I am not walking, but I am still in denial. I refuse to live the life that society expects of someone with a severe disability.

When I first experienced group therapy, I protested. Why were they putting me with *them?* I wasn't one of *them*—I wasn't disabled like *them*. I was still one of us and I was going to recover. Later, I found out that every patient has the same reaction to other patients. I had very little experience with disability before my injury. In a strange twist of fate, six months prior to my injury, I had worked with the National Organization on Disability to help plan a fund-raising event at the British Embassy. The president, Alan Reich, was a quadriplegic who used a wheelchair. I worked closely with him and was anxious in the beginning about doing or saying something wrong. What if something happened to him and no one was around but me? His assistant told me not to touch his pen. Now that I have exactly the same disability and only a few pens that I can use easily, I understand this request. Back then, I thought maybe touching the pen would trigger some sort of outburst. Within a few days, however, I appreciated how wise, accomplished and professional Alan was and I was more anxious about pleasing the top executive than I was about his disability. It took about a month after my injury to realize that them was not them but us after all. We were much more alike than different I became very close to some of the patients. Paul, two Chrises, Tracy, and Stan. We shared a bond and understanding about the task ahead of us at the hospital, about the challenge we were proving tough enough to beat.

Getting Back to Work

My professional life since my accident has been focused on increasing employment opportunities for people with disabilities. Employment is the surest way to strengthen your self-image and increase your independence through financial power. In this society, for better or worse, you are what you do. There are lots of reasons not to work—getting up and dressed and to the job is harder, you might have to train for a different job than you did before, you think (mistakenly) that you will lose your health benefits right away, and there are 200 cable channels. However, there are better reasons to work—increased self-esteem, camaraderie, financial independence, and greater dating options. Getting the courage and confidence up to face the stares and naysayers is tough, but worth it.

Many people and services are available to help retrain someone to go back to his or her former job or a new job, and there are many new technologies that will allow people with the most severe disabilities to do a variety of jobs. My home and office environments are filled with remote controls, adaptive gadgets, and software and hardware that allow me to be as productive as or more productive than anyone else. My voice recognition software enables me to write at the pace of 150 words per minute. How many people can claim that? The computer and the Internet are the most liberating tools, providing access to resources, services, people, therapies, and solutions.

To return to business school, I had the help of a vocational rehabilitation (VR) counselor and services that helped pay for school, a computer, voice recognition software and training, driving lessons, and modifications to a van. These items were not cheap, but I have given back in taxes and shopping several times the total investment in me. I had to know what I wanted, but VR delivered. I am very grateful to my counselor, who is responsible for hundreds of people becoming fulfilled, productive, contributing taxpayers, complaining like everyone else each April.

Independence

Independence—this is something that Americans learn to believe it is a guaranteed right. The loss of independence after a traumatic spinal cord injury is devastating and one of the hardest losses to accept. You will lose material things, friends, and function, but losing independence in activities of daily living is the most frustrating, affronting, and humiliating loss of all. Many people never get over needing to have others help them with the most basic life tasks. They often take it out on the people who help them. Managing your new requirements and accomplishing everything that you need to do to live, work, and have fun require defining independence in a slightly different way.

Independence should mean exercising choice over your life. If you need to hire people in order to have power over choices, then so what? Wealthy people hire help to do gardening, shopping, cleaning, driving, even dressing and bathing. They do not apologize for it and they are not ashamed of it. They think of having help as a privilege that comes with the reward of hard earned or acquired money. The wonderful nursing assistants and friends and strangers who help me are responsible for my having control and choices and I recognize, respect, and appreciate their role. Be thankful and express it often. Living the way you want to means depending on good people to do things you can't. Ideally, this is a very symbiotic relationship not a co-dependent relationship. However rewarding helping a person with a spinal cord injury may be for someone, it is extremely important to remember that this is not charity work. It is a personal service that people are paid to perform. When you require personal care from others, it also helps to abandon any sense of modesty!

Mentors and Fun

Mentors are important, too. Knowing Alan Reich when I had my accident prompted me to set high expectations for myself as I had a similar injury. He was a constant source of answers to my frequent "how do you?" questions. Immediately after coming to NRH, Ed Eckenhoff, the CEO of the hospital, visited me in my room. Mr. Eckenhoff is a paraplegic, injured in a car accident. He not only proved to me that someone with a spinal cord injury could achieve the highest success measured by our society, but he convinced me that I could have fun again. He took me to a patch of grass outside his office and began adeptly hitting golf balls out of the hospital complex, over a busy street and onto a golf course. He used a cleverly adapted crutch to balance while he swung with one arm. His golf prowess impressed me, but not nearly as much as his self-assurance that he could avoid a mis-hit that might send an unsuspecting driver into his hospital.

My long-term goals had to change at that magic two-year mark when I realized I probably wouldn't be walking or playing golf again. Replacing the activities that add fun to your life is as important as teaching yourself new ways to eat, dress and write. Seeking out activities that would supplant my love of golf opened up a new world of exciting choices and experiences I never would have pursued before my accident. Sailing, hot air ballooning, kayaking, hand-cycling, white water rafting, parasailing, paragliding, and skiing are all possible for someone with no grip. In Bucks County, Pennsylvania, there is a small airport, Van Sant, which is the home to Freedoms Wings, a soaring organization with instructors and a fleet of hand-controlled gliders. After several euphoric hours flying over farms, vineyards and rivers, I realized I could let go of the hope of playing on a golf course as long as I could fly over them. My early post-injury dreams about flying were brought to life, giving me a greater sense of freedom and independence.

Personal Relationships

What happens to personal relationships and how others react to you and your new circumstances is always a question that is uppermost in people's minds when they acquire spinal cord injury. The injury does not just affect the person who acquires it. People closest to you suffer the same sense of loss, just in a different way. I immediately questioned whether I would ever be attractive or able to date again. At the time of my injury, I was recently divorced and dating the man who pushed me into the swimming pool. We both felt it was important to maintain our relationship during my recovery to support each other. However, after four years, it was clear that we were going in different directions, and I had met someone who was more compatible and blind to my disability. I gained the confidence to date again. Like everyone else, I maximized the positive and tried to minimize the negative. I emphasized my hair and face and downplayed my skinny legs and big feet (made bigger by the larger shoes I was forced to wear to accommodate swelling). I dressed up everyday and found that people treated me more seriously and with greater respect.

Just as I thought any employer would be very lucky to have someone like me with my credentials and new skills of problem solving, perseverance, determination, and discipline, I thought any man would be very lucky to have someone so smart, humorous, and accomplished as a companion. Not everyone is open to dating someone who uses a wheelchair, though. A former work colleague came up to me after my accident and said, "I used to have the biggest crush on you," as if it was safe to admit since I was no longer dateable. Of course, he was the one who wasn't dateable with or without a disability! Fortunately, plenty of others don't care or get over the fact you use a wheelchair quickly as soon as they see you handle yourself assuredly. When you are comfortable with yourself, you put people at ease with your disability. Don't ever think that a physical limitation keeps you from contributing equally in a relationship. Disability isn't sexy, but humor, a positive attitude, and confidence are! My dating days ended last February when I got married.

Building Awareness

Since I left the hospital, I have found that a lot of my time is spent educating the world around me. I realized quickly that you represent the whole society of people with disabilities if you are the only one that someone has contact with. Your response to a situation or question may determine whether that person ever interacts with another person with a disability. True cultural change takes decades and inches forward only when an individual is touched personally. This is not to say that you have to be nice and entertain everyone's questions all the time. A former faculty member stomped over to me when I was at Georgetown business school and barked, "What happened to you?" It was clear that he saw me as my disability, not as a human. I didn't feel I had to dignify his query with a response. Now if a stranger says, "Nice handbag; what happened to you?" or "Hello, I'm Jim, do you mind if I ask you a question?" then I gladly entertain their curiosity if I have time.

And one evening, I was waiting outside a restaurant where I was meeting a friend, and a tourist rushed to me, saying loudly with an accent, "Oh you poor girl! Look at you. So many people complain about their aches and pains, but you have to live life in a wheelchair!" Looking around quickly, I desperately sought another wheelchair user who could have been the focus of his attention. I wanted to be invisible from the stares of others who heard him yell at me, but I knew I was going to have to give a mini-ADA/disability lesson on the spot. I said to him, "You must not be from this country or you wouldn't pity me. People with disabilities in the United States have a guaranteed right to all the activities and benefits everybody else has here. I work, own my own home, have a boyfriend (who I later married) and have more fun than most people."

"Do you fly?" I asked the stranger.

"Yes, of course. I flew to Washington yesterday," he replied.

"No," I said, taking a chance, "Can you pilot a plane?"

"No," he said incredulously. "Can you?"

"Yes, I'm taking lessons to get my license. When you're in this country, don't be surprised if you get on a plane and your pilot has just put his wheelchair in the hold."

I found that a lot of people who ask questions rudely and inappropriately are selfishly wondering what happened to you, so they can avoid that activity and maintain their delusion of invincibility. This primarily happens with older men. In a light-hearted way, I can poke fun at their vulnerability with a little white lie. In those circumstances, I will respond that, "I acquired an embolism in my spinal cord that usually occurs in older men when they're having sex."

I always try to answer children's questions honestly, though. Personal interaction is the only way to debunk the stereotype or prevent them from taking hold. Of course, you never know how kids will respond. I gave a presentation at nursery school. The audience ranged from two to four year-olds who had been visited all week by people in their neighborhood—a fireman, a lawyer, and a policeman. I sat in front of them in my wheelchair and said, "You've heard from a lot of people this week and everyone is different in some way. What you think is different about me?" The kids looked at me and giggled and whispered to each other, then one little girl jumped up raising her hand shouting, "I know, I know, I know! You're really old!"

Bad Days, Good Days

It is impossible not to have bad days once in a while. Everybody has them. There are days when my chronic pain is intolerable, when I come home from work, roll over a mess my dog made, and drop my entire sushi dinner on the floor. I have waited hours in the cold for shuttles because the subway elevators were down. Not that I was any good, but I miss dancing and I miss cracking my own crabs. At those times, I feel very sorry for myself. It is natural and healthy to give in to the grief briefly, even cry for a little while, but then remember your eyes will be puffy in the morning and there are so many ways your situation can be worse. I have so much joy and satisfaction in my life with my husband, friends, and family, and through my work and fun experiences. It is so much easier and energizing to stay positive and forward thinking.

Postscript

In 1999—five years after my spinal cord injury—I was in a life-threatening car accident. After two weeks in intensive care, two weeks in the hospital, and three months in a nursing home, I began the arduous process of my second rehabilitation at NRH. This time, I had complete confidence in my new abilities to do whatever was necessary to recover and cope with unknown obstacles. As soon as I was assured that I was going to live, I was elated. I couldn't wait to return to my life with a spinal cord injury! I realized how fortunate I am, how many things I love doing, how complete and fulfilling every day is.

Today, I am proud of my disability. It's like having a visible diploma that only a few people have earned and that proves you can survive and thrive after the toughest test. I believe people with severe disabilities and people who have faced traumas that others view as unthinkable are an elite crew who are wiser, tougher and more capable than everyone else.

You Can Do It, Too!

Tim Strachan

F. Scott Fitzgerald once wrote, "Show me a hero and I will write you a tragedy." In our society, many heroes have become heroes because they have successfully confronted tragedy. Likewise, whenever we see a tragic situation—one in which a person is placed in a position to overcome adversity that seems insurmountable—we tend to put that person up on a pedestal. The words "I couldn't do that if I were in that position" come so easy. However, when I became a person in a "tragic" situation, dealing with a spinal cord injury and dependent on a wheelchair, I just learned to live my life the best way that I could and to the best of my abilities. Now my message to all people, whether in a "tragic" situation or not, is "You can do it, too!"

Ever since I was five years old, my dream was to play college football. In the summer of 1993, that dream was unfolding right before my eyes. I was 17 years old and a standout quarterback at DeMatha Catholic High School, in Hyattsville, Maryland, a school that is nationally known for its outstanding basketball and football programs. At DeMatha, I was living a dream playing both varsity basketball and varsity football through my sophomore and junior years. That summer, heading into my senior year, my sights were set on only football. Along with the likes of Payton Manning and Donnovan McNabb, I was ranked as one of the top five quarterbacks in the nation. My name was in pre-season magazines as a pre-season All-American. I was getting trash bags full of recruiting letters from colleges all over the country. According to my coach, I could play football at just about any college in the country. I was even offered a scholarship by Penn State University's Joe Paterno before I ever played a down in my senior year. My dream was becoming a reality right before my eyes.

One week before football camp was to start, I took an annual trip to the beach with my family. I was never one for sitting still—I am still that way today. Thus, on August 5, 1993, after a day of jogging, lifting weights, and finally playing some beach volleyball, I decided to cool off with a swim. I ran toward the ocean and high stepped it in to where the water was nearly waist deep, then dove into an oncoming wave. My head hit the ground, I broke my neck, and I was instantly paralyzed.

With my dream of playing college football crushed and my life completely altered forever, I was faced with the biggest and most challenging obstacle I would ever face: life with a spinal cord injury and in a wheelchair. I was diagnosed with a C-5 quadriplegic incomplete injury. Stricken with severe pneumonia and paralysis, I spent five months in the hospital, three of which I spent at National Rehabilitation Hospital. My main focus was to get healthy enough to return home. However, that focus was cluttered with visions of what life would be like disabled, paralyzed, and totally dependent on a wheelchair and others. The hospital staffs did everything they could to prepare me for life after intensive care and rehab. However, nothing completely prepares you for the reality that awaits you. It seemed that the world kept moving, but that my life was suspended and full of anticipation, apprehension, and even fear. You can't help but ask questions such as: What is it going to be like? How will I be able to live like this? How are others going to react to me? Will life ever be normal again?

My first experiences in that outside world took place when, "on leave" from the hospital for a day, I attended the last three football games of the DeMatha football team—the team I was supposed to lead to the championship. On the way to the game, I remember thinking: Will everyone be looking at me? Will they be feeling sorry for me? Will I enjoy the game I once loved so much? What if it is a terrible experience? However, once I was there those questions subsided. I was just happy to be "out" and among family and friends. The game started and I was right back to being me again. Nothing else mattered. I cheered my team to victory and the day was a success. Although life had changed, I realized I was still me. Each game brought less apprehension and more excitement—not just for winning games or simply being outside the hospital, but for living.

I finally came home from the hospital on December 23. I went shopping for presents on Christmas Eve. Again came the apprehension, the questions, the anticipation of what is was going to be like. Sure it was different—especially since my perspective was from 4' rather than 6'4". I encountered frustration, problems, and some stares, but overall it was just another day. That experience and others I had made me realize that I could go on with life, that there were things I could do, that I was still the same person and enjoyed the same things as before my injury. Slowly, but surely, over the next month I got up every day and did what I had to do to get to the next. I had to get my routine down. I was forced to do things I never had to do in the hospital because there were no nurses, therapists, or doctors to do them for me. If I dropped something on the ground, I had to learn to pick it up. If I wanted to eat or drink, I had to learn to do that on my own. The next thing I knew I was doing more than I had ever thought was possible.

DeMatha had built a ramp for me to get into the main floor of the school.

Also, the school staff put all my classes on the same floor because there was no access to other floors. (Since then, DeMatha has installed an elevator and other students in wheelchairs have attended the school from the 9th through 12th grade.) At first, everything felt different and I once again was forced to learn how to get through another day, another obstacle. With each passing week, everything became more and more normal, not only because I was accepting my new place in the world, but also because the other students and faculty and staff were becoming adjusted as well. I learned that others also had apprehensions, questions, and fears about my new situation. I learned that "we"—me and all the people around me—were learning from this experience, growing together. I learned I was not alone. They accepted me just as much as I accepted them. Again, it took time and patience, and involved trial and error. The more I tried and the more I did, the easier life became and the more I was capable of doing. For example, at first I had trouble writing with a splint, but I needed to write at school, so I kept at it and eventually learned to do it. I gained confidence to do even more as time went by, and I ended up graduating from high school on time with my class.

I went on to college, but chose to go part-time to ease into the much larger campus environment and a more demanding part of my life. It was a whole new experience, a whole new place, all new people, and more apprehension. Once again, I was forced to do more and I got it done. If something didn't work the first time, I tried it a different way. At that time, I could write only about a paragraph within about 30 minutes. My first day I had no choice but to write four pages of notes in one class and a six-page essay in the next. The essay wasn't very legible, but I did it. I was forced to open doors. I was forced to ask for help (something that wasn't easy for someone who was once so independent and a big stud football player). Again, I experienced my share of frustration, failures, and disappointment. I also experienced triumphs and victories, both big and small. Some people helped and some did not. My only concern was, and continues to be, to do what I had to do no matter what it took to get it done. One challenge at a time, one victory at a time.

I went on to graduate from the University of Maryland, and in 2004 received my law degree from Georgetown University Law Center. I am a color analyst for University of Maryland football games heard on local radio stations WBAL in Baltimore and WMAL in Washington, D.C., I am a professional motivational speaker, and I do a number of other things (no need for a resume). The point is that I started off this new beginning with apprehension, anticipation, questions, and fear—all of which are normal parts of being human. In 11 years, I have responded by going after one victory at a time. Sure, sometimes things haven't worked and I've had to try and try again. Over time, I've learned what it takes to move on and not dwell on the past or what could have been.

I remember one night in the hospital when it was late, dark, and quiet, and I was alone. I began to pray and started to ask myself the question "Why me?" However, I stopped before the words were formed and had an overwhelming feeling that it was not fair to ask it. I felt that way because I had never asked why my life was so good to begin with. I had never asked why I was such a good football player. I had never asked why I had never gone without life's necessities. I had never asked why when things were fine with my life. To ask why only when things were breaking down and falling in all around me seemed wrong.

That night, I realized how much I still had to be thankful for in life, despite a devastating injury. I realized then that not being able to walk or play football were a little less significant than I had thought. I realized I had an entire life ahead of me and I had to find any way to live it the best I could. I continue down that path today. Sure, there will be failures and there will be frustration. However, there will also be victories and triumphs. I still have the same goals and dreams today, along with new ones to boot. I don't want to be put on a pedestal for that, nor do I deserve to be. I am just doing what I have to do each day. The most important thing to remember is that you can do it, too.

Family, Friends, and Lovers—Relationships of Young People with Spinal Cord Injury
Steven Ferguson

Relationships make your life fuller. You want to have someone to go to the movies with or someone to shop with at the mall. Someone you can talk to when you're depressed or lonely, who can make you smile when you're sad. Someone you can talk to at night when you most need intimacy.

No matter what your situation is, relationships can be a challenge—even hard work. Dealing with them may be more difficult when you have a disability and find that you depend on others for help with eating, grooming, and basic care. Getting around to see people can be more complicated. You might need to move farther away from your family and friends, and at times you might feel lonely as you become acquainted with your new environment. Also, when you experience life from sitting down, you no longer look at people at eye level. People might stare at you because of your chair, and when they talk to you it's often about how you got in the chair. Sometimes the challenge is more within you—you don't think others will want to deal with you in your new situation, or you feel you'll burden them or that you're less of a person than you used to be when you're with them.

Family Relationships

You might find that changes happen not only in your relationships with friends or co-workers, but also within your family. You might live somewhere else now, and it might take a while to get used to your new mobility, to figure out how you can use transportation to see your family. On the other hand, you might find that it's best to move back into your family's home after having been on your own. This may require adjustments and some getting used to, for everyone involved.

Having your family more involved in your life can also have benefits. For example, your parents and siblings might be able to help you sort out practical matters and give you the emotional support you need. You might also find that your relationships don't change very much, or that they improve. As one young man with spinal cord injury explained, "Your family is going to be your family regardless. My family shows me love and support. You have your different tribulations that go on in your life, but you've got to look outside of the negative things and think positively."

Particularly challenging may be changes in your relationships with your own or other children. Depending on their ages at the time of your injury, children may not understand what has happened to you, and they have to learn about changes in your mobility. It may be difficult for you to accept these changes and to find ways to explain what is happening. And, as children get older, they might have more questions. A young mother told me that helping her four-year-old daughter to understand her situation was challenging. "She accepted it when she was younger, but now she's getting older and she's starting to wonder why mommy can't get up and go and we can't run like we used to," she said.

Most kids cope with challenges and changes very well after learning about and coming to terms with what has happened. Many parents with disabilities agree that their kids are a great source of support, and often they show a greater degree of maturity compared to kids of the same age with parents who do not have a disability.

Friendships and Romance

Friendships can also change after a spinal cord injury. Many people find disappointment and increased distance on the part of their friends, but that new and more focused friendships can also emerge. Sometimes keeping friends is a matter of helping them adjust to your new circumstances. Let them know that you are still you and that you want to keep the friendship going.

The biggest relationship challenge for many young people with spinal cord injury is romance. Romance is difficult when you are first injured, and many relationships change or even end as a result. Whether you have lost a relationship or not, you might not feel ready for romance when you're first dealing with other changes, such as where to live.

It seems that the best hope for keeping a romantic relationship going is to involve your partner in the rehabilitation process right from the beginning. The road to recovery is long, so your partner will need to learn everything about your injury and care. That way, when you leave the hospital he or she will know as much as you do about your injury and care, and will be able to assist you much better. The process can be very stressful for everybody involved, and by itself it cannot guarantee that the relationship will work out.

The good news is that new romantic relationships and friendships are not only possible, but they will happen. One young man I talked with reflected that after you deal with the changes, the crying and saying that you're not going to date anymore, and the belief that you won't find anybody else in the condition you're in, then something changes. You might meet a new girl or someone will say hi to you on a bus. "You get the spark of joy," he said. "You realize there is someone out there for you. You start to hold your head up. You start speaking to people more, you start putting what happened to you in the past. Then hopefully things will get better with time."

Meeting New People

You'll also meet or cross paths with new people after your injury. People who don't know you may not understand what has happened to you or what you are experiencing. They may be curious and want you to explain why you are using a wheelchair and how you got injured. Some will remain at a distance and avoid contact. You'll probably develop strategies over time to deal with too much attention or inappropriate questions. It's important that you feel you can control the information you're willing share with others. Not everybody needs to know all the details. In fact, most people's curiosity can be satisfied quickly with some short answers. If you feel it's none of their business to inquire about why you're using a wheelchair, let them know that.

However, some people may ask you because they aren't sure what to do and whether they can be of assistance or not. They're not experienced in dealing with people who use wheelchairs and might be afraid of making mistakes. They need your help. You can disperse a lot of their concerns by answering their questions frankly and by giving them very detailed instructions when you need their assistance.

Whether you're trying to re-fit your old relationships into your new life or looking for new relationships, the most important step is the one you take within yourself. As one person recommended, "Get yourself together. Take care of yourself. Get out. Start doing things you did before. Get back into your hobbies. Don't sit around and mope."

As you move on in your life, here are some strategies for success that is based on the experiences of many people with spinal cord injury.

Keep active and pursue your interests, whether through hobbies, education, or work. It is one of the healthiest things you can do—to keep old relationships strong, to meet new people and make new connections, and to enable yourself to grow as a person. You will find it is often easier to plan things with friends when you take the initiative, when you call them and suggest a place to meet or an activity to do.

Be creative and find new ways to do things. You can share many hobbies with old and new friends, people in wheelchairs and without wheelchairs. If you are into sports, there are many ways you can do sports when you are in a wheelchair. If you are into music, computers today make it a lot easier today to compose and perform. Computers can also help you to keep in touch with friends and family through e-mail and the Internet. You don't even have to have a computer yourself. You can sign up with a free Internet e-mail service and you can access the Web in schools, at the hospital, and in public libraries. Your public library's staff can be very helpful in getting you started.

Be clear about your needs, and be assertive in communicating them to others. You know best what your wishes and needs are. Nobody can take that away from you. Make sure that other people, whether friends, family, or strangers, know what your needs are. Talk to them about what you want to do and how you want to do it. Let them know how they can assist you. Be open about your disability—it will strengthen your ability to deal with situations and make it easier for others to assist you according to your needs and not theirs.

Look at your situation and plan ahead. When you arrange to meet other people, make sure the meeting place is accessible. Be clear about the support and assistance you need to meet someone in a new location. Call ahead to be sure that your wheelchair can fit through doorways and that there are ramps that allow you to negotiate steps. Plan to have the right assistance waiting for you. Explore how public or private transportation will get you from one place to the next in time. Order paratransit services well ahead of time. Allow extra time for broken-down elevators and escalators that would require you to wait for and use shuttle services between subway stations.

Take a second look, be flexible, and move on. Most certainly, you will encounter glitches along the way. You can plan a meeting well ahead of time, but then something will go wrong. The paratransit service won't show up on time or you'll get to a building with stairs and no ramp. This can be frustrating, but most likely where there is a plan A, there is also a plan B, C, and D. Re-evaluate the situation and think about what can be done about it next time. You may need to ask for immediate assistance. For the long term, you might find ways to avoid a similar situation by planning slightly differently. For example, you might schedule the meeting elsewhere, and you can be sure you have the phone number of the person you're going to see so you can call him or her in case you run into problems.

This essay is adapted from a peer-to-peer brief, "Family, Friends, Lovers: Relationships of Young People with Violently Acquired Spinal Cord Injuries," published by the National Rehabilitation Hospital's Center for Health and Disability Research. The author, who was a patient at NRH and then an intern at the NRH Center for Health and Disability, gathered information for the brief from conversations with other young adults with violently acquired spinal cord injury.

Adapting and Adjusting: It's All About Family
Robert Marsteller

My life was literally turned upside down when I was walking down the sidewalk in Washington, D.C., several years ago. As I walked along the G Street sidewalk, a woman floored her gas pedal and zoomed across the sidewalk and directly into my path. In an effort not to be mowed over, I jumped onto the hood of her car and held on for dear life. Before swerving and hitting two other cars, she threw me straight into the side of a parked delivery truck. Still alert, but immobile, I was not yet able to process all of the changes that my C5-C6 spinal cord injury would cause for me and for my family.

Before my accident, I might have described myself in many roles—husband, friend, banker, tennis player, etc., but perhaps being a parent was my favorite role of all. So, after my injury, having my seven-year-old son, Wiley, and my five-year-old daughter, Emily, taken care of was utmost in my mind. My wife, Maralyn, spent most of her days and many nights helping me at George Washington University Hospital, Washington Hospital Center, and the wonderful National Rehabilitation Hospital. From the moment that Maralyn was told about my accident, friends and family helped take over the day-to-day logistics of the children's lives. Our small but close in-town family dropped everything to help. Maralyn's mother manned our home front and fielded the endless incoming calls of concern. Maralyn's brother relieved Maralyn at the hospital and used his architectural skills to adapt our house for my homecoming. I consider myself very lucky that my brother is a neurologist and could help guide us through the myriad of medical decisions during those early weeks and beyond.

Our incredible friends drove the children to and from school and organized their activities, making sure that their lives were as normal as possible. The children's lunches were made for the entire school year. Birthday gifts for the children to take to parties were purchased and wrapped by anonymous friends. Even cookie dough appeared at Christmas time from a mysterious angel. Several friends even offered their nannies' services to help fill up some holes in the schedule. We can never thank our many friends and family enough for saving us during this really complicated period.

Our children's school, the Norwood School, and its unbelievable community also made this scary time as easy as possible for Maralyn and the children. Since Emily was still a quiet, new kindergartener, her teacher took lots of extra time and energy to greet Emily at the front door with a hug each day. She also monitored play dates and ensured that Emily only go home with families that she considered comfortable for Emily. Wiley's second grade teacher encouraged our quiet and careful son to talk about his dad's accident and promoted discussion of the "superhero" element of my jumping on the hood of the car. The administrators of our lovely school also let us know that whatever we needed would be done for us. Our children's school lives would retain their wonderful normalcy. Without that our family's burden might have been too heavy to bear.

The immediate challenge that Maralyn faced was to inform the children of my situation without scaring them. Friends advised us to be as honest as possible so we could maintain trust in the future. Maralyn chose to tell Wiley and Emily the facts with a superhero twist – Wiley especially enjoyed this part of the story! We also used my high fitness level as an example of how I managed to jump onto the car and survive such an assault. Children are very malleable. They were most concerned with my being alive and that their lives would not be altered to too great a degree.

Maralyn remembers that a huge hurdle was when the children first saw me about a week after the accident. I was out of the ICU, but still had a lot of tubes connected to me.Emily was in a particularly awkward stage and Maralyn so worried that she'd bump into her still brittle father. Actually, seeing me appeared to make them more comfortable with their new reality.

Ed Eckenhoff, the most able president of NRH, was so incredibly supportive of our family. Since I was hospitalized for three months, he realized that my wife and my children were my lifeline. He even allowed Maralyn and the children to occasionally spend the night at the hospital. I could share the video of Emily's premier as a pink bunny in the school's Halloween program and Wiley scoring home runs in baseball games. The nurses made them feel comfortable and complimented their homemade Christmas gifts, which they constructed in the corner of my room. My fabulous NRH room was lively with walls filled with children's cards and holiday decorations.

I wouldn't say that any part of my journey has been easy. But, knowing that my most significant role as a parent was still intact, I have maintained a positive attitude throughout. In the months that followed my homecoming, I continued to coach baseball, learned to use my voice-activated computer software, and was taught how to drive my accessible van. I became a regular in the school carpool, although I'm sure this was met with initial hesitation! I became a show-and-tell item and have maintained my relationships with my children's friends and teachers. I can't use my fingers, but I can help with homework. I ask my children for help when I need it and these jobs are now just part of their daily chores. I help my wife whenever and however I can and since she is a softie, I am the chief disciplinarian of the family!

We have lived through this adventure for almost four years now. Recently, Emily was asked if her life is different because her dad is in a wheelchair. She responded, "Of course! We have an elevator!"

Becoming paralyzed has cost me many things, but it has also given me a unique perspective. What children most need from their parents are unconditional love, unlimited time, and the knowledge that we will be there for them unfailingly. The paramedics told my wife that they were amazed that I survived. I have been given the gift of time with my family. That has been a gift indeed.

Having a Baby
LaShonne T. Williams-Fraley

I am 34 years old, I have had a C7 spinal cord injury since July 1990, and I am the mother of a wonderful four-year-old son who was born about 10 years after my injury. Let me start by saying that this was not a planned pregnancy. Before actually finding out that I was pregnant, I had symptoms like those of an ulcer or really bad heartburn. My stomach had a burning feeling that I could not explain. I just knew I had developed an ulcer and for the first several weeks I drank ginger ale and ate crackers and Tums. When I went to see my primary care physician to find out what was going on, she sat down and asked me what my symptoms were and when was my last cycle. After answering her questions, she examined me and drew blood for testing. She told me that she was including a pregnancy test and that the results would be back in about three days.

For the next three days, I was a nervous wreck because I couldn't understand how I got an ulcer. Then I received a message from my doctor stating that my test results were in and that I needed to give her a call back as soon as possible. Hearing those words made me even more nervous, so I picked up the phone and called the office. When she finally answered she said, "Congratulations. It seems that you could be six to eight weeks pregnant, so you need to contact your ob/gyn as soon as possible."

I took a deep breath and made my first appointment with my ob/gyn doctor. At that appointment, he went through the normal routine, and when he got to the part about me being pregnant he was more than happy to do a sonogram so we could confirm the pregnancy and see the baby for the first time. While looking at the sonogram, I didn't know exactly what I was seeing. The doctor turned to me and said, "There is your baby," and I said, "That looks like a lima bean!" We laughed and he turned back to the screen and pointed out the baby's heartbeat. By this time, I had tears welling up in my eyes. I was excited, nervous, and scared, and a whole list of other emotions started pouring in.

After leaving the doctor's office, I started thinking to myself, "What are you going to do? How are you going to take care of a baby when you're in a wheelchair yourself?" All kinds of questions came to me so fast that I contemplated having an abortion even though I don't believe in them. My life had changed instantly when I saw that little tiny lima bean. My thoughts went from me to the baby. I went home and with tears in my eyes told my mother, and she said to me "It's gonna be OK. You're almost 30 and you know we will help you." Immediately, I started to feel better. My family was so excited that I was having a baby. A lot of them thought that I would never be able to have children.

I found my ob/gyn through my primary care physician, who told me that the ob/gyn had seen another woman in a wheelchair. At my first visit with him, the ob/gyn explained that he had never had a patient with a spinal cord injury, that his other patient in a wheelchair had multiple sclerosis. He was patient and understanding about my needs and I felt very comfortable with him. I have been his patient for about 10 years now.

During my pregnancy, I had good days and bad days, which I think is normal for every woman. The only difference I can remember is the frequency of urinary tract infections due to the high protein level in my body.

My son was delivered at 33 weeks. I was admitted into the hospital on a Monday because of premature contractions. When they examined me, they told me that I had not dilated but the baby's head was real low. My doctor successfully stopped the contractions but they wanted to keep me an extra day for observation. On Tuesday, I was having my bath in bed when the nurse rolled me too far and I slid out of the bed and onto the floor. I had to stay for X-rays to make sure none of my bones were fractured (I didn't hit the floor that hard, but they had to take precautions). They also did a sonogram and placed me on a monitor to make sure there was no injury to the baby.

Tuesday night into Wednesday I started contracting again so they gave me some medicine to stop the contractions again. On Thursday—maybe because of all the excitement—I started to feel a shortness of breath, and that's when they found out that the oxygen level in my blood was low. By this time, my doctor said if the contractions started again he was going to go ahead and let me deliver because he wasn't sure what was going on and why my oxygen level was low. Sure enough, my son heard that and started the contractions again.

That night, they gave me an epidural to help prevent dysreflexia, and my doctor examined me to see how much I had dilated, if any. I was 2_ centimeters so they gave me some Pitocin to increase my contractions. On Friday morning, my doctor came in to check on my progress but found there was no change. I was still 2 _ centimeters and the baby was low enough but hadn't move down into the birth canal. At 10:45 a.m., my doctor decided to break my water, and he told me that around 5:00 or 6:00 that evening the baby should be in position and I would begin to push.

In the meantime, I was lying there praying and listening to the baby's heartbeat, I was experiencing some dysreflexia (through sweating) so I asked the nurse if I could get a dry gown because I was getting cold from being wet. Around 12:40 p.m. the nurse helped me wash and change my gown, rolling me to the left and right. When we were done around 12:45, I rolled onto my back and my son was in the bed with me! With all the rolling, he had worked his way down and out on his own. I was so afraid because there was no doctor in the room to check him. He was crying, and that of course was a good sign. I was crying, he was crying, and I was so happy to hear him crying. The doctors came in and examined me and my son and they took him off to the neonatal intensive care unit because he was premature. It was a good experience in spite of everything that took place during that week.

My son is five years old now, and being a parent during those five years has been a remarkable journey—just as it is for all new parents. In fact, the whole process has been easier than I expected it would be. It's been tiring, but that's true for any new parent, able-bodied or disabled. Because of my disability, I've had to make some adjustments like sleeping partially upright in an adjustable bed so I could get to him when he woke up at night as a baby. Before that, I found that lying flat would not work because as we know when you first wake-up and try to sit-up your muscle spasms are very strong and will throw you. This would especially happen to me when I was startled and woke up at night. I also made up little tricks like undoing the sticky tapes on the disposable diapers before instead of after laying him on top.

It's been a joy watching my son develop from stage to stage—it's totally amazing watching him grow, listening to him learn words, helping him learn, and having him want me to read to him. A lot of people think it's cute when they see us when we're out together. In this day and time, people have gotten used to seeing people in wheelchairs, but a lot of people assume he was born before I was in the chair.

Fortunately, I come from a large family that lives nearby, and I've had my mom and plenty of other support around me to help when needed. This kind of support is very, very important, and parents with disabilities should seek out support from others, including family and friends. My advice is to let friends and family know when you need help or if there's something that you're not comfortable with, but don't depend totally on others' support in case it's not there right when you need it. If you get support from others, be sure to thank them for it. I also suggest that new moms, especially those with disabilities, be sure to take time for themselves. When the child is asleep, get some rest and do things for yourself because you need quiet time for yourself. This is true for all new mothers, but even more so for mothers with disabilities. Most importantly, be patient and seek out help when you need it.

How Does Spirituality Transcend Disability?
Rev. Rob McQuay

Whenever we face adversity in life, we all handle it differently. From the first moment to years later, we each adjust physically, emotionally, mentally, and spiritually at different paces and in different ways. There appears to be no single answer to how to deal with a life change. And yet, we know that the mind plays a significant role in the way in which we manage adversity. It is said that a positive attitude can overcome many things. I would agree that a positive attitude will see you through many problems in life, but where does that attitude come from? Can we just turn it on? Are we born with a positive or negative attitude?

At age 28, some 14 years ago, I went into the ocean and came out a quadriplegic. Mere seconds after the impact of the wave broke my neck in two places, as I was floating helplessly in the turbulent surf, I had a vision. I saw myself and my son on a running track and I was in a wheelchair. I immediately prayed to God saying, "I can deal with being a paraplegic, just let me live." Seconds later, a woman came running into the surf and pulled me out. From that moment on, I have never asked, "Why me?" You see, I have come to learn that there was and is a reason for this happening to me, not the least of which is fulfilled even as I write this essay.

I have had to adjust physically, emotionally, and mentally, but the constant in all of these adjustments has been spiritually. If we are guided spiritually, then everything else can and will follow. It is amazing to me that when we ground our being spiritually, how easy it is to have that positive mental, emotional and yes, even physical perspective. We can begin to see how we as individuals play a part in a larger play.

To consider how spirituality can help someone with a disability, we need to consider the terms spirituality and disability. When one becomes disabled, that person becomes acutely aware of his or her own body, how it functions, and how it cannot function any longer. We begin to see the world in a very different way. Just days after my accident, as I was lying in my hospital bed in the ICU, the movie "Tootsie" was playing on the television. There is a scene when Dustin Hoffman, having been transformed into a woman, is walking down the streets of New York City. There is a mass of people walking in the streets. As I watched the scene, I began to see those people as being special, lucky, as being beyond the norm because they could walk. This, of course, was a distortion of reality. However, it is an example of how we "shrink" ourselves down to the basis of our own experience. We become focused only on our own bodies and what we can or cannot do. It is a selfish, yet very necessary, phase to go through. The world that we knew is gone or, at the very least, greatly altered.

Spirituality, then, involves transcendence. Many of us believe that as we pray, we are transcending the physical world and communicating in a mystical way with God. I believe, and in my experience have found that—regardless of one's faith—spirituality is capable of raising us beyond our physical, disabled world and allowing us to function in the "normal" world by the way in which we project ourselves, physically, emotionally, and mentally. When we tap into our spirituality, we are able to see past our own limitations and into the wonderful possibilities that are available to us only because of our disability. For example, as an assistant pastor of a church, my witness and testimony is strengthened by the mere visual fact of my disability. Many times I have heard, "A minister in a wheelchair? Hmm." This immediately challenges the person to reassess his or her perceptions and pre-conceived notions of who people are or can be. This has given me the opportunity to speak to many groups with which I would not have interfaced, or at least not in the same capacity, because of my disability. I see this as God's perfect plan in my life—a spiritual transcendence of who I was and was to become, to who I have become.

Even the Apostle Paul dealt with a physical disability in his ministry. He was given a "thorn in the flesh". We do not know what exactly that "thorn in the flesh" was, but we do know that it was important enough for Paul to cry out to God three times, "pleading with the Lord to take it away…" (2 Corinthians 12:8), but the Lord replied, "My grace is sufficient for you, for my power is made perfect in weakness" (2 Corinthians 12:9).

Let us delve into our spirituality so that we can move beyond our immediate physical world and limitations, and affect a positive change in the world around us by how we act and transcend our disability. This is how I believe your spirituality will take you far beyond your physical, emotional, and mental reality and transcend you in this world even before you are finally transcended in body and soul in Paradise.

Rev. Rob McQuay is a Minister of the Methodist Episcopal Church, USA.

Spinal Cord Injury and Substance Abuse: A Cautionary Tale
Steven A. Towle

My name is Steve Towle; I am a quadriplegic. I am also an alcoholic and a drug addict. Of the two disabilities, I think I prefer the spinal cord injury. Spinal cord injury (SCI) did not cause my addiction; it did exacerbate and accelerate the disease process. With hindsight, I'm sure I exhibited addictive behavior before I was injured. And while I'm certain that there will one day be a cure for paralysis, I'm equally certain that the only cure for substance abuse is, and will forever be, complete, life-long abstinence.

This is in part a cautionary tale. Statistics relating spinal cord injury to substance abuse are scary. If you even think that you have a problem, you probably do. When I sustained my cervical spinal cord injury in 1974, I was active duty military. In those days, many rehabilitation hospitals, not just veterans hospitals, did a good job of rehabilitation and an equally good job of cranking out addicts. Folks needed pain pills, sleeping pills, and muscle relaxers. Some needed them more than others. For five bucks you could always buy a half-pint of vodka from the right orderly. Keep in mind that it was a different time in a different culture. I was hospitalized almost exactly a year, not unusual for a C5-6 injury in 1974. Lots of time to sit around with the old hands and learn the ropes. Damn near enough ropes to hang yourself.

Ten years later, I went to Walter Reed Army Medical Center because I was incredibly miserable and because I knew that I was completely out of control; I was using large quantities of codeine, Valium, sleeping pills, street drugs including heroin, Dilaudid, and Percocet. I was seeing lots of doctors (Rush Limbaugh did not invent doctor shopping.) and studying amateur pharmacology on the side.

I had an appointment with a doctor whom I had never met before. I explained that I was taking heavy doses of narcotic drugs, that I was sick of it, and that I wanted to quit. I don't really remember how the conversation progressed, but a plan evolved. I would take 18 Percocets a day for two days, then 16 pills for two days, and so on. In this way, I could titrate myself off the drugs, and I would be cured. Finally! I could see the light at the end of the tunnel. As you have probably already surmised, that light was a train.

The doctor gave me a bottle of 100 or 200 pills, I don't remember how many, to take home. I was back too soon with my sad story: I had lost some, the dog had eaten the pills, my roommates had stolen some, whatever. She gave me another bottle of pills. Or two.

The next time I went in for a refill, another doctor spotted me for the addict that I was. He knew the pattern. Some quads and all addicts are first class manipulators: They have to be to survive. The doctor was certain that I had other doctors writing prescriptions, but he would make certain that no additional prescriptions were written for me at Walter Reed. I had two choices: I could go home or I could go into detox. After 10 days or so on methadone, the treatment of choice for junkies at the time, they backed an ambulance up to the door and took me directly to the Richmond Veterans Administration (VA) hospital, where I spent about 45 days doing a 30-day program.

Except for a brief period last summer after I fractured my femur parasailing (yeah, I know—we don't have time to go into that here), I have not taken a mood-altering "drug" since that day. But by early 1994 my life had become manageable. I had gone back to school and gotten a couple of degrees. I was an officer in several non-profit organizations and had started one of my own. One of the groups asked me to represent them at a conference in New Orleans. I had stopped going to the meetings of a certain anonymous fellowship a couple of years before; the only reason I went was to pick up an annual chip. I had nine. I hadn't had a drink or a drug for nine years, almost 10 actually. People trusted me. I was president of this and vice president of that; I was cured, I was in control.

I relapsed in a Gentleman's Club in New Orleans, and so I never picked up my 10-year chip. When I'd come through the VA program in 1984, narcotics were my drug of choice. But I was quickly drinking at least two liters of vodka a day, often much more. I needed serious help. In 1984 the VA inpatient program was 30 days, but as a person with a spinal cord injury, I had had to live on the spinal cord unit and visit the drug and alcohol (D&A) unit as a day patient. It had worked to a point, but I was excluded from much of what went on because I was a visitor to the unit, not quite a full participant. This only served to reinforce my uniqueness, a dangerous quality for an addict.

One year prior to my current recovery, in a failed try at getting sober, I tried to repeat what had worked for me 17 years earlier; the program had been reduced to 21 days and everything was different. After about a week of this I was drinking every evening; after a couple weeks I gave up and went home.

During a rare lucid period a year later, I began by searching out every inpatient alcohol treatment program in the D.C. area. I contacted the 32 programs listed and was unable to locate a single inpatient program that was wheelchair accessible and could offer the personal assistance services I would need to get in and out of bed, bathe, get dressed, and take care of my other personal care needs. Then I expanded the list to programs outside of Maryland. I didn't even get to pursue the access question with many of these programs, as they simply couldn't accept anyone outside the state/region. The few private programs in Minnesota, Florida, and California all said they could not provide personal assistance services.

At this point, I gave up. I could not drink and make the calls, and I wasn't sure I wanted to work so hard to get sober anyway. My friends and my family didn't give up. They contacted board members from the National Association on Alcohol, Drugs, and Disability (NAADD), and enlisted their help. They called hospitals and community programs, and queried friends in recovery who are also in the business. They called our state Governor's Office for Disability Services, the Maryland Alcohol and Drug Administration, the governor's and lieutenant governor's offices, 10 different offices within the federal and regional Veterans Administration, several offices within the state mental health system, and several more offices within the state health department. Then they called their county offices.

Virtually all places they called needed to be called repeatedly; none returned calls, other than the governor's offices. The others never returned the calls, ever. When the governor's office returned the calls, they referred us to many of the same places already called.

I don't want you to think that there is no help out here. It is hard to find, but the alternative is not pretty. If you are spinal cord injured and you think you have a substance abuse problem, you are not alone. Substance abuse is as much 300 percent higher in people with SCI, as compared with the general population. As many as 80 percent of SCIs are drug and/or alcohol related. [Substance Abuse Resources & Disability Issues (SARDI)]

Allow me to get on my soapbox for just a moment. People with disabilities—Americans "created equal"—who are seeking treatment for alcoholism and drug addiction should not be required to depend on a series of random events to receive the care to which they are entitled. The Americans with Disabilities Act is more than 13 years old. Its mandates and their effects ripple throughout our society. There is, however, virtually no compliance with this common sense federal law when it comes to drug and alcohol treatment for people with disabilities. This is particularly disturbing since many people acquire their disability as a direct result of drug and alcohol abuse, or begin self-medicating after becoming disabled, and become addicted as a result. Clearly, people with disabilities need access to high quality drug and alcohol treatment, just like everyone else.

As angry as the lack of response made me, I understood it. The office we called were unresponsive because there weren't any programs available to meet the accessibility and personal assistance service needs of people with disabilities. They weren't holding out on me—the programs simply didn't exist in anything like the demand or our laws would have predicted. It's been over three years. Things are only marginally better, but there is help if you will ask for it.

In my case, it was clear I was not going to be able to find the disability-related inpatient care that I needed and the treatment for alcoholism in the same facility. My options for an accessible program were almost non-existent, particularly when geography and my insurance were thrown into the mix. I decided I would present myself at a local hospital for treatment. If I hadn't then said that I was depressed and suicidal they would not have admitted me. I spent five days on the sixth floor A&D unit.

The hospital's A&D folks could not provide the nursing and personal assistant services that I needed. I had to arrange for and pay a nurse to come in every morning and evening to get me dressed and ready to participate in the program. My nursing needs are not unusual for a person with quadriplegia. Generally an hour in the morning and an hour at night is all that's needed to meet all of my personal care needs.

I was discharged after six days of detoxification. With the guidance from a certain anonymous recovery program, a great sponsor, family, and friends, and nearly 10 years of previous experience to tell what not to do, I now have over three years sober. One day at a time. But the "system" did not help much. I somehow never lost my positions as president of this and vice president of that, but I sure was not giving my best. It's good to be back. And I've added a part time job with the National Association on Alcohol, Drugs, and Disability.

Steven A. Towle is president of the Spinal Cord Injury Network of Metropolitan Washington, an Washington, DC, regional chapter of the National Spinal Cord Injury Association.

Appendix B: Glossary

activities of daily living (ADL): routine activities a person does every day, such as standing, sitting, walking, eating, bathing, and grooming
activities of daily living: routine activities a person does every day, such as standing, sitting, walking, eating, bathing, and grooming
acute care hospital: a hospital that provides acute medical care
acute medical care: medical care that is meant to stabilize one's medical condition and minimize complications; usually received before rehabilitation
acute rehabilitation: medical services that include both general medical care and medical rehabilitation services
adaptive equipment: equipment that helps a person become as independent and functional as possible
ambulation: walking
Americans with Disabilities Act (ADA) of 1990: a civil rights act protecting persons with disabilities against discrimination in the workplace, housing, transportation, and other aspects of life
anemia: a condition in which the blood is deficient in red blood cells, in hemoglobin, or in total volume
ASIA Impairment Scale: A scale developed by the American Spinal Injury Association that is widely used by doctors and other health care providers to identify and standardize the level and extent of a spinal cord injury and to assist in predicting functional outcomes (what the person eventually should be able to do)
assistive equipment (assistive technology): any equipment or device, such as a wheelchair, braces, walker, or speech aids that help a person to become more independent, function better, or perform activities of daily living or mobility
autonomic function (autonomic activities): the automatic (or not under conscious control) functions of the body such as breathing, the heart beating, sweating, etc.
autonomic dysreflexia: a potentially dangerous complication of spinal

cord injury in which blood pressure rises to dangerous levels; if not treated, autonomic dysreflexia can lead to stroke, seizure, and possibly death

benefits: services or equipment that a health insurance plan will pay for

case manager: a professional who works for an insurance company, hospital, or rehabilitation facility to make sure that all aspects of treatment comply with the rules of an individual's health plan

catheterization (of the bladder): insertion of a small tube into the bladder to empty urine

cauda equina: a collection of nerves at the bottom of the spinal cord, below the L2 level

Center for Independent Living (CIL): a community-based organization that provides services to and advocates for persons with all types of disabilities to assist them in achieving their maximum potential; CILs often are private, non-residential, and consumer-controlled

Centers for Medicare and Medicaid Services (CMS): The federal government agency that administers the Medicare program and works in partnership with the states to administer Medicaid, the State Children's Health Insurance Program, and health insurance portability standards

cervical: the part of the spine in the neck region

circulatory system: the body system that sends nutrients from food and oxygen from the lungs to other parts of your body; includes the heart, arteries, veins, and capillaries

clinical psychologist (see psychologist)

complete injury: a spinal cord injury that results in no voluntary movement and no feeling below the level of injury and through the sacral area

constipation: a common bowel problem that involves having infrequent, difficult bowel movements

copayment: a small, fixed-dollar amount paid by the patient for a doctor's visit, prescription drugs, or other health care services

day treatment: rehabilitation care that provides a full range of intensive services, but allows patients to stay at home overnight

decubitus ulcer (see pressure sore)

deductible: a yearly dollar amount that an insured person must pay before an insurance company begins paying for any services

digestive system: the body system that is responsible for breaking down food and liquid into nutrients for your body to use; includes the mouth, esophagus, stomach, small intestine, and large intestine

disability: a problem or limitation with a human activity, such as not being able to walk

discharge: departure (or to depart) from an inpatient hospital or other facility

durable medical equipment (DME): equipment that has a medical purpose, can be used repeatedly, and is appropriate for use in the home; examples include wheelchairs, walkers, and hospital beds

edema: swelling

embolus: a blood clot (thrombus) that has broken loose and is moving through the bloodstream

environment control unit (ECU): technology that allows greater control over one's indoor environment, such as to control lights, telephones, entertainment systems, and other equipment

extremity: an arm or leg; the upper extremities include the arms, forearms, and hands, and the lower extremities include the thighs, lower legs, and feet

fee-for-service: a method of payment for medical services in which a specific fee is charged for each individual service; the method of payment used under traditional indemnity policies

functional ability: how well a person is able to perform activities of daily living, such as eating, bathing, or dressing, communicating

handicap: disadvantage experienced by an individual as a result of an impairment, such as a spinal cord injury

health maintenance organization: a type of managed care plan in which people can only see doctors who are a part of their health maintenance organization network of providers; referrals from a primary care provider typically are needed in order to see specialists or to get other health care services within the network

helpful technology: technology that help a person control things in his or her environment or interact with a computer

heterotopic ossification: development of bone in abnormal areas, usually in soft tissues

home health care: health care services provided in your home by a visiting health care professional, such as a nurse or therapist

hydronephrosis: a condition in which the kidney's urine-collecting system becomes stretched and distended because the free outflow of urine from the kidney to the bladder is blocked

impairment: a physical problem with a body or organ function, such as paralysis

incomplete injury: a spinal cord injury in which there is some feeling or voluntary movement below the level of the injury and through to the sacral area

incontinence: having a bowel or bladder accident

inpatient rehabilitation: rehabilitation services received as an inpatient in a hospital setting

lumbar: the part of the spine in the middle back, between the thoracic and sacral vertebrae

managed care: a health insurance plan that delivers comprehensive health care services at a reduced price for members who agree to use certain providers and facilities

Medicaid: a health insurance program run by individual state governments that provides health coverage primarily for low-income families and people with significant disabilities

Medicare: a health care insurance program administered by the federal government that provides health insurance for people over age 65, some people with disabilities, and others who qualify

mobility: the ability to move from one place to another

myelopathy: disease of or around the spinal cord causing spinal cord dysfunction

neurogenic: arising or originating from the nervous system

neurogenic pain: pain that results from nervous system malfunction

neurologist: a doctor who specializes in diagnosis and treatment of problems with the nervous system

nursing home: a facility where patients stay to receive rehabilitation services, long-term care, or skilled nursing care

occupational therapy (OT): therapy that teaches skills and adaptations to improve one's ability to do tasks at home, at work, and in the community so that they are as independent as possible; an occupational therapist or occupational therapy assistant may provide occupational therapy service

orthotics (orthoses): devices designed to support or supplement a weakened joint or limb

orthotist: a professional who helps make, fit, and repair adaptive devices, such as orthopedic braces (orthoses)

outpatient rehabilitation: rehabilitation services provided to a person who lives at home; intensity of outpatient services can vary from once a week to daily

paralysis: the inability to control movement of a part of one's body, such as an arm or a leg

paraplegia: a condition involving complete paralysis of the legs

paratransit services: alternative, accessible transportation services for persons who cannot use regular, fixed-route public transportation systems, such as bus lines, because of a disability or health condition; paratransit providers typically offer door-to-door van or mini-bus transportation services that can be scheduled for doctor's appointments, shopping, social activities, or other purposes

peer mentor: a peer who is willing to share his or her knowledge about and experiences with spinal cord injury

personal care assistant (PCA): an individual who is hired to take care of the daily routine needs of a person with a disability

physiatrist: a doctor who specializes in physical medicine and rehabilitation

physical medicine and rehabilitation (PM&R): a medical specialty dedicated to diagnosing, treating, and preventing disability, and to improving patients' functional ability, quality of life, and independence.

physical therapy (PT): therapy that restores and maximizes movement and function; services provided by a physical therapist

point-of-service (POS) option: an option with a health maintenance organization plan that allows a person to receive care from specialists who have not joined the health plan network.

preferred provider organization (PPO): a type of health maintenance organization (HMO) that offers more freedom of choice in selecting health care providers; may require larger co-payments to doctors in the plan's network than would be made in a traditional HMO plan.

pressure relief: changing positions in a wheelchair or bed to increase blood flow in areas of pressure

pressure sore (decubitus ulcer, pressure ulcer, bed sore): a reddened area or open skin sore caused by unrelieved pressure on the skin over bony areas such as the hip bone or tail bone, or areas of external pressure (such as a tight shoe)

primary care physician: a doctor who provides non-specialist medical care, such as an internist, family practitioner or pediatrician

prosthesis: an artificial limb or body part

prosthetist: a professional who helps make, fit, and repair adaptive devices, such as artificial limbs (prostheses)

psychologist: A mental health professional who can help people understand and adjust to disability; clinical psychologists teach coping skills, such as stress management and pain control, and offer individual, family, or group counseling

pulmonary: having to do with the lungs and breathing

quadriplegia (see tetraplegia)

quality of life: a person's level of satisfaction with all aspects of his or her world, including self-esteem, personal and family relationships, social activities, financial conditions, employment status, spiritual activities, and anything else that influences satisfaction with life

range of motion: an arc of movement of one of the body's joints

rehabilitation: treatment received as part of a program to enhance functional ability following disease, illness, or injury; rehabilitation services include medical care, nursing care, physical therapy, occupational therapy, speech-language therapy, therapeutic recreation, vocational rehabilitation, counseling, and other activities prescribed to increase a patients independence and functional abilities

rehabilitation case manager: a health care professional who makes sure that a person receives needed services, coordinating care across health care providers and facilities, and ensuring that all aspects of treatment comply with the rules of the person's insurance coverage.

rehabilitation engineer: a specially trained engineer who helps select, modify, and design assistive equipment for mobility, communication, work, recreation, and therapy needs.

rehabilitation nurse: a specially trained nurse who works with other rehabilitation professionals to personalize a plan of care, and teaches individuals about disability, medications, and treatment

rehabilitation services: individual medical or rehabilitation treatments received as part of a medical or rehabilitation program. Rehabilitation services include medical and nursing care, laboratory tests, rehabilitation therapies such as physical, occupational, recreational, speech and vocational therapy, counseling sessions, recreational activities, and anything else prescribed to increase a patient's independence

rehabilitation team: a group of health care professionals from different fields who work with the patient and family to plan and provide rehabilitative care

respiratory system: the body system involved in intake and exchange of oxygen and carbon dioxide; includes the nose, mouth, trachea, bronchial tubes, lungs, and diaphragm

respiratory therapist: a health care professional who tests one's ability to breathe and designs a personalized breathing program

sacral: the part of the spine in the hip area

sensation: physical feelings of touch, pain, heat and cold, vibration, and awareness of where a body part is in space

shearing: skin damage caused by the skin being pulled in one direction (for example, by a bed or transfer surface) while the body moves in the opposite direction; similar to rug burn

skilled nursing facility (SNF): a facility that provides patients with a high level of nursing care and meets certain industry accreditation standards

Social Security Administration: the government agency that manages the nation's social insurance program, consisting of retirement, disability, and survivors benefits

Social Security Disability Income (SSDI): a federal government disability program that pays benefits to a person with a disability and certain members of his or her family if the person has worked long enough and paid Social Security taxes.

social worker: a professional who provides social work services to help with the transition from an acute care setting to rehabilitation, and then back to the family and community. A social worker will work with you, your family, and community agencies to make arrangements for support services that may be needed during and after rehabilitation.

spasm: a sudden, uncontrolled muscle contraction

spasticity: involuntary movement of one's arms and legs

speech therapy (speech-language pathology, speech-language therapy): therapy to restore and develop communication skills and abilities; services provided by a speech-language pathologist

spinal cord: a rope-like bundle of millions of nerves that carry information between the brain and other parts of the body, such as the arms, legs, and organs

spinal cord injury: an injury to the spinal cord that can lead to paralysis

splint: a device used to support a body part or to hold a body part in place

subacute rehabilitation: rehabilitation services that include daily nursing services, supervision by a rehabilitation doctor, and medical care as needed; these services are less intensive and generally las longer than acute rehabilitation services

Supplemental Security Income (SSI): a federal government program that pays benefits to persons who are aged, blind, or disabled and have little or no income; provides cash to meet basic needs for food, clothing, and shelter

tetraplegia (quadriplegia): a condition involving complete paralysis of the legs and partial or complete paralysis of the arms

therapeutic recreation: therapy to regain as much independence as possible in one's leisure activities, pastimes, and hobbies; therapeutic recreation specialists (recreation therapists) help to evaluate individuals' leisure and pastime needs, abilities, and interests, and to develop a treatment program.

thoracic: the part of the spine in the chest to mid-back area

thrombus: a blood clot that stays in the veins of a person's leg

transfer: the process of moving safely from one surface to another, such as from a bed to a wheelchair or from a wheelchair to a car

urinary system: the body system that turns wastes into urine, stores the urine, and releases the urine from the body; includes the kidneys, ureters, bladder and urethra

urinary tract infection (UTI): an infection anywhere along the urinary tract, including in the kidneys, the ureters (the tubes that take urine from each kidney to the bladder), the bladder, or the urethra (the tube that empties urine from the bladder to the outside)

vertebrae: the hollow bones that make up the spine, through which the spinal cord passes

vocational rehabilitation: services that help to figure out a person's job strengths, and provide guidance for employment or education planning; **vocational rehabilitation specialists (counselors)** work with an individual's employer or school, or helps plan for future employment or education

Appendix C:
Rescources and
Additional Reading

National Organizations and Information Resources

ABLEDATA
8630 Fenton Street, Suite 930
Silver Spring, MD 20910
800-227-0216
TTY: 301-608-8912
E-mail: abledata@orcmacro.com
www.abledata.com
A federally funded project that provides assistive technology information, including product descriptions, an online library, other disability-related resources, and a consumer forum.

Adaptive Driving Alliance
4218 W. Electra Lane
Glendale, Arizona 85310
623-434-0722
www.adamobility.com
A nationwide group of vehicle modification dealers who provide van conversions, hand controls, wheelchair lifts, scooter lifts, tie downs, conversion van rentals, paratransit, and other adaptive equipment for disabled drivers and passengers.

AgrAbility Project
University of Wisconsin-Cooperative Extension
460 Henry Mall
Madison, WI 53706
866-259-6280 or 608-262-5166
www.agrabilityproject.org
A federally funded project that provides practical education and assistance to promote independence in agricultural production and rural living.

American Association of People with Disabilities
1629 K Street NW, Suite 503
Washington, DC 20006
800-840-8844 or 202-457-0046 (voice and TTY)
E-mail: aapd@aol.com
www.aapd.com

Member Services
258 Main Street, Suite 203
Milford, MA 01757
866-241-3200 or 508-634-3200 (voice and TTY)
    A nonprofit, cross-disability member organization that works with other disability organizations to ensure economic self-sufficiency and political empowerment for Americans with disabilities.

Canadian Abilities Foundation
340 College Street, Suite 650
Toronto, ON M5T 3A9
416-923-1885
E-mail: info@enablelink.org
www.enablelink.org
    A Canadian disability organization. Website offers information, chat rooms, message boards, classifieds, and other resources. Also publishes Abilities, a quarterly magazine.

Center for Research on Women with Disabilities
Department of Physical Medicine and Rehabilitation
Baylor College of Medicine
3440 Richmond Ave, Suite B
Houston, TX 77046
800-44-CROWD (800-442-7693) or 713-960-0505
E-mail: crowd@bcm.tmc.edu
www.bcm.tmc.edu/crowd
    A research center that promotes, develops, and disseminates information to expand the life choices of women with disabilities so that they may fully participate in community life.

Center for Universal Design
College of Design
North Carolina State University
50 Pullen Road, Brooks Hall, Room 104
Campus Box 8613

Raleigh, NC. 27695-8613
800-647-6777 or 919-515-3082
E-mail: cud@ncsu.edu
www.design.ncsu.edu/cud
Collects, updates, publishes, and distributes resource information about construction and home modifications for accessibility. Provides information and technical assistance on universal design and accessible housing.

Centers for Independent Living
(see Independent Living Resource Utilization Program)

Christopher & Dana Reeve Paralysis Resource Center
800-539-7309 or 973-379-2690
E-mail: info@paralysis.org
www.paralysis.org
A program of the Christopher Reeve Paralysis Foundation formed through a cooperative agreement with the Centers for Disease Control and Prevention. Serves as a comprehensive, national source of information for people living with paralysis and their caregivers to promote health, foster involvement in the community, and improve quality of life.

Community Technology Centers' Network (CTCNet)
1436 U Street, NW, Suite 104
Washington, DC 20009
202-462-1200
www.ctcnet.org
Brings together agencies and programs providing opportunities for people of all ages to learn to use technologies, offers resources to enhance capacity to provide technology access and education, and serves as an advocate for equitable access to computers and related technologies.

Consortium for Citizens with Disabilities
1331 H Street, NW, Suite 301
Washington, DC 20005
202-783-2229
E-mail: Info@c-c-d.org
www.c-c-d.org/about.htm
A coalition of national consumer, advocacy, provider and professional organizations headquartered in Washington, D.C. Since 1973, the CCD has advocated on behalf of people of all ages with physical and mental disabilities and their families. Products include the Opening Doors newsletter.

Consortium for Spinal Cord Medicine
Clinical Practice Guidelines
Paralyzed Veterans of America
801 Eighteenth Street, NW
Washington, DC 20006-3517
www.scicpg.org
scicpg@pva.org

Disability Resources
www.disabilityresources.org
A non-profit organization that promotes and improves awareness, availability, and accessibility of information to help people with disabilities live independently. Its Web site includes information about government agencies and non-profit organizations, publications, databases, and online guides.

Independent Living Resource Utilization Program
The Institute for Rehabilitation and Research
2323 South Shepherd, Suite 1000
Houston, TX 77019
713-520-0232 (voice and TTY)
TTY: 713-520-5136
www.ilru.org
A national center for information, training, research, and technical assistance in the area of independent living. The ILRU Website offers a national directory of independent living centers and information about living independently with a disability.

Job Accommodation Network
West Virginia University
P.O. Box 6080
Morgantown, WV 26506-6080
800-526-7234 (voice and TTY in United States)
800-232-9675 (for ADA Info)
304-293-7186 (V/TTY worldwide)
E-mail: jan@jan.icdi.wvu.edu
www.jan.wvu.edu
A free, federally funded consulting service designed to increase the employability of people with disabilities by providing individualized worksite accommodations solutions, providing technical assistance regarding the ADA and other disability related legislation, and educating callers about self-employment options.

Miami Project to Cure Paralysis
1095 Northwest 14 Terrace
Miami, FL 33137
800-782-6387 or 305-243-6001
www.miamiproject.miami.edu
A comprehensive research center at the University of Miami School of Medicine, dedicated to finding more effective treatments and ultimately a cure for paralysis.

Model Spinal Cord Injury System
National Center for the Dissemination of Disability Research
Southwest Educational Development Laboratory
211 East 7th Street, Suite 400
Austin, TX 78701-3253
www.ncddr.org/rpp/hf/hfdw/mscis/index.html
Sponsored by the National Institute on Disability and Rehabilitation Research (NIDRR) of the U.S. Department of Education, provides assistance to establish innovative projects for the delivery, demonstration, and evaluation of comprehensive medical, vocational, and other rehabilitation services to meet the needs of individuals with spinal cord injury. Model System Centers nationwide work together to demonstrate improved care, maintain a national database, participate in independent and collaborative research, and provide continuing education relating to spinal cord injury.

National Association for Home Care and Hospice
228 7th Street, SE, Washington, DC 20003
(202) 547-7424
www.nahc.org
The nation's largest trade association representing the interests and concerns of home care agencies, hospices, home care aide organizations, and medical equipment suppliers.

National Association of Protection and Advocacy Systems, Inc.
900 Second Street, NE, Suite 211
Washington, DC 20002
202-408-9514
E-mail: info@napas.org
www.napas.org
A national voluntary membership association of Protection and Advocacy Systems and Client Assistance Programs, which make up the nationwide network of congressionally mandated, legally based disability rights agencies. Assumes leadership in promoting and strengthening the role

and performance of its members in providing quality legally based advocacy services.

National Center on Accessibility
2805 East 10th Street, Suite 190
Bloomington, IN 47408-2698
812-856-4422
TTY: 812-856-4421
E-mail: nca@indiana.edu
www.ncaonline.org
A collaborative program of Indiana University and the National Park Service, promotes access for people with disabilities in recreation, increases awareness of inclusion of people with disabilities in parks, recreation and tourism, and focuses on universal design and practical accessibility solutions.

National Council on Independent Living
1916 Wilson Blvd, Suite 209
Arlington, VA 22201
877-525-3400 or 703-525-3406
TTY: 703-525-4153
E-mail: ncil@ncil.org
www.ncil.org
A membership organization that advances the independent living philosophy and advocates for the human rights of, and services for, people with disabilities to further their full integration and participation in society.

National Dissemination System for Children with Disabilities
P.O. Box 1492
Washington, DC 20013
(800) 695-0285 (voice and TTY)
E-mail: nichcy@aed.org
www.nichcy.org/index.html
Offers information about disabilities in infants, toddlers, children, and youth; the Individuals with Disabilities Education Act (IDEA, the law authorizing special education); No Child Left Behind (as it relates to children with disabilities), and research-based information on effective educational practices. Website provides information about organizations, conferences, publications, and more.

National Family Caregivers Association
10400 Connecticut Ave, Suite 500
Kensington, MD 20895-3944

800-896-3650 or 301-942-6430
E-mail: info@thefamilycaregiver.org
www.thefamilycaregiver.org/
Supports, empowers, educates, and speaks up for the more than 50 million Americans who care for chronically ill, aged, or disabled loved ones.

National Mobility Equipment Dealers Association
11211 N. Nebraska Avenue, Suite A-5
Tampa, FL 33612
(800) 833-0427 or (813) 977-6603
E-mail: nmeda@aol.com
www.nmeda.org
A membership organization dedicated to providing safe and quality adaptive transportation and mobility for consumers with disabilities.

National Organization on Disability
910 16th Street, NW, Suite 600
Washington, DC 20006
202-293-5960
TTY: 202-293-5968
Email: ability@nod.org
www.nod.org
Seeks to expand the participation and contribution of America's 54 million men, women, and children with disabilities in all aspects of life by raising disability awareness through programs and information.

National Rehabilitation Information Center
4200 Forbes Boulevard, Suite 202
Lanham, MD 20706
800-346-2742 or 301/459-5900 (voice)
301/459-5984 (TTY)
E-mail: naricinfo@heitechservices.com
www.naric.com
A federally funded library and information center that provides brochures, resource guides, and fact sheets, and collects and distributes results of federally funded research projects concerned with disabilities and rehabilitation.

National Spinal Cord Injury Association
6701 Democracy Blvd, Suite 300-9
Bethesda, MD 20817
800-962-9629 or (301) 214-4006

E-mail: info@spinalcord.org
www.spinalcord.org
Works to educate and empower survivors of spinal cord injury and disease to achieve and maintain the highest levels of independence, health, and personal fulfillment by providing a Peer Support Network and by raising awareness about spinal cord injury and disease.

Nursing Home Compare
www.medicare.gov/nhcompare/home.asp
A Website that helps consumers find nursing homes in specific geographic areas. Created by the federal Centers for Medicare and Medicaid Services, which runs the Medicare and Medicaid programs.

Paralysis Care Network
3320 North Clinton Street
Fort Wayne, IN 46805
219-483-2100
Implements programs concerned with injury prevention and provides information and support services to individuals with SCI and their families.
Paralyzed Veterans of America
801 18th Street NW
Washington, DC 20006-3517
800-424-8200 or 202-872-3000
E-mail: info@pva.org
www.pva.org
A veterans service organization devoted to maximizing the quality of life for people with spinal cord injury or spinal disease through research, education, advocacy, and recreation programs.

Rehabilitation Research and Training Center on Secondary Prevention through Exercise in Individuals with Spinal Cord Injury
National Rehabilitation Hospital
102 Irving Street, NW
Washington, DC 20010-2949
202-877-1038
www.sci-health.org
A federally funded center that focuses on development of knowledge about and prevention of selected secondary conditions found in people with spinal cord injury. The Center is a collaborative effort of clinicians and researchers at the National Rehabilitation Hospital and experts in the field from the University of Miami School of Medicine/Miami Project to Cure Paralysis; Independent Living Resource Utilization at the Institute for

Rehabilitation and Research; and the National Spinal Cord Injury Association and its Washington, D.C., metropolitan chapter, the Spinal Cord Injury Network.

Spinal Cord Injury Information Network
619 19th Street South, SRC-529
Birmingham, Al 35249
205-934-3283
TTD: (205) 934-4682
E-mail: sciweb@uab.edu
www.spinalcord.uab.edu
A project of the federally funded Rehabilitation Research and Training Center on Secondary Conditions of SCI, offers numerous materials and links to resources concerned with spinal cord injury.

Spinal Cord Injury Network International
3911 Princeton Drive
Santa Rosa, CA 95405-7013
800-548-2673 or 707-577-8796
E-mail: spinal@sonic.net
www.spinalcordinjury.org
A non-profit organization dedicated to facilitating access to high-quality health care by providing information and referral services to spinal-cord-injured individuals and their families. Its Information Center has books, journals and clippings files; information sheets; and a video lending library.

Tetra Society of North America
Box 27, Suite A304
Plaza of Nations
770 Pacific Boulevard South
Vancouver, British Columbia
CANADA V6B 5E7
1-877-688-8762 or 604-688-6464
Email: info@tetrasociety.org
www.tetrasociety.org
Recruits skilled volunteer engineers and technicians to create assistive devices for persons with disabilities.

United Spinal Association (formerly Eastern Paralyzed Veterans Association)
Executive Office
75-20 Astoria Boulevard

Jackson Heights, NY 11370
718-803-3782
Services Office
245 West Houston Street
New York, NY 10014
800-807-0192
E-mail: info@unitedspinal.org
www.unitedspinal.org
   Seeks to enhance the lives of individuals with spinal cord injury or disease by assuring quality health care, promoting research, advocating for civil rights and independence, and educating the public.

Federal Government Resources

DisabilityInfo.gov
   As a gateway to the federal government's disability-related information and resources, serves as a directory of government Web links relevant to persons with disabilities, their families, employers, service providers and other community members.

Centers for Medicare and Medicaid Services
U.S. Department of Health and Human Services
7500 Security Boulevard
Baltimore MD 21244-1850
877-267-2323 or 410-786-3000
TTY: 866-226-1819 (toll-free) or 410-786-0727
www.cms.gov
   The federal government agency responsible for the Medicare and Medicaid health insurance programs. CMS offers information about Medicare and Medicaid coverage.

National Institute on Disability and Rehabilitation Research
U.S. Department of Education
400 Maryland Avenue, SW
Washington, DC 20202-7100
202-245-7640
TTY: 202-245-7316
www.ed.gov/about/offices/list/osers/nidrr
   A part of the Office of Special Education and Rehabilitation Services, provides leadership and support for research related to the rehabilitation of people with disabilities.
A federally funded center offering free health information for women.

Website features a section focused on women with disabilities, including spinal cord injury.

National Institute of Neurological Disorders and Stroke
National Institutes of Health
P.O. Box 5801
Bethesda, MD 20824
800-352-9424 or 301-496-5751
TTY: 301-468-5981
Conducts, fosters, coordinates, and guides research on the causes, prevention, diagnosis, and treatment of neurological disorders and stroke, and supports basic research in related scientific areas.

National Institute on Disability and Rehabilitation Research
U.S. Department of Education
400 Maryland Ave., S.W.
Washington, DC 20202-7100
202-245-7640
TTY: 202-245-7316
www.ed.gov/about/offices/list/osers/nidrr
Provides leadership and support for a comprehensive program of research related to the rehabilitation of individuals with disabilities, with a focus on improving the lives of individuals with disabilities from birth through adulthood.

National Women's Health Information Center
U.S. Department of Health and Human Services
8550 Arlington Blvd., Suite 300
Fairfax, VA 22031
800-994-WOMAN (800-994-9662)
TDD: 888-220-5446
www.4woman.gov/wwd

Office of Disability Employment Policy
U.S. Department of Labor
Frances Perkins Building
200 Constitution Avenue, NW
Washington, DC 20210
866-633-7365
TTY: 877-889-5627
www.dol.gov/odep
Works to increase employment opportunities for adults and youth with

disabilities. Its Web site includes facts sheets and other publications about employment of persons with disabilities, links to employers that wish to hire persons with disabilities, and information about employment-related programs.

Office of Special Education and Rehabilitation Services
U.S. Department of Education
U.S. Department of Education
400 Maryland Ave., S.W.
Washington, DC 20202-7100
202-245-7468
www.ed.gov/about/offices/list/osers
Reports on current developments in research, policy, practice and legislation with regard to education and employment of people with disabilities. OSERS includes the National Institute on Disability and Rehabilitation Research, the Office of Special Education Policy, and the Rehabilitation Services Administration (see separate listings for contact information).

Office of Special Education Policy
U.S. Department of Education
400 Maryland Ave., S.W.
Washington, DC 20202-7100
202-245-7459
www.ed.gov/about/offices/list/osers/osep
Works to improve education results for infants, toddlers, children, and youth with disabilities ages birth through 21 by providing leadership and financial support to assist states and local districts.

Rehabilitation Services Administration
U.S. Department of Education
400 Maryland Ave., S.W.
Washington, DC 20202-7100
202-205-5482
www.ed.gov/about/offices/list/osers/rsa
Oversees programs that help people with disabilities live independently by providing counseling, job training, and other services.

Social Security Administration
Office of Public Inquiries
Windsor Park Building
6401 Security Boulevard
Baltimore, MD 21235

800-772-1213
TTY: 1-800-325-0778
www.ssa.gov (includes a locator for local Social Security Administration offices)

Offers information about Social Security Disability Insurance (SSDI) and other benefits that persons with disabilities may be eligible for. For lists of service providers, visit: www.ssa.gov/work/ServiceProviders/rehabproviders.html.

State Vocational Rehabilitation Agencies

State vocational rehabilitation agencies offer information about state programs for people with disabilities, as well as job and rehabilitation information. Each state offers different services and resources. For a list of the contact information for each of the 50 states and the District of Columbia, visit: www.jan.wvu.edu/sbses/vocrehab.htm.

Rehabilitation Professional Organizations

American Academy of Physical Medicine and Rehabilitation
One IBM Plaza, Suite 2500
Chicago, IL 60611-3604
312-464-9700
E-mail: info@aapmr.org
www.aapmr.org

A professional organization of physiatrists, who are specialists in physical medicine and rehabilitation. The AAPM&R Web site includes a searchable database that helps users to find physical medicine and rehabilitation specialists (www.e-aapmr.org/imis/imisonline/findphys/ find.cfm).

American Association of Spinal Cord Injury Psychologists and Social Workers
75-20 Astoria Blvd.
Jackson Heights, NY 11370
718-803-3782
E-mail: aascipsw@unitedspinal.org
www.aascipsw.org

Advances and promotes psychosocial care of persons with spinal cord injury, and develops and advances education and research in that area.

American Congress of Rehabilitation Medicine
6801 Lake Plaza Drive, Suite B-205

Indianapolis Indiana 46220
317-915-2250
www.acrm.org
   A professional organization for professionals who work in rehabilitation
fields that promotes the art, science, and practice of rehabilitation care for
people with disabilities. The ACRM Web site includes resources and links to
other organizations.

American Occupational Therapy Association
4720 Montgomery Lane
PO Box 31220
Bethesda, MD 20824-1220
301-652-2682
TDD: 1-800-377-8555
www.aota.org
   A professional organization for occupational therapy professionals. Its
Web site provides consumers with general information about occupational
therapy; tip sheets about health and disability issues, conditions, and daily
living; resource listings; and a searchable directory of occupational therapy
specialists.

American Paraplegia Society
75-20 Astoria Boulevard
Jackson Heights, NY 11370
718-803-3782
E-mail: aps@unitedspinal.org
www.apssci.org
   Convenes an annual scientific conference to report state-of-the-art techniques, disseminate information about scientific and technological break-
throughs, and discuss advances in research and the latest standards for
achieving optimal health care of the individuals with spinal cord impairment.

American Physical Therapy Association
1111 North Fairfax Street
Alexandria, VA 22314-1488
800-999-2782 or 703-684-2782
TDD: 703-683-6748
www.apta.org
   Fosters advancements in physical therapy practice, research, and education. Offers consumers information about physical therapy, including
research, fitness guides, and an online directory of certified therapists that is

searchable by state and specialty.

American Speech-Language-Hearing Association
10801 Rockville Pike
Rockville, MD 20852
800-638-8255 (voice and TTY)
E-mail: actioncenter@asha.org.
www.asha.org
   A professional organization that provides callers with referrals to certified speech-language therapists, and audiologists, and helps consumers to find accredited speech, language, and hearing programs.

American Spinal Injury Association
2020 Peachtree Road, NW
Atlanta, GA 30309-1402
404 355-9772
www.asia-spinalinjury.org
   ASIA is a multidisciplinary professional organization whose membership is composed of physicians and allied health professionals specifically involved in spinal cord injury management.

American Therapeutic Recreation Association
1414 Prince Street, Suite 204
Alexandria, Virginia 22314
703-683-9420
atracommunications@atra-tr.org
www.atra-tr.org
   A professional organization of recreational therapists, health care providers who use recreational therapy interventions to improved the functioning of individuals with illness or disabling conditions.

Association for Driver Rehabilitation Specialists
711 S. Vienna Street
Ruston, LA 71270
800-290-2344 or 318-257-5055
www.driver-ed.org
   Supports professionals working in the field of driver education/driver training and transportation equipment modifications for persons with disabilities through education and information dissemination.

Association of Rehabilitation Nurses
4700 West Lake Avenue

Glenview, IL 60025-1485
800-229-7530 or 847-375-4710
E-mail: info@rehabnurse.org
www.rehabnurse.org
Promotes and advances professional rehabilitation nursing practice through education, advocacy, collaboration, and research to enhance the quality of life for persons affected by disability and chronic illness.

International Spinal Cord Society (IScoS)
National Spinal Injuries Centre
Stoke Mandeville Hospital
Aylesbury
Bucks
HP21 8AL, UK
Phone: +44 1296 315 866
Fax: +44 1296 315870
E-mail: admin@iscos.org.uk
http://iscos.org.uk
An international impartial, non-political, non-profit association that seeks to study all problems relating to traumatic and non-traumatic lesions of the spinal cord. This includes causes, prevention, basic and clinical research, medical and surgical management, clinical practice, education, rehabilitation and social reintegration.

Rehabilitation Engineering and Assistive Technology Society of North America (RESNA)
1700 N. Moore St, Suite 1540
Arlington, VA 22209-1903
703-524-6686
TTY: 703-524-6639
E-mail: info@resna.org
www.resna.org
An interdisciplinary association of professionals with an interest and skills in technology and disability.

Rehabilitation Psychology Division, American Psychological Association
Division 22 Administrative Office
American Psychological Association
750 First Street, NE
Washington, DC 20002-4242
202-336-6013
www.apa.org/divisions/div22

Brings together American Psychological Association members concerned with the psychological aspects of disability and rehabilitation, educates the public on issues related to disability and rehabilitation, and develops high standards and practices for professional psychologists who work in rehabilitation.

Volunteers for Medical Engineering
2301 Argonne Drive
Baltimore, MD 21218
410-243-7495
E-mail: vme@toad.net
www.toad.net/~vme

An organization made up of volunteers, engineers, and medical professionals who work to improve the independence of individuals with disabilities and elderly persons through custom design of new products and modifications to existing devices. Also loans computers to individuals with disabilities.

Health Care Facility Accreditation Organizations

Joint Commission on Accreditation of Healthcare Organizations (JCAHO)
One Renaissance Boulevard
Oakbrook Terrace, IL 60181
630-792-5000
www.jcaho.org

Looks at how well health care programs, including rehabilitation programs, meet standards of quality in care. JCAHO's Website includes a comprehensive guide to the more than 15,000 JCAHO-accredited health care organizations and programs throughout the United States (http://www.jcaho.org/quality+check).

Commission on Accreditation of Rehabilitation Facilities (CARF)
4891 East Grant Road
Tucson, AZ 85712
(888) 281-6531 or 520-325-1044 (voice and TTY)
www.carf.org

An independent, not-for-profit organization that reviews and accredits rehabilitation facilities to help ensure high-quality care and the best possible outcomes. CARF's Web site includes a list of accredited rehabilitation programs that can be searched by state and program type.

Periodicals

New Mobility
P.O. Box 220
Horsham, PA 19044
888-850-0344
E-mail: info@newmobility.com
www.newmobility.com
A monthly magazine providing current information on current issues relevant to persons with disabilities and includes a wealth of information on resources, legal rights, and equipment. Also publishes the book, *Spinal Network*.

PN/Paraplegia News
PVA Publications
2111 E. Highland Avenue, Suite 180
Phoenix, AZ 85016-4702
888-888-2201 or (602) 224-0500
E-mail: pvapub@aol.com
www.pvamagazines.com/pnnews
This monthly magazine published by the Paralyzed Veterans of America covers the latest on spinal cord injury research, new products, legislation, people with disabilities, accessible travel, computers, and more.

Pushin' On
619 19th Street South, SRC 529
Birmingham, AL 35249-7330
205-934-3283
TDD: 205-934-4642
E-mail: sciweb@uab.edu
www.spinalcord.uab.edu/show.asp?durki=21396
A free annual newsletter published by the University of Alabama at Birmingham Model Spinal Cord Injury System of Care and the Spinal Cord Injury Information Network. Covers health, research, and other various issues related to secondary conditions of SCI.

Resourceful Woman
(312) 238-1051
www.rehabchicago.org/community/hrcwd.php
A free newsletter distributed by the Health Resource Center for Women with Disabilities at the Rehabilitation Institute of Chicago, that provides women and health care professionals current information and in-depth

analyses of issues relevant to women with disabilities.

Spinal Cord Injury Update
Box 356490
Seattle, WA 98195-6490
206-685-3999
E-mail: rehab@u.washington.edu
http://depts.washington.edu/rehab/sci/update.shtml
   Quarterly newsletter published by the University of Washington, Rehabilitation Medicine that contains articles on SCI for health care providers and consumers, as well as summaries of current literature on SCI.

Sports 'n Spokes
PVA Publications
2111 East Highland Avenue, Suite 180
Phoenix, AZ 85016-4702
(888) 888-2201 or (602) 224-0500
www.pvamagazines.com/sns
   Published by the Paralyzed Veterans Association, provides information on a variety of sports and competition events.

Online Information and Communication Resources

Dimenet.com

Disabled Individuals Movement for Equality Network (Dimenet) provides accessible access to the information infrastructure to people with disabilities through Independent Living Centers.

DisabilityGuide.org
301-528-8664

Produced by Access Information, Inc., offers information about accessibility, transportation, museums, malls, theaters, restaurants, and hotels in the Washington area.

DisabilityInfo.gov

A comprehensive federal Web site of disability-related government resources. It offers information about employment, housing, transportation, technology, and other topics.

iCan.com

Offers a wide range of resources, information, and a message board.

New Mobility.com

Website includes a message board, a chat room, classifieds, a bookstore, an "Ask the Expert" page, and links to other organizations. Book titles include: From There to Here: Stories of Adjustment To Spinal Cord Injury; Spinal Network: The Total Wheelchair Resource Book; Kids on Wheels; Enabling Romance: A Guide to Love, Sex, and Relationships for People with Disabilities (and the People who Care About Them); and The Complete Product Guide for People with Disabilities.

NRHhealthtown.org

An online resource of the National Rehabilitation Hospital that includes a library, employment center, shopping and community services resources, personal pages, and more.

Quad Link
www.2tim.net/

Connects people with spinal cord injury and offers resources.

Quad-List
http://come.to/quadlist

Provides a discussion forum for quadriplegics (tetraplegics) to communicate with others who share the same condition.

Vent-Users List
www.makoa.org/ventuser.htm

Provides a discussion forum for people who require a ventilator (respirator) to breathe to communicate with others who share the same condition.

Health and Income Supports (Chapter 6)

Additional Reading

Beatty, P. B. (2002, Spring). To your health: An overview on health and managed care issues on SCI. SCI *Life*, pp. 8-10, 11.

Hess, D. W., Ripley, D. L., McKinley, W. O., & Tewksbury, M. (2000). Predictors for return to work after spinal cord injury: A 3-year multicenter analysis. *Archives of Physical Medicine and Rehabilitation*, 81, 359-363.

Jones, G. C. (2002, November). *Rural Medicaid managed care for people with disabilities: Recommendations for smooth sailing. Policy Brief*. Washington, DC: NRH Center for Health & Disability Research.

Kongstvedt, P. R. (2001). *The essentials of managed health care*. (3rd ed.). Gaithersburg, MD: Aspen Publishers, Inc.

Meyer, D. R. (1995). Supplemental security income. In R. L. Edwards (Ed.-in-Chief). *Encyclopedia of social work* (19th ed., pp. 2379-2385). Washington, DC: National Association of Social Workers.

NRH Center for Health & Disability Research. *Keys to managed care: A guide for people with physical disabilities*. Washington, DC: Author.

Social Security Administration. (2002, January). *2002 Red Book on Employment Support: A Summary Guide to Employment Support Available to People with Disabilities under the Social Security Disability Insurance and Supplemental Security Income Programs*. SSA Pub. No. 64-436900.

Social Security Administration. (2003, February). *Disability benefits*. SSA Publication No. 05-10029. http://ssa.gov/pubs/10029.html. First retrieved 7/10/03.

Social Security Online. (2003). *Automatic Increases: Substantial Gainful Activity*. http://www.ssa.gov/OACT/COLA/SGA.html. First retrieved June 9, 2004.

Tracy, M. B., & Ozawa, M. N. (1995). Social security. In R. L. Edwards (Ed.-in-Chief). *Encyclopedia of social work* (19th ed., pp. 2186-2195). Washington, DC: National Association of Social Workers.

Getting Ready to Go Home (Chapter 7)

Additional Reading

Able Data. (January, 1995). *Informed Consumer's Guide to Accessible Housing*.

Available at: www.abledata.com/Site_2icg_hous.htm.

Corbet, B., & Dobbs, J. (Eds.). (2002). *Spinal Network: The Total Wheelchair Resource Book.* Horsham, PA (VERFIFY): Nine Lives Press.

Medical Rehabilitation Research and Training Center in Secondary Complications in Spinal Cord Injury, University of Alabama. (2004). Adjustment to Spinal Cord Injury (SCI InfoSheet #20). Available at: www.spinalcord.uab.edu.

Medical Rehabilitation Research and Training Center in Secondary Complications in Spinal Cord Injury, University of Alabama. (1998). Caregivers for SCI (SCI InfoSheet #17). Available at:: www.spinalcord.uab.edu.

Medical Rehabilitation Research and Training Center in Secondary Complications in Spinal Cord Injury, University of Alabama. (1995). Personal Care Assistants (SCI InfoSheet #6). Available at: www.spinalcord.uab.edu.
National Endowment for Financial Education, Paralyzed Veterans of America, National Spinal Cord Injury Association. (2002). *On The Move, A Financial Guide for People with Spinal Cord Injury.*

Opening Doors: A Housing Publication for the Disability Community. (June 2000). *Accessible Housing for People with Disabilities.* Issue 10.

Ulicny, Gary R., Adler, Amy B., Kennedy, Sara E., Jones, Michael L., (1987). *A Step-By-Step Guide to Training and Managing Personal Attendants.* Volume1: Consumer Guide. Research and Training Center on Independent Living (RTC/IL). University of Kansas, Lawrence, KS 66045.

Physical Activity and Recreation (Chapter 8)

Sports Organizations for Athletes with Disabilities

America's Athletes with Disabilities, Inc.
8630 Fenton Street, Suite 920
Silver Spring, MD 20910
800-238-7632 or 301-589-9042
E-mail: aadhdq@aol.com
www.americasathletes.org
   Promotes and sponsors sports, recreation, fitness, and leisure events for children and adults with physical disabilities.

BlazeSports Clubs of America
U.S. Disabled Athletes Fund, Inc.
280 Interstate North Circle, Suite 450
Atlanta, GA 30339
770-850-8199
E-mail: blazesports@blazesports.com
www.blazesports.com

A comprehensive sports and fitness program founded by the U.S. Disabled Athletes Fund, Inc., in partnership with the National Recreation and Park Association. Offers wheelchair tennis, basketball, racing, rugby, and swimming programs for children and adults with physical disabilities that involve Paralympic athletes, coaches, and other nationally ranked disabled athletes. Website includes a list of local clubs.

Disabled Sports USA
451 Hungerford Dr, Suite 100
Rockville, MD 20850
301-217-0960
E-mail: information@dsusa.org
www.dsusa.org

A non-profit organization offering nationwide sports rehabilitation programs to anyone with a permanent physical disability. Activities include winter skiing, water sports, summer and winter competitions, fitness, and special sports events.

National Center on Physical Activity and Disability
1640 W. Roosevelt Road
Chicago, IL 60608-6904
800-900-8086 (voice and TTY)
E-mail: ncpad@uic.edu
www.ncpad.org

An information center concerned with physical activity and disability that promotes the substantial health benefits that can be gained from participating in regular physical activity. Offers resources ranging from guidelines for starting an exercise program to fact sheets on many popular activities, games, recreational pursuits, and sports that have been adapted for persons with disabilities.

Wheelchair Sports, USA
1668 320th Way
Earlham, IA 50072
515-833-2450

E-mail: wsusa@aol.com
www.wsusa.org
   A volunteer organization of athletes who use wheelchairs at the local,
regional, national, and international levels.

Aquatics

United States Wheelchair Swimming
229 Miller Street
Middleboro, MA 02346

USA Swimming
One Olympic Plaza
Colorado Springs, CO 80909
719-578-4578
www.usa-swimming.org

Archery

American Wheelchair Archers
Road 2, Box 2043
West Sunbury, PA 16061
United Foundation for Disabled Archers
E-mail: chad@evl.net

Wheelchair Archery, USA
c/o Wheelchair Sports, USA
3595 East Fountain Boulevard, Suite L10
Colorado Springs, CO 80910
719-574-1150

Basketball

National Wheelchair Basketball Association
6165 Lehman Drive, Suite 101
Colorado Springs, CO 80918
719-266-4082
E-mail: toddhatfield@nwba.org
www.nwba.org

Boating/Rowing/Sailing

Access to Sailing
19744 Beach Blvd., Suite 340
Huntington Beach, Ca 92648
949-722-5371

American Canoe Association (canoeing and kayaking)
8580 Cinderbed Road
Newington, VA 22122
703-550-7495

National Ocean Access Project GET MORE INFO
P.O. Box 10726
Rockville, MD 20849-0726

The Parasail Vision Quest
305-361-9191
E-mail: info@parasail.com
www.parasail.com

U.S. Association of Disabled Sailors
Southern California Chapter
P.O. Box 15245
Newport Beach, CA 92659
U.S. Rowing Association
11 Hall Place
Exeter, NH 03833
U.S. Sailing Association: Sailors With Special Needs
PO Box 1260, 15 Maritime Drive
Portsmouth, RI 02871-0907
401-683-0800
http://ussailing.org/swsn

Bowling

American Wheelchair Bowling Association
N54 W15858 Larkspur Lane
Menomonee Falls, WI 53051
414-781-6876

Flying

International Wheelchair Aviators

1117 Rising Hill Way
Escondido, CA 92025
619-746-5018

Golf

Association of Disabled American Golfers
P.O. Box 280649
Lakewood, CO 80228-0649
303-922-5228
E-mail: adag@usga.org
www.toski.com/golf/adag
Handcycling

United States Handcycling Federation
P.O. Box 3538
Evergreen, CO 80437
303-679-2770
E-mail: info@ushf.org
www.ushf.org

Hockey

American Sled Hockey Association
21 Summerwood Court
Buffalo, NY 14223
716-876-7390
E-mail: rich_deglopper@kenton.k12.ny.us
www.sledhockey.org

USA Wheelchair Hockey Association
7216 39th Avenue. North
Minneapolis, MN 55427
763-535-4736
E-mail: hockey@usewha.org
www.usewha.org

Motorcycling

National Handicap Motorcyclist Association
404 Maple Street
Upper Nyack, NY 10960

914-353-0747
Wheelchair Motorcycle Association
108 Torrey St
Brockton, MA 02401
508-583-8614

Powerlifting

USCPAA Powerlifting Sports Technical Officer
8420 West Chester Pike
Upper Darbe, PA 19082
610-356-1910
Rugby

United States Quad Rugby Association
101 Park Place Circle
Alabaster, Alabama 35007
205-868-2281
E-mail: supersports@mindspring.com

United States Quad Rugby Association
2418 West Fallcreek Court
Grand Forks, ND 55201
701-772-1961

Scuba Diving

Handicapped Scuba Association
1104 El Prado
San Clemente, CA 92672-4637
714-498-6128
www.hsascuba.com

Shooting

National Wheelchair Shooting Federation
102 Park Avenue
Rockledge, PA 19046

NRA Adaptive Shooting
11250 Waples Mill Road
Fairfax, VA 22030

215-663-0102

Outdoor Buddies Hunting Program
P.O. Box 37283
Denver, CO 80237
303-771-8216
E-mail: outbud@juno.com
www.outbud.freeservers.com

Snow Skiing
Adaptive Sports Center
800-544-8448, ext. 2296; (970) 349-2296

Breckenridge Outdoor Education Center
970-453-6422

Challenge Aspen
970-923-0578

Ski for Light Inc.
Mobility Impaired Coordinator
1400 Carole Lane
Greenbay, WI 54313
414-494-5572

United States Disabled Ski Team
P.O. Box 100
Park City, UT 84060
801-619-0909

Softball

National Wheelchair Softball Association
1616 Todd Court
Stamford, CT 55033

Tennis/Racquet Sports

International Foundation for Wheelchair Tennis
2203 Timberloch Place, Suite 126
The Woodlands, TX 77380
National Foundation of Wheelchair Tennis

2380 McGinley Road
Monroeville, PA 15146
Fax: 714-361-6603

940 Calle Amanecer, Suite B
San Clemente, CA 92672

National Wheelchair Racquetball Association
535 Kensington Road, Apartment #4
Lancaster, PA 17603
719-635-5396

Track and Field/Road Racing

Achilles Track Club
212-354-0300
www.achillestrackclub.org

Achilles Track Club of Greater Washington
301-649-4909

International Wheelchair Road Racers Club
30 Myano Lane
Stamford, CT 06902
Rolling Thunder Runners Club
http://run.to/rollingthunder

Triathlon for the Disabled
PO Box V-16
Pal Alto, CA 94304
Wheelchair Athletics of the USA
1475 West Gray #161
Houston, TX 77019
Phone: 713-522-9769

Wheelchair Sports USA
719-574-1150
www.wsusa.org

Volleyball

Disabled Sports USA

451 Hungerford Drive, Suite 100
Rockville, MD 20850
301-217-0960
www.dsusa.org

Water Skiing

American Waterski Association – Disabled Ski
681 Bailey Woods Road
Dacula, GA 30211
404-995-8528

Disabled Ski Committee
Camp ASCCA
PO Box 21
Jackson, AL 36861
1-800-THECAMP
www.campascca.org

Weightlifting

United States Wheelchair Weightlifting Federation
39 Micheal Place
Levittown, PA 19057
215-945-1964

Wilderness Adventures and Hiking

Follow-Me-Outdoors
Wilderness on Wheels
7125 Jefferson #155
Lakewood, CO 80235
303-988-2212
www.wildernessonwheels.org

National Sports Center for the Disabled
303-293-5711
www.nscd.org

Physically Challenged Access to the Woods
53W Park
PO Box 357

Empire, CO 80438
303-569-2106
www.outdoors4all.org

Wilderness Inquiry
808 14th Avenue SE
Minneapolis, MN 55414-1516
800-728-0719; 612-676-9400
TTY: 612.676.9475
Email: info@wildernessinquiry.org
www.wildernessinquiry.org

Wilderness on Wheels
P.O. Box 1007
Wheat Ridge, CO 80034
303-403-1110

Sources of Adaptive Equipment for Recreation

Access to Recreation
8 Sandra Court
Newbury Park, CA 91320-4302
800-634-4351
www.AccessTR.com

Dynamic Living, Inc.
P.O. Box 370249
West Hartford CT 06137-0249
888-940-0605

Flaghouse
601 Flaghouse Drive
Hasbrouck Heights NJ 07604-3116
800-793-7900
www.flaghouse.com

Sammons Preston Enrichments
P.O. Box 178
Ortonville, MI 48462-0178
800-323-5547

S & S Healthcare
P.O. Box 513
Colchester, CT 06415-0513
800-243-9232
www.ssww.com

SPORTAID
770-554-5033 (customer service)
800-743-7203 (to order)
www.SportAid.com

Sexuality (Chapter 10)

Additional Reading

Annon, JS, *The Behavioral Treatment of Sexual Problems*. Vol. 1: Brief Therapy. Hawaii: Enabling Systems, 1974.

Bennett, C, High Tech Fertility. In: Maddox, S., ed. *Spinal Network, The Total Wheelchair Book, Second Edition*, Malibu, CA: Miramar Communications, Inc., 1994.

Dahlberg, J, Sex, Etc., for Men. In: Maddox, S.,ed. *Spinal Network, The Total Wheelchair Book, Second Edition*, Malibu, CA: Miramar Communications, Inc., 1994. VERIFY – MAY NOT BE CURRENT EDITION

Ducharme, SH, Gill, KM, *Sexuality after Spinal Cord Injury*, Baltimore, MD: Paul H. Brookes Publishing Co.,1997.

Duffy, Y, *All Things are Possible*, Ann Arbor, MI: A.J.Garvin and Associates, 1981.

Halstead, LS, Seager, SWJ, Electroejaculation and its Techniques in Males with Neurologic Impairments. In: Hazelton, F, Cole, S, Gray, D, eds. *Reproductive Issues for Persons with Physical Disabilities*, Baltimore, MD: Brooks Press, 1993.

Hanson, M, Kurinczuk, JJ, Bower, C. Webb, S. The risk of major birth defects after intracytoplasmic sperm injection and in vitro fertilization. New Eng J Medicine 2002, 346: 725-730.

Kaufman, M., Silverburg, C., & Odette, F. (2002 VERIFY). *The Ultimate*

Guide to Sex and Disability: For All of Us Who Live with Disabilities, Chronic Pain and Illness. San Francisco: Cleis Press.

Klebine, P. Sexuality for Women with Spinal Cord Injury. Office of Research Services, 619 19th St, South – SRC 529, Birmingham, AL, 35249, 2002.

Kroll, K., & Klein, EL. (2001). *Enabling Romance: A Guide to Love, Sex, and Relationships for People with Disabilities (and the People who Care About Them)*. Horsham, PA: No Limits Communications.
Lindsey, L, Klebine, P. Sexuality for Men with SCI. Office of Research Services, 619 19th St, South – SRC 529, Birmingham, AL, 35249, 2000. Email: rtc@uab.edu

McDonald, SE, Lloyd, WM, Murphy, D, Russert, MG, *Sexuality and Spinal Cord Injury*, Milwaukee, WI: Froedtert Memorial Lutheran Hospital, 1993.

Mooney, TO, Cole, TM, Chilgren, RA, *Sexual Options for Paraplegics and Quadriplegics*, Boston, MA: Little, Brown and Company, 1975.

Sipski, ML, Spinal Cord Injury and Sexual Function: An Educational Model. In: Sipski, ML, Alexander, CJ, eds. *Sexual Function in People with Disability and Chronic Illness*, Gaithersburg, MD: Aspen Publishers, Inc., 1997.

Sipski, M, Alexander, CJ. Basic Sexual Function over Time. In: Sipski, ML, Alexander, CJ,eds. *Sexual Function in People with Disability and Chronic Illness*, Gaithersburg, MD: Aspen Publishers, Inc., 1997.

Whipple, B, McGreer, KB, Management of Female Sexual Dysfunction. In: Sipski, ML, Alexander, CJ, eds. *Sexual Function in People with Disability and Chronic Illness*, Gaithersburg, MD: Aspen Publishers, Inc., 1997.

Whipple, B, Richards, E,Tepper, M, Komisaruk, BR, Sexual response in Women with Complete Spinal Cord Injury. In: Krotoski, DM, Nosek, M, Turk, M, eds. *Women with Physical Disabilities: Achieving and Maintaining Health and Well-Being*, Baltimore, MD: Paul H. Brookes Publishing Co., 1996.

Weiner, DN, Rosen, RC. Medications and their Impact. In: Sipski, ML, Alexander, CJ, eds. *Sexual Function in People with Disability and Chronic Illness*, Gaithersburg, MD: Aspen Publishers, Inc., 1997.

Other Resources

American Association of Sex Educators, Counselors, and Therapists
P.O. Box 5488
Richmond, VA 23220-0488
Website: www.aasect.org
E-mail: aasect@aasect.org
Phone: 804-644-3288

Sexuality Information and Education Council of the United States
130 West 42nd Street, Suite 350
New York, NY 10036-7802
Phone: 212/819-9770
Website: www.siecus.org
E-mail: siecus@siecus.org

Parenting and Having a Baby (Chapter 11)

Additional Reading

BabyCenter. Ob-Gyn or Family Physician Interview Sheet. Available at:
www.babycenter.com/general/pregnancy/childbirth/3432.html

Baker E, Cardenas D. Pregnancy in spinal cord injured women. Archives of
Physical Medicine & Rehabilitation. 1996;77:501-7.

Briggs, GC, Freeman, RK, Yaffe, SJ. (2001). *Drugs in Pregnancy and Lactation
(6th Ed.)* Baltimore?: Lippincott Williams & Wilkins.

Garee B (Ed.). *Parenting Tips for Parents (Who Happen To Have a Disability)
on Raising Children,* Bloomington, IL: Accent Special Publications, Cheever
Publishing, Inc., 1989.

Jackson, A. B. Pregnancy and delivery. (1996). In: D. Krotoski, M. Nosek,
and M. Turk, eds. *Women With Physical Disabilities Achieving and Maintaining
Health and Well-Being,* Baltimore: Paul Brooks Publishing Company.

Kirshbaum M. Parents with physical disabilities and their babies. Zero Three
1988; 8(5): 8-15.

Kirshbaum M., Olkin R. Parent with Physical, Systemic, or Visual
Disabilities. Sexuality and Disability 2002; 20(1):7-28.

Neurological and Psychiatric Disorders. In: F. G. Cunningham, N. F. Grant, K. J. Leveno, L. C. Gilstrap III, J. C. Hauth, K. D. Wenstrom, eds. *Williams Obstetrics – 21st Edition,* New York: McGraw-Hill Medical Publishing Division, 2001:1417.

Neville H, Johnson DC. *Temperament Tools: Working With Your Child's Inborn Traits.* Seattle, WA: Parenting Press, Inc., 1998.

Organization of Teratology Information Services Fact Sheets. These fact sheets answer frequently asked questions about drug exposures, herbal products, infections and vaccines, material medical conditions, illicit exposures, and other exposures during pregnancy. Available at: www.otispregnancy.org or call (866) 626-OTIS, or (866) 626-6847

Rogers JA. (in press). *Disabled Women's Guide To Pregnancy and Birth Pregnancy and Birth,* New York: Demos Publications.

Stanford P. You poor old soul. Disability, Pregnancy and Parenthood International 2001; 33: 17-19.

Tuleja C, DeMoss A. Babycare assistive technology. *Technology and Disability* 1999; 11: 71-78.

Tuleja C, Rogers J, Vensand K, DeMoss A. *Continuation of Adaptive Parenting Equipment Development,* Berkeley, CA: Through the Looking Glass, 1998.

Vensand, K., Rogers, J., Tuleja, C., & De Moss, A. *Adaptive Baby Care Equipment: Guidelines, Prototypes, and Resources.* Berkeley, CA: Through the Looking Glass, 2000.

Organizations

American College of Obstetricians and Gynecologists
(Website includes a tool to identify obstetricians/gynecologists by Zip code)
409 12th Street, SW, P.O. Box 96920
Washington, D.C. 20090-6920
202-638-5577
www.acog.org

Assistive Technology Services Division
Occupational Therapy Department,
Woodrow Wilson Rehabilitation Center

(800) 345-9972
www.wwrc.net/menuroot/AT-over-view.htm

Charlotte Institute of Rehabilitation
Charlotte, NC
(704) 355-4300.
Website: www.carolinas.org/services/rehab/CIR/index.cfm

Consultation Resource Services for Women with Disabilities
School of Nursing, University of British Columbia
Phone: (604) 822-7444
www.school.nursing.ubc.ca/faculty/memberBio.asp?c=70.2993598832877

Disabled Adoption Listserv
groups.yahoo.com/group/disabledadoptiveparents

Health Resource Center for Women with Disabilities
Rehabilitation Institute of Chicago
Phone: 1-800-354-REHAB (7342); (312) 238-1000
Website: www.rehabchicago.org

Through the Looking Glass: The National Resource Center for Parents with Disabilities
2198 6th Street, Suite 100
Berkeley, CA 94710-2204
800-644-2666; 510-848-1112
E-mail: tlg@lookingglass.org
www.lookingglass.org

Tree of Life Adoption Center
9570 SW Barbur Boulevard, Suite 304
Portland, OR 97219
503-244-7374
www.toladopt.org

Baby Care Equipment/Product Manufacturers

Arm's Reach® Concepts, Inc.
800-954-9353
www.armsreach.com

Offers the Co-Sleeper®, a portable, accessible bassinet that attaches to the side of a parent's bed.

Baby Tech® International, Inc.
949-760-6009
www.babytechint.com
Offers the Pacifier Plus® Fever Indicating Pacifiers.

Gerber®
800-4-GERBER
www.gerber.com
Offers the Harness and Hand Strap, a fanny pack worn by the child with an attached tether that allows the adult keep the child nearby.

Little Wonders
800-639-2984
www.littlewonders.com
Offers the Baby Bundle bottle holder.

One Step Ahead® Online Store
800-274-8440 or 800-950-5120
www.onestepahead.com
Offers the Kid Keeper, a child's chest harness with a tether that allows the adult to keep your child nearby.

Snugli Early Care Sling™
800-233-5921
www.snugli.com

Sammons Preston Rolyan (an AbilityOne Company)
(Offers a Rehab Catalog)
800-323-5547
www.sammonspreston.com

School Aids, Toys, Games, and Outdoor Recreation Equipment

Abilitations
800-850-8602
www.abilitations.com

Ablenet, Inc.
800-322-0956; 651-294-2200

www.ablenetinc.com

Enabling Devices (a division of Toys for Special Children, Inc.)
800-832-8697 or 914-478-0960
www.enablingdevices.com

Grounds For Play
800-552-7529; 817-477-5482
www.groundsforplay.com
    Creates accessible playgrounds that meet the needs of children and parents for safe, stimulating outdoor experiences.

Hotshot Products
888-663-5911 or 310-533-5911
www.hotshotproducts.org

Offers beach and other all-terrain wheelchairs, including the Beach Cruzr.

IntelliTools®, Inc.
800-899-6687
www.intellitools.com
    Designs computer products for people who face challenges ranging from learning disabilities to significant physical disabilities.

Recreation Dynamics, Inc.
866-221-6999
www.recreationdynamics.com
    Offers Mobi-Mat, a rollout mat that provides wheelchair accessibility on any type of terrain. Makes parks, beaches, riverbanks, campgrounds, golf courses, and nature trails more accessible.

Roleez® Wheels, Inc.
800-369-1390; 707-751-3999
www.roleez.com
    Offers wheels that are interchangeable with manual wheelchair wheels that allow transport over soft, sandy, muddy, and environmentally sensitive terrain.

The World Playground, Parks, and Recreation Accessible Products and Services Web Directory
800-352-1137; 604-929-7771
www.playgrounddirectory.com/accessible.htm

An online directory of manufacturers of disability-accessible playground equipment, accessories, components, and products.

Parenting Publications

The DPPi Journal
020 7263 3088 (in London)
www.dppi.org.uk/journal/index.html
A quarterly journal published by Disability, Pregnancy, and Parenthood International that promotes better awareness and support of persons with disabilities during pregnancy and parenting.

Parenting with a Disability
(800) 644-2666; (510) 848-1112
www.lookingglass.org/newsletter
A free newsletter distributed by the Through the Looking Glass that provides current information about issues relevant to parents with disabilities.

Parenting Videotapes

Adaptive Baby Care Equipment for Parents with Physical Disabilities (10 minutes, VHS)
Available from Through the Looking Glass
(800) 644-2666
www.lookingglass.org/publications
Demonstrates how parents with physical disabilities have successfully used adaptive baby-care equipment and adaptive baby-care techniques.

Disability and Motherhood (25 minutes, VHS or DVD)
Available from Films for the Humanities and Sciences
(800) 257-5126
www.films.com/Films_Home/item.cfm?s=1&bin=5407
Three mothers with physical disabilities share their experiences of motherhood and disability and discuss public attitudes.

Appendix D: My Baby Care Planner

1. Which baby care activities do I most want to do?

2. Which baby care activities do I think I can do?

3. Which baby care activities do I want someone else to do or will I need help with ?

4. Ideas on who can adapt or create my baby care equipment.
(wheelchair repair shops, woodworkers, handy men/women, shoe repair shops, sail makers, occupational therapists [students], rehabilitation engineers [students], upholsterers)

5. Ideas on who can be "mommy and daddy helpers"
(Extended family, pre-teen or retired neighbors, occupational therapy, physical therapy, or nursing students)

6. What do I need in my home in order to care for my baby?
(child-proofing, child's bedroom on the first floor, accessible and safe outdoor play area)

My Baby Care Planner—Tricks and Equipment

Baby Care Activities	Tricks and Adaptive Strategies	Equipment and Accessories to Buy	Equipment to Make or Change
Holding/Supporting My Child Near Me • lifting and placing baby on my lap or seat			
Changing Positions: • lying down to sitting up • rolling on your side • turning over			
Carrying/ Moving baby: • inside the house (short distances) • outside of the house (longer distances)			
Breastfeeding: • lift and place into arms or supportive seat • feeding positions • burping techniques			

My Baby Care Planner—Tricks and Equipment (continued)

Baby Care Activities	Tricks and Adaptive Strategies	Equipment and Accessories to Buy	Equipment to Make or Change
Bottle feeding: • lift and place into arms or sup-portive seat • preparing bot-tles • securing/feed-ing bottle • burping			
Spoon feeding: • lift and place into highchair • food prepara-tion • spoon food up to mouth • clean face/hands			
Diapering: • lift and place onto diapering surface • bottoms off/on • diaper off/on • cleaning bot-tom			
Bed/nap time: • lift and place in crib or bassinet			
Bathing: • fill bath water • lift/place into baby tub, or guide into tub • wash hair and body • dry body			

My Baby Care Planner—Tricks and Equipment (continued)

Baby Care Activities	Tricks and Adaptive Strategies	Equipment and Accessories to Buy	Equipment to Make or Change
Health/safety: • get baby out of the • house in an emergency • in and out of infant car seat • child-proofed home • take child's temperature • give medicine			
Play: • Play areas or surface. • Activities			

Helper(s) Schedule

	Mon.	Tue.	Wed.	Thu.	Fri.	Sat.	Sun.
Morning							
After-noon							
Evening							
During the night							

Index